TECHNIQUES IN SURGICAL CASTING AND SPLINTING

Kent K. Wu, M.D.

Department of Orthopaedic Surgery
Henry Ford Hospital
Detroit, Michigan

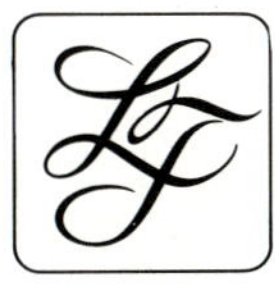

LEA & FEBIGER 1987 *Philadelphia*

Lea & Febiger
600 Washington Square
Philadelphia, PA 19106-4198
U.S.A.
(215) 922-1330

Library of Congress Cataloging-in-Publication Data

Wu, Kent K.
Techniques in surgical casting and splinting.

Includes bibliographies and index.
1. Plaster casts, Surgical. 2. Splints (Surgery)
I. Title. [DNLM: 1. Casts, Surgical. 2. Splints.
W0 170 W959t]
RD114.W82 1987 617'.93 87-2894
ISBN 0-8121-1076-5

PRINTED IN THE UNITED STATES OF AMERICA

Print No. 4 3 2 1

TECHNIQUES IN SURGICAL CASTING AND SPLINTING

Dedicated to my wife, Judith Nelson Wu, and my children, Jonathan, Richard, and Kimberly Nelson Wu, whose love, understanding, and constant encouragement enabled me to complete this orthopedic textbook and several similar textbooks.

Foreword

Having personally applied tens of thousands of casts of various types and having thumbed through many orthopedic textbooks during the past 30 years, I have been constantly amazed by the paucity of books providing in-depth descriptions of surgical casting techniques. In addition, over the years I have been asked by numerous highly qualified orthopedic surgeons to apply various spica casts, cast-braces, and body casts for them because they were not familiar with the newest and best methods of applying these casts.

The desperate need for a complete and up-to-date book on casts is finally fulfilled by Dr. Wu's *Techniques of Surgical Casting and Splinting*, which I expect will become the bible of surgical casting techniques. Dr. Wu's book shows how to make every kind of cast, from the simplest to the most difficult, and for each cast it describes the indications, required cast materials, patient position, and the techniques for executing it, either in plaster or fiberglass. Drawings and photographs illustrate each step in the process of making each cast. This thorough and systematic presentation should enable orthopedists, other physicians, and even paramedical people to apply casts with confidence, simply by following the instructions. For instance, a first-year orthopedic resident who had never seen a patellar-tendon-bearing (PTB) cast was able to complete a fairly satisfactory PTB cast all by himself by following the sequential illustrations contained here.

I am deeply honored to have been afforded the opportunity to work with Dr. Wu on the compilation of the technical material contained in his book and to have been able to contribute my knowledge and expertise.

Harold L. Brady, Chief Orthopaedic Technician
Department of Orthopaedic Surgery,
Henry Ford Hospital
Detroit, Michigan

Preface

It is well known that casts are the foundation as well as the bread and butter of orthopedic surgery. My frequent observation of the inferior quality of the more technically demanding casts, such as patellar-tendon-bearing, supracondylar, hip spica, Risser, and Minerva casts, and various long-arm and long-leg cast-braces applied by some orthopedic residents and practicing orthopedic surgeons made me feel that what was urgently needed was a comprehensive textbook on casts, cast-braces, and splints, written in a "cookbook" style and illustrated with step-by-step pictures and drawings.

My wish for a cookbook on casts started to become reality when Lea & Febiger of Philadelphia asked me to write a cast book and Harold Brady, Chief Orthopaedic Technician in the Department of Orthopaedic Surgery at Henry Ford Hospital, agreed to serve as my technical advisor. I consulted with numerous partially and fully trained orthopedic surgeons and decided to make it a reference book for all, from the experienced orthopedic surgeon to the paramedic. Accordingly, I decided to write the book in plain English, avoiding highly technical terms, to include a brief description of the history of cast techniques, a description of cast materials and equipment, the fundamentals of casting techniques, and complications of casts. I decided to discuss both plaster and fiberglass casts, including the exact amount of all materials needed for each cast, and to progress from the simplest casts to the most difficult and complicated casts, like the Minerva and Risser casts.

My greatest thanks go to Harold Brady, who gave invaluable technical advice throughout the writing of this book. In addition, Mr. Brady and his colleague, Willie Bender, made all the casts illustrated in this book. I also wish to thank Shari Morency, Dawn Robinson, Sherie Johnson, Theresa Cunningham, Karen Schwartz, and my wife, Judith Nelson Wu, for their willingness to serve as cast models. I am very much obliged to my chairman, Dr. Henry H. Sprague, for his constant encouragement and support; to Nardina Nameth, Valerie Reid, Fern Cheek, Hildegard Joseph, Lisa Costello, and Janet Sparks for providing me with hundreds of references; to Jim Latif for taking the cast pictures and making prints for me; to Jay Knipstein for providing me with his superb drawings which can be seen throughout this book; and to the Orthopedic Product Division of 3M Company for paying the modeling expenses. Finally, I am indebted to my secretary, Justine

Frankfurth, who not only tirelessly and meticulously typed the whole manuscript, but also skillfully managed my busy orthopedic practice at the same time.

Detroit, Michigan Kent K. Wu, M.D.

Contents

CHAPTER 1. CASTS AND CAST-BRACES: GENERAL CONSIDERATIONS

HISTORY OF CASTS

The need to immobilize a fractured extremity in order to provide pain relief and restore useful function was obvious even in prehistoric times. The earliest historical records indicate that the ancient Egyptians immobilized fractured extremities with primitive casts made of linen bandages stiffened with gum.

The main principles of closed treatment of fractures were established in 350 B.C. by Hippocrates, who recommended that the fractured extremity should first be pulled in opposite directions by "two strong men" to reduce the fracture before bandages made rigid with waxes and resins were applied to the injured extremity. William Cheselden (1688–1752) used rags dipped in egg albumen and wheat flour to make casts for fracture treatment. Similarly, the famous French army physician Baron Larrey treated fractures with linen that had been soaked in a mixture of spirits of camphor, egg white, and lead acetate.

The Arabs were probably the first to use gypsum to treat fractures, but its use was unknown to Europeans until a Mr. Eton, a former British consul in Bassora, Arabia, reported it in 1798. In 1816, Hubinthal mixed equal parts of plaster of Paris and ground-up blotting paper to immobilize fractures, and Koyl and Kluge poured liquid plaster of Paris into a mold that surrounded a fractured extremity to immobilize the fracture. However, the above-mentioned casts were either not strong enough or too cumbersome for practical use.

The technique of plaster application was dramatically changed in 1852, when a Dutch army surgeon named Antonius Mathysen treated battle wounds with mesh cotton bandages impregnated with plaster-of-Paris powder, which could be easily and effectively applied to the injured extremities. These bandages could be prepared far in advance and could be transported with ease, but the plaster powder could easily fall away from the cotton mesh during transportation or application.

In 1927 the modern hard-coated plaster-of-Paris rolls were developed. In these rolls a binder, usually consisting of starches, gums, and resins, is used to adhere the plaster of Paris to the cloth. In addition, different additives are blended into modern plaster-of-Paris bandages to produce bandages with different physical properties. For example, additives such as salicylic acid, zinc, magnesium, copper, iron, or aluminum speed up the setting process, whereas glue or gum slows it down.

HISTORY OF CAST-BRACES

Medieval armor can be considered a special type of cast-brace. The metallic plates protected the wearer from being injured by sharp weapons, and the hip, knee, ankle, shoulder, elbow, wrist, and finger hinges allowed the wearer to walk, use weapons, and ride a horse. Nevertheless, the use of cast-braces in treating fractured extremities is relatively recent. For example, Benjamin Gooch (1709–1776) made wooden leg splints by gluing a piece of wood about one-tenth of an inch thick to leather and then making parallel longitudinal cuts in the wood down to the leather so that it could be used to wrap around a fractured extremity to provide external support. A femoral fracture could be treated by applying this flexible wooden splint to the thigh; and a tibial fracture, by applying the same splint to the lower leg. Gooch also devised an ingenious metallic brace with a foot piece and two knee hinges to be used with the thigh and lower-leg splints for simultaneous treatment of femoral and tibial fractures. Robert Chessher (1750–1831) also used a primitive form of cast-brace to treat tibial fractures.

In the late eighteenth century, William Sharp used a modular cast-brace system of three different sizes to treat tibial fractures. His system consisted of two strong medial and lateral pasteboards, which were molded closely around the medial and lateral femoral condyles and malleoli and were strapped to the fractured lower leg to allow knee motion but to prevent significant rotation of the tibia on the femur. In 1801, Benjamin Bell invented a below-knee amputation prosthesis made of hardened leather. The upper part of the prosthesis was carefully molded around the femoral condyles and the patella to provide pressure relief for the amputation stump, just as the modern patella-tendon-bearing cast does.

Sarmiento (1967, 1974) has popularized the use of different cast-braces that allow immediate joint motion and early rehabilitation of the injured extremities. Furthermore, having been invited by the Chinese Medical Association to be a visiting professor to the People's Republic of China on two occasions, I have seen an interesting Chinese cast-bracing system. It is inexpensive and can be used in treating different extremity fractures. The injured bone is immobilized with three or four padded wooden splints around the injured portion of the limb, and weight-bearing is begun as soon as the patient can tolerate it. Since no joint is immobilized, loss of joint motion usually does not occur. The rate of union is extremely high, but some angulation and shortening of the fractured bones may take place (Figs. 1-1–1-5).

PHYSICAL AND CHEMICAL PROPERTIES OF PLASTER OF PARIS

Plaster of Paris is derived from gypsum, or calcium sulfate dihydrate ($CaSO_4 \cdot 2H_2O$, a naturally occurring rocklike substance commonly found with rock salts. When gypsum is heated to approximately 128°C, a chemical reaction takes place during which most of the water of crystallization is driven off, resulting in a powdery substance commonly known as plaster of Paris.

$$\underset{\text{Gypsum}}{CaSO_4 \cdot 2H_2O} + \text{Heat} \rightleftarrows \underset{\text{Plaster of Paris}}{CaSO_4 \cdot {}^1/_2H_2O} + 1^1/_2H_2O$$

When water is added to plaster of Paris, the water molecules go from the liquid state into a solid state by incorporating themselves into the crystalline lattice of the calcium sulfate hemihydrate molecules, thus giving up most of their kinetic energy in the form of heat. This hydration process again converts the weak and powdery plaster of Paris into a homogeneous rock-hard mass, which has to undergo a curing process over a period of several days, during which excess water is removed by evaporation, which can be accelerated by low humidity, high ambient temperature, and fast air circulation around the cast.

When the plaster is being transformed from a liquid into a solid, it reaches a critical period during which any motion can interfere with the proper formation of the crystalline network of calcium sulfate dihydrate, resulting in a significant weakening of the plaster. Schmidt and Somerset (1973) have shown that plaster reaches its optimal mechanical strength when its water content has decreased to 21% of its initial hydrated level (it usually takes at least 24 hours to reach this level). While a cast is being cured, it should be protected from excessive stress such as weight bearing until its much stronger dry state has been reached.

Because the chemical process involved in the formation of plaster of Paris is reversible, the hardened plaster can be degraded easily by soaking the cast in water for a period of time, after which often the cast can be removed simply by unwrapping the softened plaster bandages. The reversibility of the process of formation of plaster enables parents to soak and remove corrective casts the night before their children's orthopedic appointments so that they can be spared the frightening experience of hearing loud and unpleasant noises and feeling the tingling vibrations produced by the cast saws during removal of the cast in the office.

ADVANTAGES AND DISADVANTAGES OF PLASTER AND SYNTHETIC CASTS

The so-called synthetic casts are usually made of fiberglass, but other synthetic fibers and plastic sheets (e.g., Orthoplast) have also been used. The accompanying table shows the advantages and disadvantages of plaster and synthetic casts.

	Plaster cast	Synthetic cast
Cost	Low	Relatively high
Strength and durability	Average	Superior
Radiolucency	Poor	Good
Ease of molding	Excellent; the material of choice for fresh fractures	Average; usually used in subsequent casts
Water resistance	Poor	Excellent

	Plaster cast	Synthetic cast
Weight	Heavy	Relatively light
Drying and curing time	Prolonged	Relatively short, thus allowing immediate weight bearing
Usefulness in treating open fractures and large soft-tissue wounds	Limited	Very useful, especially when soaks and whirlpool therapy have to be used
Usefulness in treating common congenital deformities with frequent cast changes	Very useful: easily molded and may be removed by soaking	Limited
Possible undesirable effects on castroom instruments and personnel and the wearer	Perhaps some health hazard from inhaling the dust	Rapid dulling of the cast saw blade, frequent damage to the wearer's clothes because of the rough texture, and possible health hazard from inhaling the dust
Chance of producing thermal burn	Has been known to occur	Unlikely
Allergenicity	Very low	Relatively high

PRACTICAL USES OF CASTS

Fractures and dislocations of bones and joints.

Injuries of muscles, tendons, fasciae, and ligaments.

Correction of congenital and acquired deformities.

Treatment of infections of bones, joints, and associated soft tissues.

Joint fusions.

Protection of vascular or nerve repairs.

Treatment of cutaneous ulcers (e.g., diabetic foot ulcers) by distributing body weight over a much wider area.

Treatment of inflammatory diseases (e.g., rheumatoid arthritis) with bone, joint, or soft somatic tissue involvement.

Application around amputation stumps to speed up stump maturation for early prosthetic fitting and to facilitate early weight-bearing.

Protection of avascular bones (e.g., femoral head in Legg-Calvé-Perthes disease, autogenous and cadaveric bone grafts in limb salvage procedures) until revascularization has taken place.

Temporary immobilization of one or more extremities so that a pedicle skin graft can be moved from one part of the body to another.

Casts make it possible for patients to be taken care of at home and thus reduce the cost of hospitalization.

A carefully applied cast can be used to produce a replica of almost any part of the body, from which a corresponding prosthesis, orthosis, or brace can be fashioned.

Prevention of progressive deformities (e.g., inhibition cast in managing patients with cerebral palsy).

Treatment of joint effusion or hemarthrosis (e.g., hemophiliac hemarthrosis).

ADVANTAGES AND DISADVANTAGES OF CASTS AND CAST-BRACES

The accompanying table shows the advantages and disadvantages of casts and cast-braces.

	Cast	Cast-brace
Cost	Low	Relatively high
Ease of application	Fairly easy	Technically demanding
Stretching of injured or repaired ligaments	Minimal	Can be considerable if range of motion is not limited
Muscle atrophy	Often	Minimal
Disuse osteoporosis	Very common	Minimal
Rate of fracture healing	Average	Accelerated
Patient acceptance	Average	Higher than average
Chance of fracture angulation and shortening	Average	Higher than average
Weight	Heavy	Usually lighter than comparable cast
Duration of hospitalization	Average	Short
Rehabilitation time	Slow	Rapid
Time required to achieve independence	Variable, depending on site and nature of injury	Usually relatively short

BIBLIOGRAPHY

Austin, R.T.: Robert Chessher of Hinckley (1750–1831), First English Orthopaedist. Leicester, Leicestershire Libraries, 1982.

Austin, R.T.: Treatment of broken legs before and after the introduction of gypsum. Injury, *14:* 389, 1983.

Bagby, G.W.: Compression bone-plating: Historical considerations. J. Bone Joint Surg. [AM.], *59:* 625, 1977.

Bell, B.: A System of Surgery. 7th Ed. Edinburgh, Bell, Bradfute and Dickson, 1801.

Camerson, D.M.: Plaster-of-paris—a history. Am. J. Orthop., *3:* 8, 1961.

Cooper, A.: A Treatise on Dislocations and on Fractures of the Joints. 3rd Ed. London, Longman, 1824.

Dehne, E.: Treatment of fractures of the tibial shaft. Clin. Orthop., *66:* 159, 1969.

Gibson, D., and Lindsey, R.W.: Plaster-of-paris—its history, functional properties and potential complications. Conn. Med., *49:* 525, 1985.

Gooch, B.: Medical and Chirurgical Observations. London, G. Robinson, 1773.

Hunt, D.M.: New materials for the immobilization of fractures. Br. J. Hosp. Med., *24:* 273, 1980.

Luck, J.V.: Plaster-of-paris casts—an experimental and clinical analysis. JAMA, *124:* 23, 1944.

Mathysen, A.: Plaster-of-paris in the treatment of fractures. Liege, Grandmont-Doners, 1854.

Monro, G.K.: The history of plaster of paris in the treatment of fractures. Br. J. Surg., *23:* 257, 1935.

Nielsen, K., and Lauritzen, J.: A new thermoplastic casting material. A comparison between plaster of paris and hexelite. Acta Orthop. Scand., *52:* 27, 1981.

Petit, J.L.: A Treatise of the Diseases of the Bones. London, T. Woodward, 1726.

Sarmiento, A.: A functional below the knee cast for tibial fractures. J. Bone Joint Surg. [AM.], *49:* 373, 1967.

Sarmiento, A.: Functional bracing of tibial fractures. Clin. Orthop., *105:* 1974.

Schmidt, V.E., and Somerset, J.H.: Mechanical properties of orthopaedic plaster bandages. J. Biomec., *6:* 173, 1973.

Sharp, W.: An account of a new invented instrument for fractured legs. Philos. Trans. R. Soc. Lond., *57:* 80, 1767.

Watson-Jones, R.: Fractures and other bone and joint injuries. Edinburgh, Livingstone, 1940.

Wiseman, R.: Several Chirurgical Treatises. Bath, Kingsmead Press, 1676.

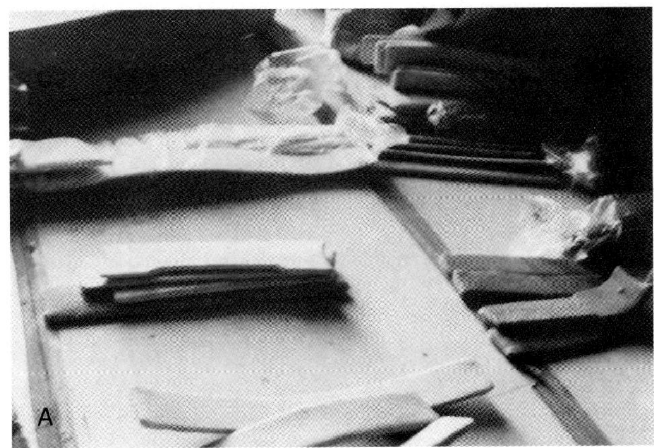

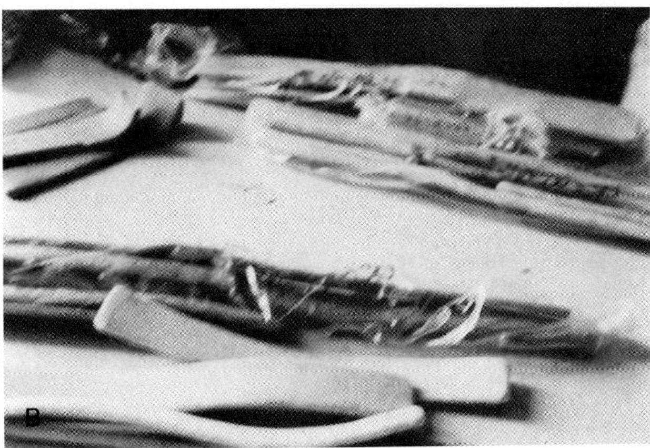

Fig. 1–1. *A, B,* Padded wooden splints of various lengths and widths. These splints are currently used by Chinese physicians in the treatment of extremity fractures. Photographs made in a medical clinic in the People's Republic of China.

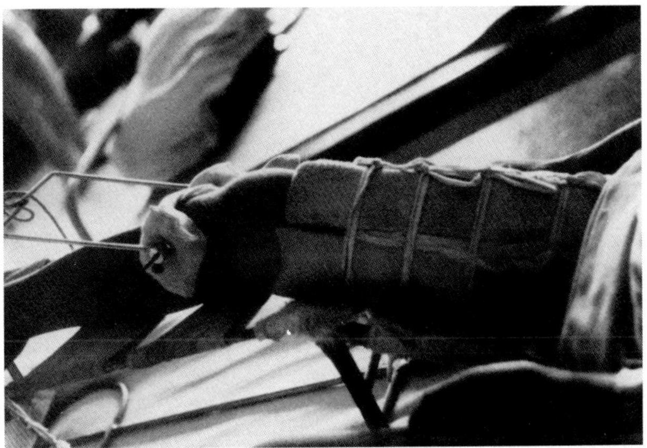

Fig. 1–2. A Chinese patient with a femoral fracture is being treated with both skeletal traction through the tibial tubercle region and padded wooden splints around the thigh. As soon as the femoral fracture is sticky, patient will start progressive weight-bearing until the femoral fracture is firmly united. The padded wooden splints are the sole means of immobilization throughout the fracture-healing process. Photographed in a medical clinic in the People's Republic of China.

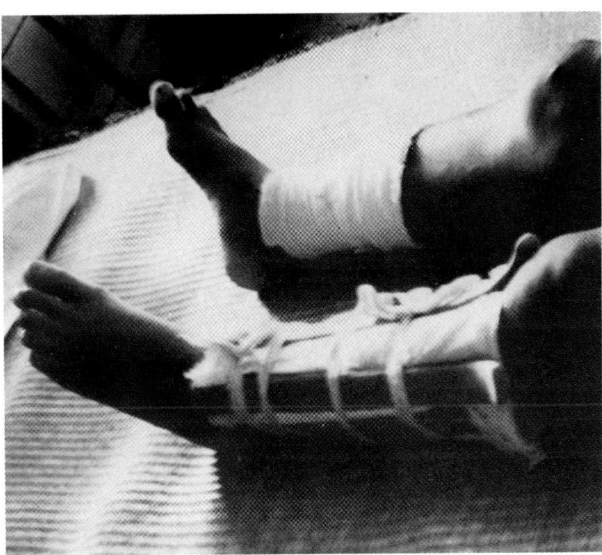

Fig. 1–3. A Chinese patient with a tibial fracture is being treated with only four padded wooden splints around the lower leg to allow full range of motion of the knee and ankle joints. Partial weight-bearing is commenced as soon as the patient can tolerate it and is gradually advanced to full weight-bearing. Photographed in a medical clinic in the People's Republic of China.

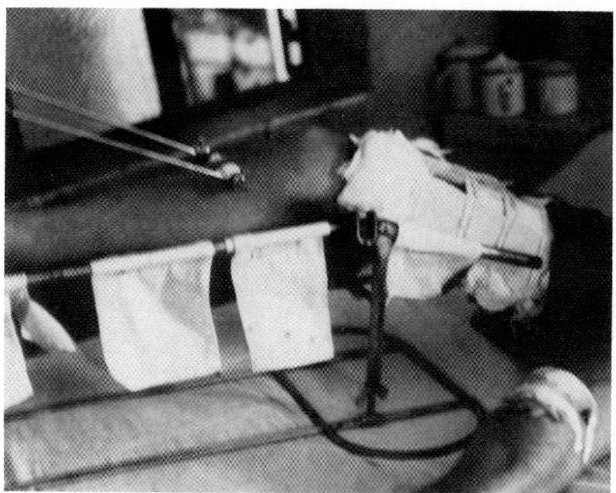

Fig. 1–4. A Chinese patient with a compound fracture of his right femur is being treated in a manner similar to that shown in Fig. 1–3, except that an opening has been left between two adjacent padded wooden splints so that the wound can be inspected and dressed daily. Photographed in a medical clinic in the People's Republic of China.

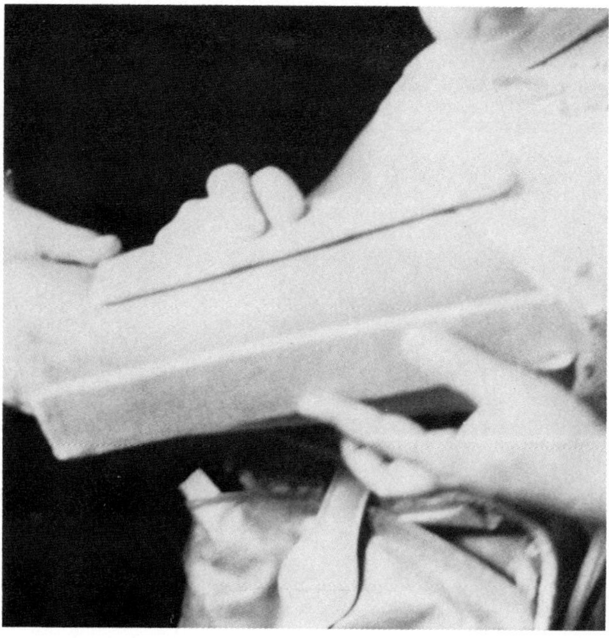

Fig. 1–5. Demonstration of the proper method of treating a humeral fracture by means of padded wooden splints. Longitudinal traction is applied to the humerus to reduce the humeral fracture before the padded wooden splints are wrapped around the upper arm. Photographed in a medical clinic in the People's Republic of China.

CHAPTER 2. MATERIALS AND EQUIPMENT USED IN MAKING CASTS, CAST-BRACES, AND SPLINTS

MATERIALS USED IN MAKING CASTS, CAST-BRACES, AND SPLINTS

Stockinet. Stockinet (Fig. 2-1) comes in widths of 2″, 3″, 4″, 8″, 10″, and 12″ and is in contact with the body.

Soft Cotton Bandage (Webril). Soft cotton bandage (Fig. 2-2) comes in widths of 2″, 3″, 4″, and 6″ and is usually wrapped directly around the stockinet.

Felt Padding. Felt padding (Fig. 2-3) is usually $^1/_2$ inch thick and is used to pad bony prominences.

Plaster Bandage. Plaster bandage (Fig. 2-4) comes in widths of 2″, 3″, 4″, and 6″ and gives the cast shape and strength.

5″ × 30″ Plaster Splints. Plaster splints (Fig. 2-5) greatly increase the strength of a cast. Splints are packaged in boxes of 10.

Fiberglass Bandage. Fiberglass bandage (Fig. 2-6) comes in widths of 2″, 3″, 4″, and 5″ and is the main component of a fiberglass cast.

Prefabricated Plaster Splints. Prefabricated plaster splints (Fig. 2-7) contain all the necessary plaster and padding materials and can be applied directly to the injured extremity.

Fiberglass Splint and Foam Padding. A fiberglass splint and its associated foam padding are shown in Fig. 2-8. After the fiberglass splint has been soaked in water and the foam padding has been applied to the injured extremity, the splint is applied over the padding.

Elastic Bandages (Ace). Elastic bandages (Fig. 2-9) come in widths of 2″, 3″, 4″, and 6″ and have wide applications in cast work. For example, they can be wrapped around bivalved casts, splints, bulky compression dressings, and cast windows.

Adhesive Tape. Adhesive tape (Fig. 2-10) is frequently used to line the margins of a bivalved cast.

Stockinet Toe Cap. A stockinet toe cap (Fig. 2-11) can be used to keep the toes warm and clean.

Bulky Cotton Roll. Bulky cotton rolls (Fig. 2-12) are frequently used in postoperative dressings to apply even compression to an extremity and thereby minimize edema.

Aluminum Splints with Foam Padding. Padded aluminum splints (Fig. 2-13) can be used to treat finger fractures or can serve as toe guards for long-leg or short-leg casts.

Polycentric Knee Hinges. Polycentric knee hinges (Fig. 2-14) allow knee motion in a long-leg cast-brace.

Polycentric Knee Hinges with Motion-Limiting Cables *Knee hinges with cables (Fig. 2-15) allow only a limited range of knee motion in order to protect injured or repaired knee ligaments from being stretched out.*

Polycentric Elbow Hinges. Polycentric elbow hinges (Fig. 2-16) permit elbow motion in a long-arm cast-brace.

Ankle Hinge with Heel Cup. Ankle hinges with heel cups (Fig. 2-17) allow ankle motion and are frequently used with short-leg or long-leg cast-braces.

Cast Cushions. Cast cushions (Fig. 2-18) are applied to the plantar aspect of a leg cast to allow weight-bearing.

Webbing and Buckle. Webbings and buckles (Fig. 2-19) are usually used to hold bivalved casts together.

Shoulder Immobilizer. A shoulder immobilizer (Fig. 2-20) is commonly used to immobilize a shoulder or to support a long-arm cast.

Cast Shoes. Cast shoes (two different types are shown in Fig. 2-21) permit weight-bearing and keep the bottom of a cast clean.

Postsurgical Shoes. Like cast shoes, postsurgical shoes (Fig. 2-22) permit weight-bearing and keep the bottom of a cast clean.

Cast Wedges. Cast wedges (Fig. 2-23) are used to keep the cut edges of a cast apart during wedging of the cast to correct fracture angulation and malalignment.

Plastic Adhesive. Plastic adhesive (Fig. 2-24) is usually painted on the edges of a bivalved cast before moleskin is applied in order to make the bivalved cast last a long time.

Moleskin. Moleskin (Fig. 2-25) is routinely used to line the rough edges of a bivalved cast.

Finger Splints. Finger splints (Fig. 2-26) are used to treat fractures, dislocations, tendon injuries of the distal portion of a finger.

Knee Immobilizer. A knee immobilizer (Fig. 2-27) is frequently used in treatment of mild to moderate disorders of the knee.

Wrist Immobilizer. A wrist immobilizer (Fig. 2-28) is used in treatment of mild to moderate wrist afflictions.

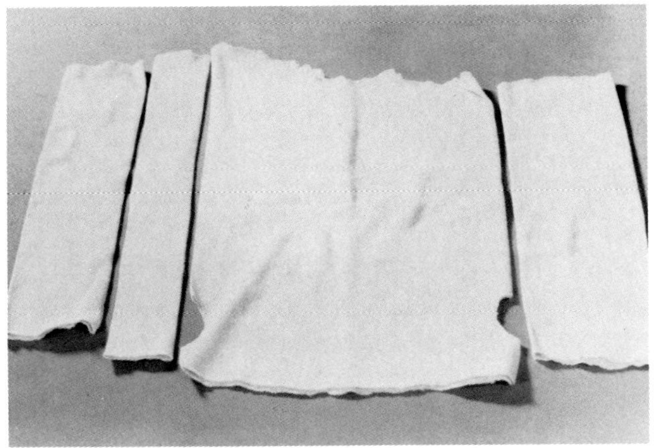

Fig. 2–1. Stockinet.

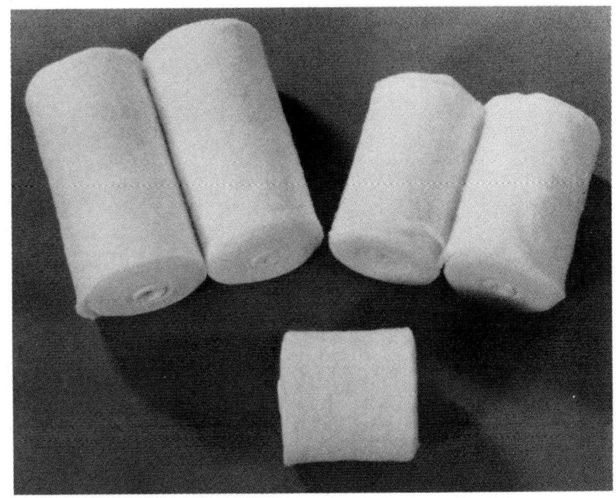

Fig. 2–2. Soft cotton bandage (Webril).

Fig. 2–3. Felt padding.

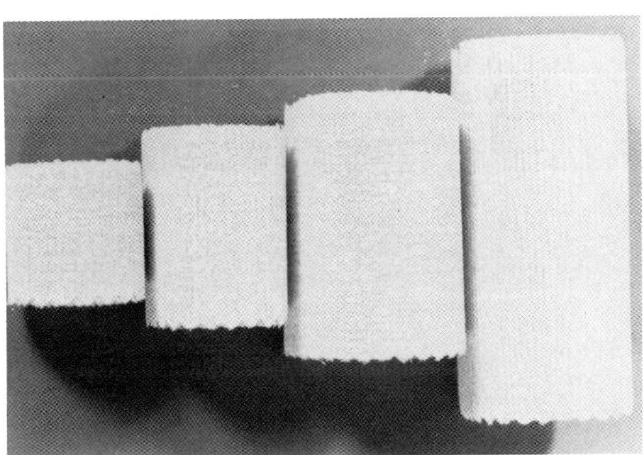

Fig. 2–4. Plaster bandages.

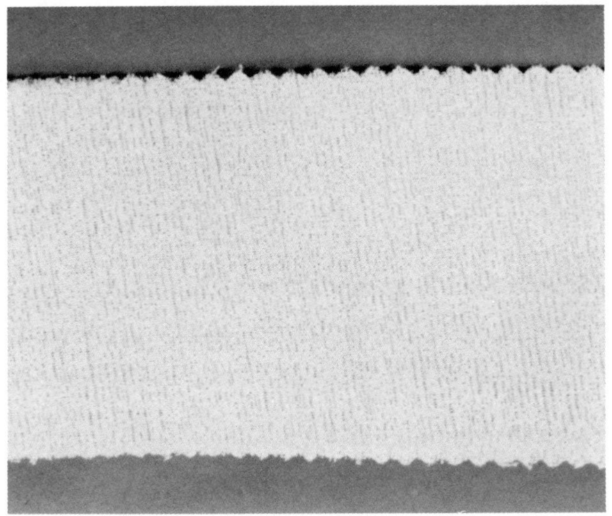

Fig. 2–5. 5″ × 30″ plaster splint.

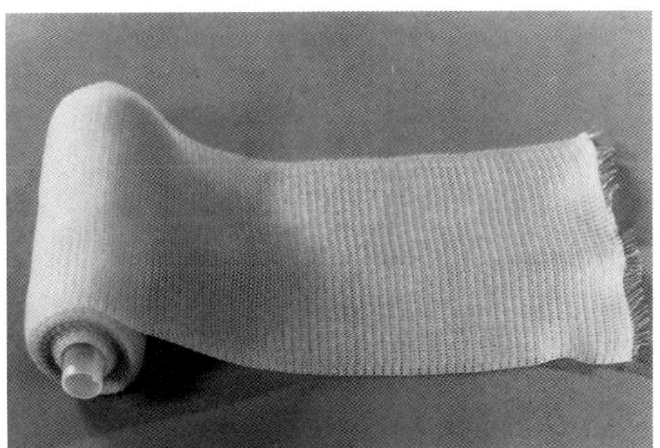

Fig. 2–6. Fiberglass bandage.

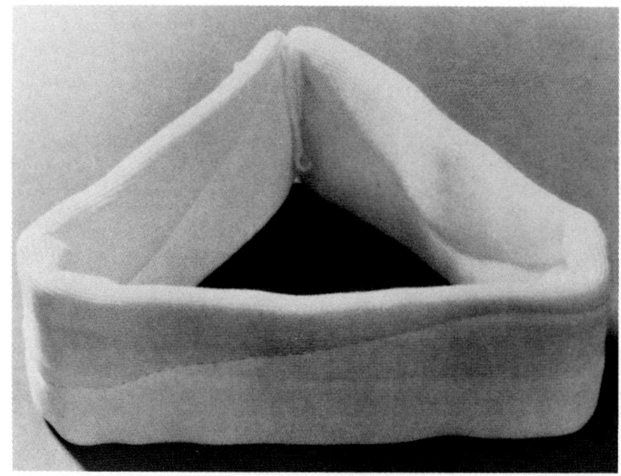

Fig. 2–7. Prefabricated plaster splint.

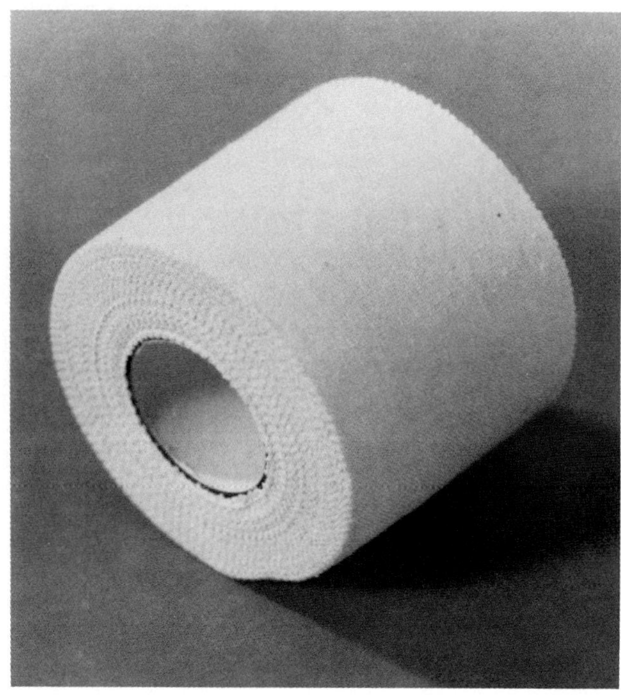

Fig. 2–10. Adhesive tape.

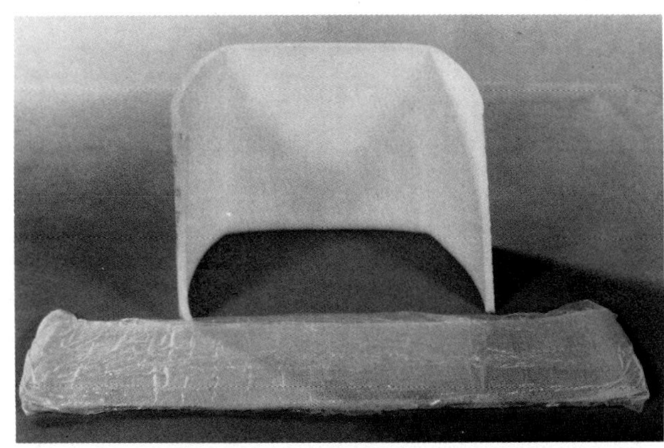

Fig. 2–8. Fiberglass splint and foam padding.

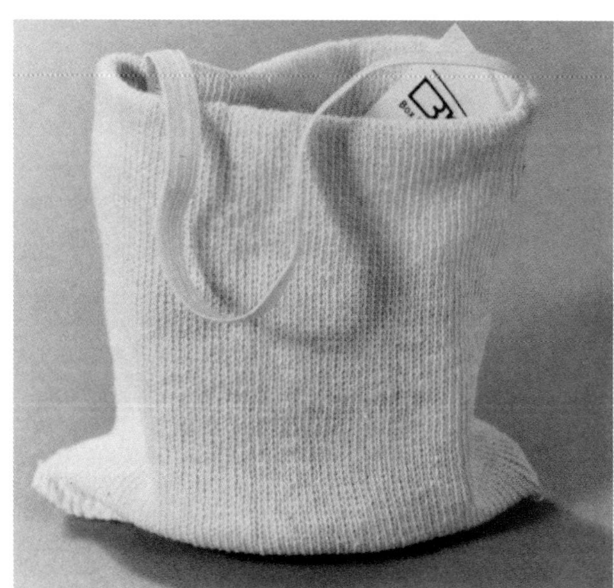

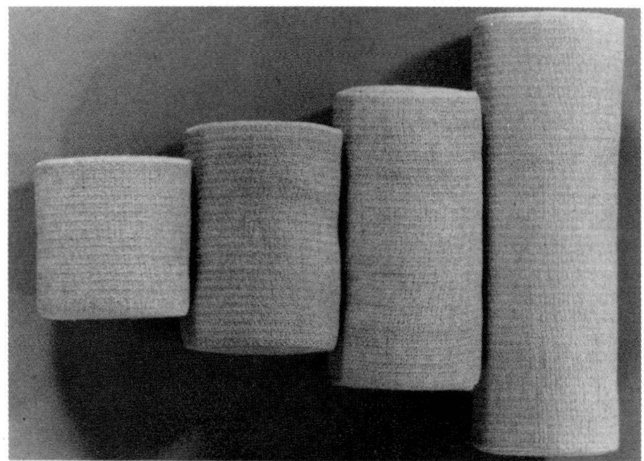

Fig. 2–9. Elastic (Ace) bandages.

Fig. 2–11. Stockinet toe cap.

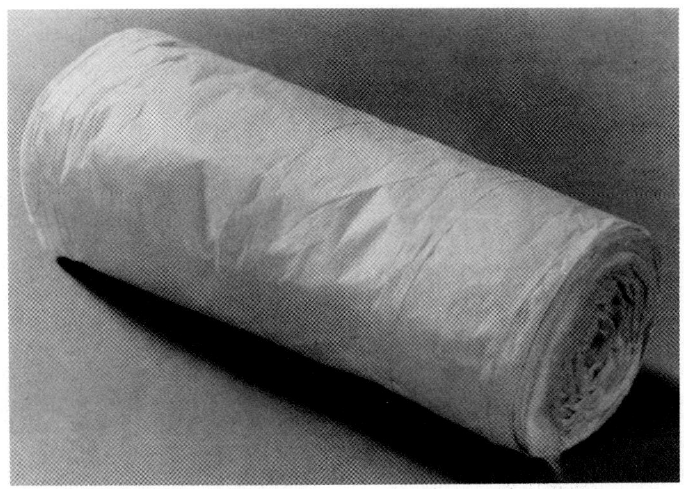

Fig. 2–12. Bulky cotton roll.

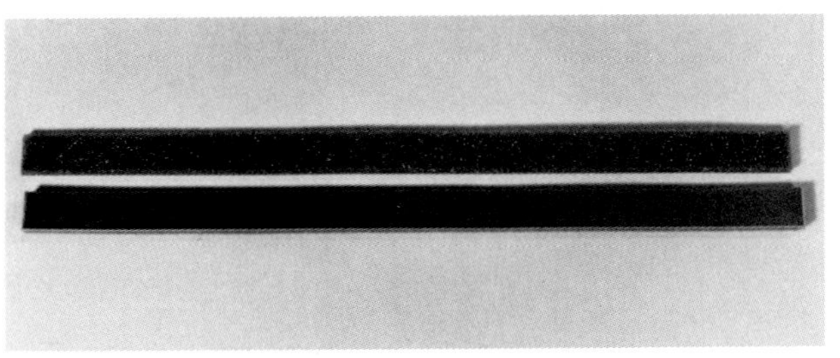

Fig. 2–13. Aluminum splints with foam padding.

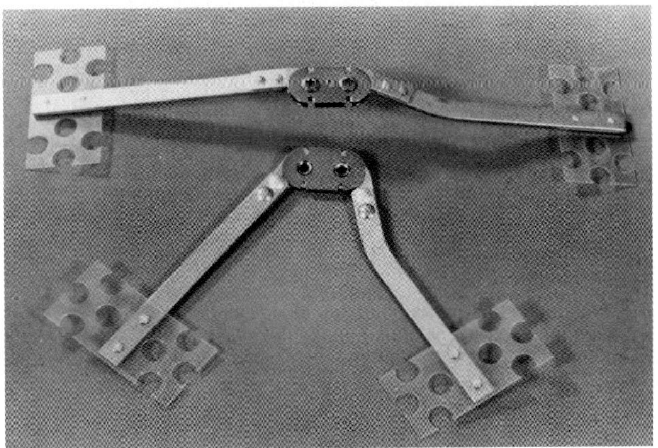

Fig. 2–14. Polycentric knee hinges.

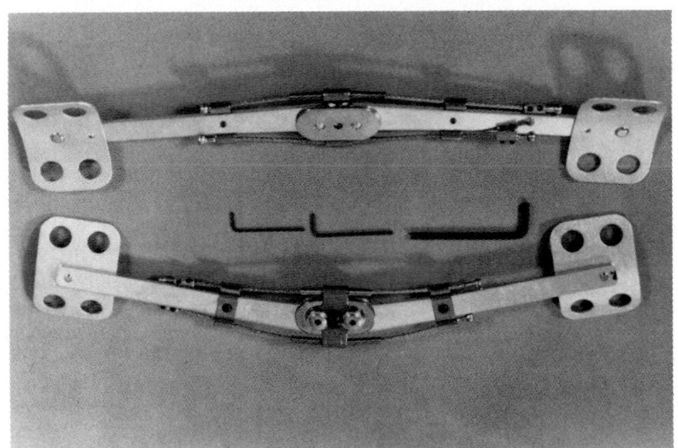

Fig. 2–15. Polycentric knee hinges with motion-limiting cables.

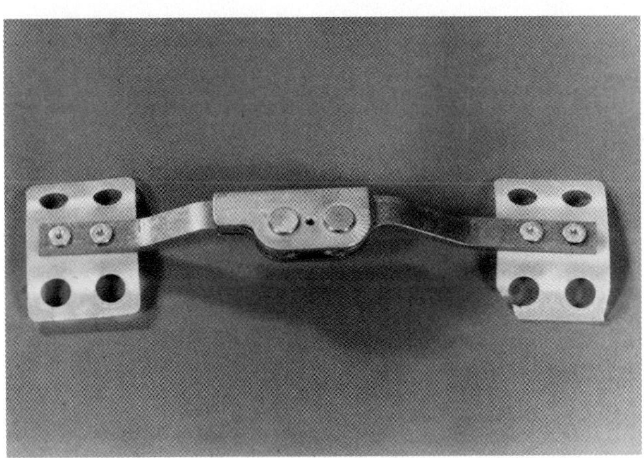

Fig. 2–16. Polycentric elbow hinge.

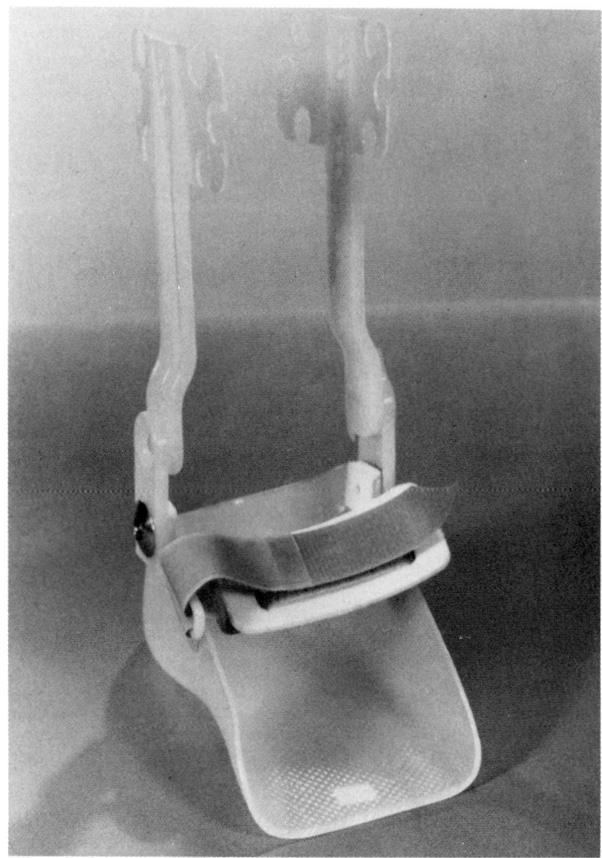

Fig. 2–17. Ankle hinge with heel cup.

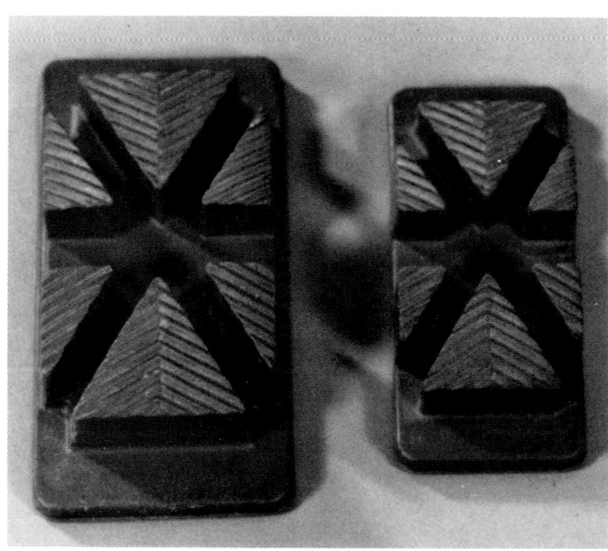

Fig. 2–18. Cast cushions.

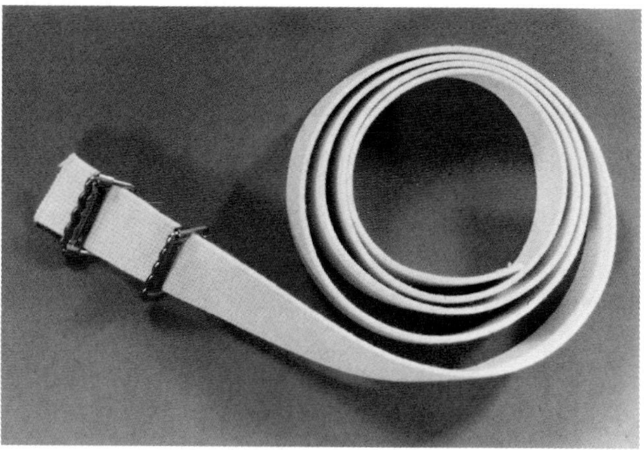

Fig. 2–19. Webbing and buckle.

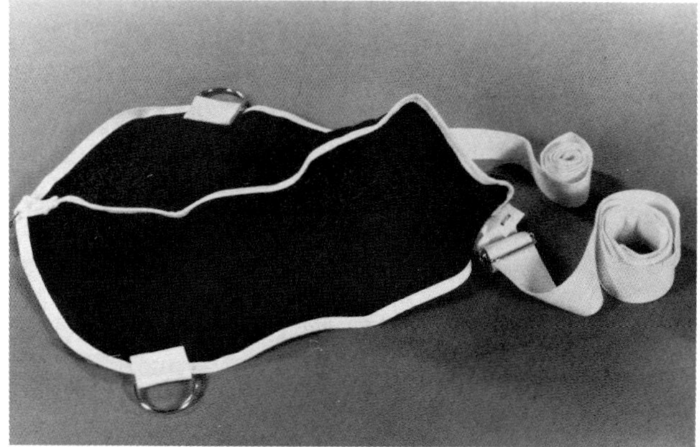

Fig. 2–20. Shoulder immobilizer.

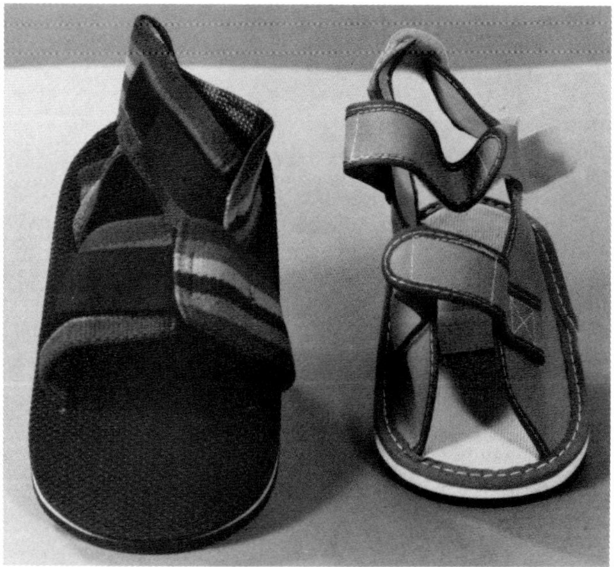

Fig. 2–21. Two different cast shoes.

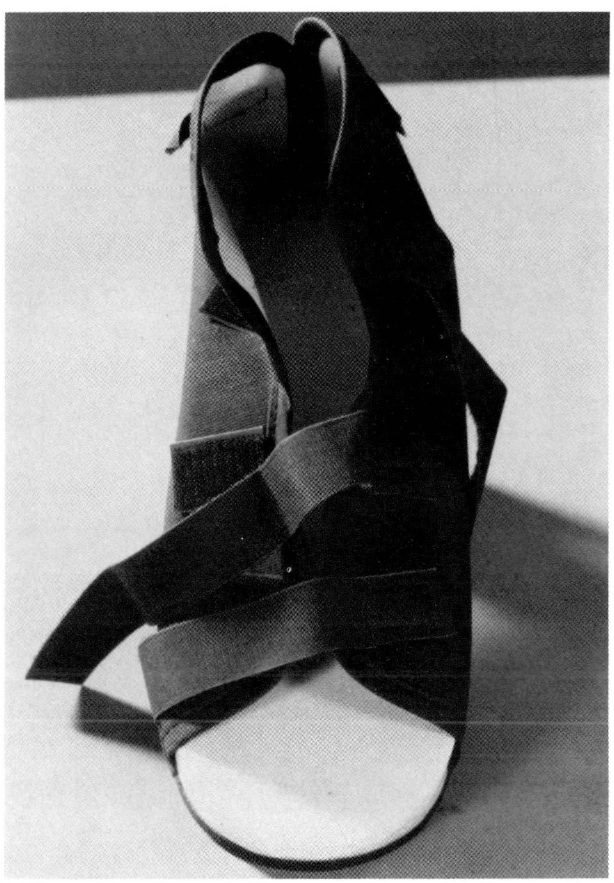

Fig. **2–22.** A postsurgical shoe.

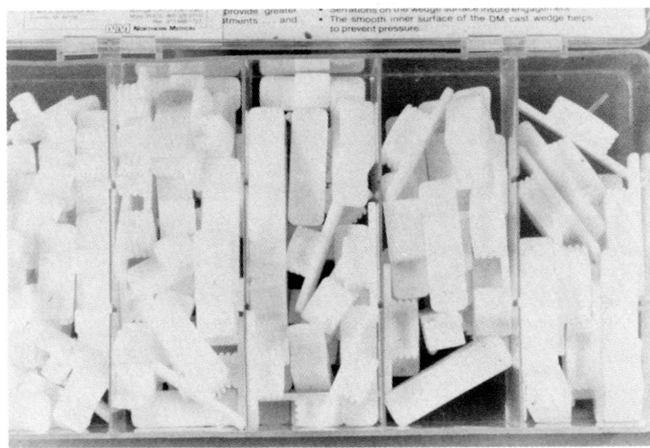

Fig. 2–23. Cast wedges.

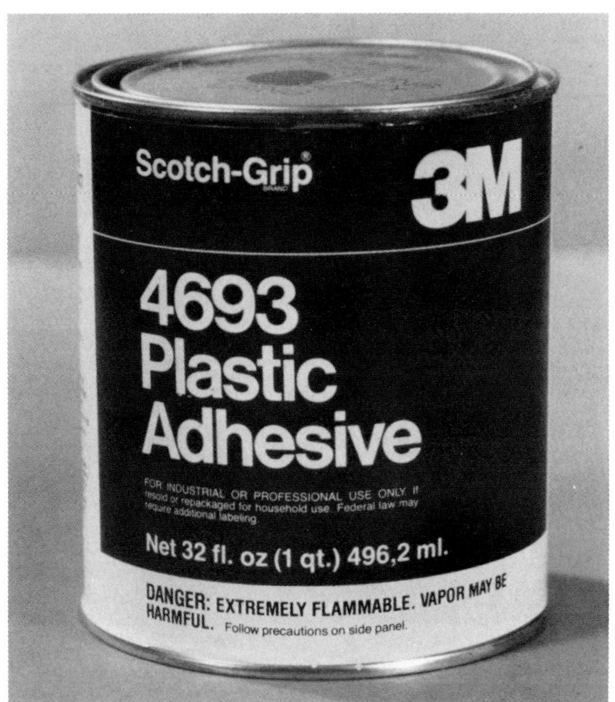

Fig. 2–24. Plastic adhesive.

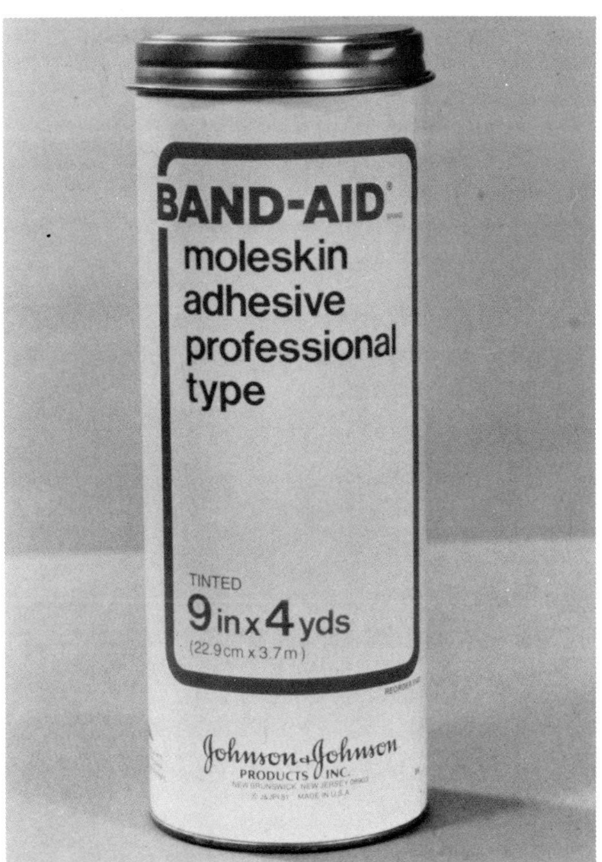

Fig. 2–25. Moleskin.

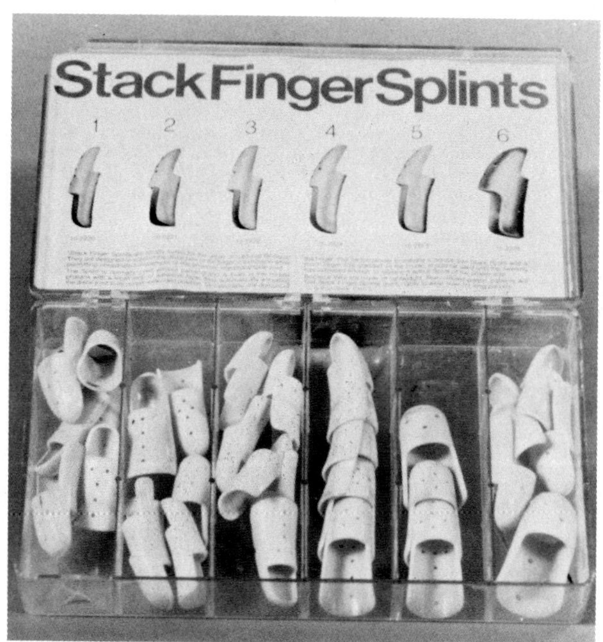

Fig. 2–26. Finger splints.

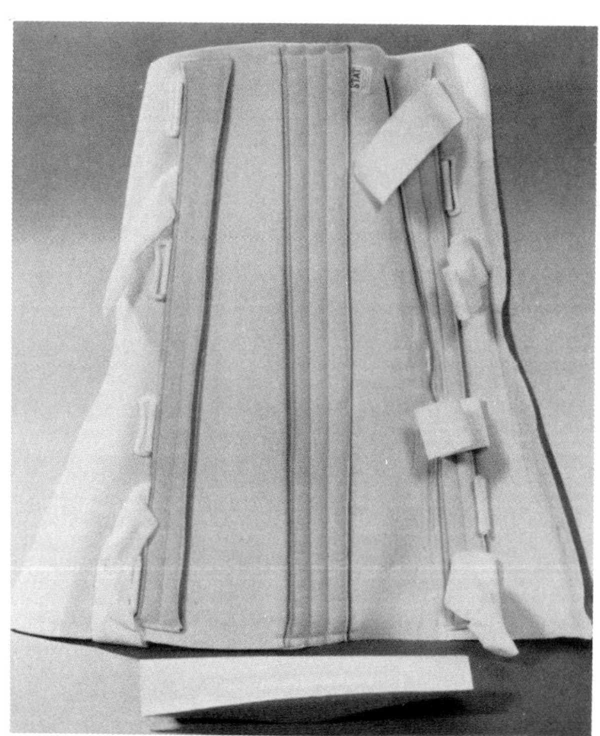

Fig. 2–27. Knee immobilizer.

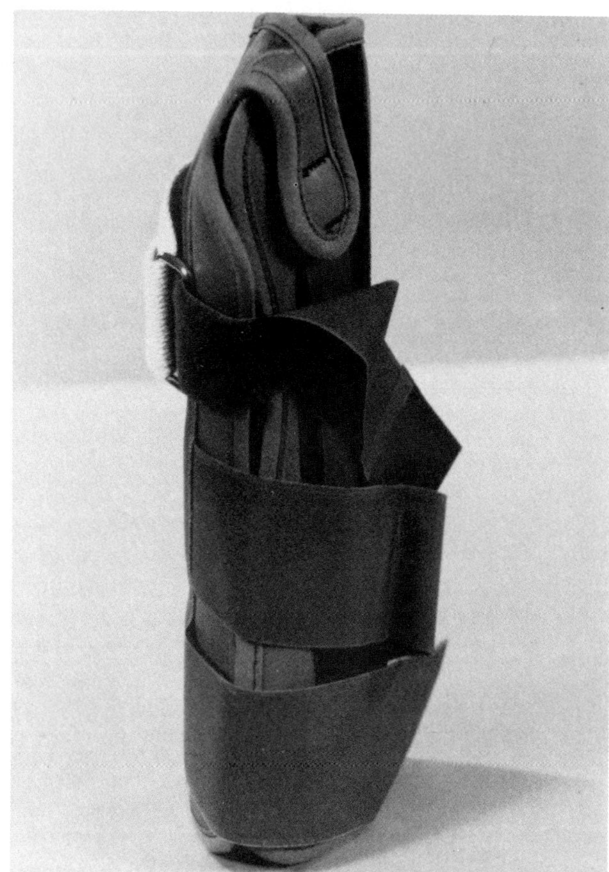

Fig. 2–28. Wrist immobilizer.

EQUIPMENT USED IN MAKING CASTS, CAST-BRACES, AND SPLINTS

Rubber Gloves. Rubber gloves (Fig. 2-29) are used to smooth off casts and to prevent plaster and chemicals from fiberglass bandages from sticking to the hands.

Face Masks. Face masks (Fig. 2-30) prevent inhalation of harmful plaster and fiberglass dust into the lungs.

Shoe Covers. Shoe covers (Fig. 2-31) protect shoes from plaster, water, and chemicals.

Stainless Steel Bucket. A stainless steel bucket (Fig. 2-32) is used for wetting plaster bandages.

Plastic Pan. A plastic pan (Fig. 2-33) is used for wetting fiberglass bandages because the chemicals from fiberglass bandages stick to metal but not to plastic.

Plaster Scissors. Plaster scissors (Fig. 2-34) are used to cut all cast materials.

Cast Spreader. A cast spreader (Fig. 2-35) is employed to separate the two halves of a bivalved cast.

Hatchet Cast Spreader. A hatchet cast spreader (Fig. 2-36) is used to separate the two halves of a bivalved cast.

Cast Knife and Scalpel. A cast knife and scalpel (Fig. 2-37) are used to trim the excess portion of a wet plaster or fiberglass cast.

Cast Breaker. A cast breaker (Fig. 2-38) is used to bend the edges of a cast to provide pressure relief.

Chinese Finger Traps. Chinese finger traps (Fig. 2-39) are applied to the fingers or toes to reduce fractures and dislocations of hand, wrist, or foot.

Wedging Separator. A wedging separator (Fig. 2-40) is used to separate the cut edges of a cast that is being wedged.

Leg Stand. A leg stand (Fig. 2-41) is used to support either the foot or the lower leg while a cast is being applied.

Foot Stand. A foot stand (Fig. 2-42) keeps the ankle in a neutral or even in a dorsiflexed position while a leg cast is being applied.

Solid Rubber Block. A solid rubber block (Fig. 2-43) is used to flatten the bottom of a leg cast to facilitate weight-bearing.

Fracture-Brace Alignment Fixture. A fracture-brace alignment fixture (Fig. 2-44) is used to line up poly-centric hinges with the center of rotation of an elbow or knee joint.

Bending Irons. Bending irons (Fig. 2-45) are used to bend knee or elbow hinges to fit a long-leg or long-arm cast.

Rivet Machine. A rivet machine (Fig. 2-46) is used to fasten buckles to webbing and to fasten webbing to bivalved casts.

Hand Drill. A hand drill (Fig. 2-47) is used to insert or remove Kirschner wires (K-wires) and Steinmann pins.

Pin Cutter. A pin cutter (Fig. 2-48) is used to cut K-wires and Steinmann pins.

Wrenches for Hoffmann Apparatus. These wrenches (Fig. 2-49) are used to remove or tighten the Hoffmann apparatus.

Cast Saw. A cast saw (Fig. 2-50) is used to remove, trim, or modify casts.

Cast-Saw Blade and Wrench. A cast-saw blade is shown in Fig. 2-51 together with the wrench used for it.

Manual Cast Cutter. A manual cast cutter (Fig. 2-52) is used to remove a cast by hand.

Plaster Vacuum. A plaster vacuum machine (Fig. 2-53), attached to the cast saw, sucks most of the plaster or fiberglass dust into its canister to minimize inhalation of dust by plaster-room personnel and patients.

Safety Goggles. Safety goggles (Fig. 2-54) protect the eyes from plaster and fiberglass dust.

Pediatric Spica Table. A pediatric spica table (Fig. 2-55) is used for making hip and body spica casts for young children.

BIBLIOGRAPHY

Bleck, E.E.: Atlas of Plaster Cast Techniques. Chicago, Year Book Publishers, 1956.

Cannon, N.M. (ed.): Manual of Hand Splinting. New York, Churchill Livingstone, 1985.

Connolly, J.F.: DePalma's The Management of Fractures and dislocations. 3rd Ed. Philadelphia, W.B. Saunders, 1981.

Lewis, R.C.: Handbook of Traction, Casting and Splinting Techniques. Philadelphia, J.B. Lippincott, 1977.

Malick, M.H.: Manual on Static Hand Splinting. 4th Ed. Pittsburgh, Harmarville Rehabilitation Center, 1980.

Mears, D.C. (ed.): Materials in Orthopaedic Surgery. Baltimore, Williams & Wilkins, 1979.

Niehuss, J.E.: An improved method to attach straps to plaster splints. Phys. Ther., *45:* 1059, 1965.

Sarmiento, A.: Functional bracing of tibial and femoral shaft fractures. Clin. Orthop., *82:* 2, 1972.

Sarmiento, A., and Latta, L.L.: Closed Functional Treatment of Fracture. Berlin, Springer-Verlag, 1981.

Sarmiento, A., et al.: Functional bracing of fractures of shaft of the humerus. J. Bone Joint Surg., *59:* 596, 1977.

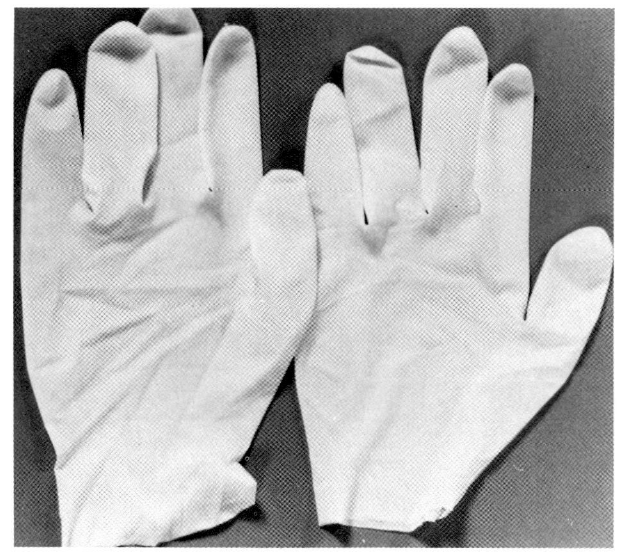

Fig. 2–29. Rubber gloves.

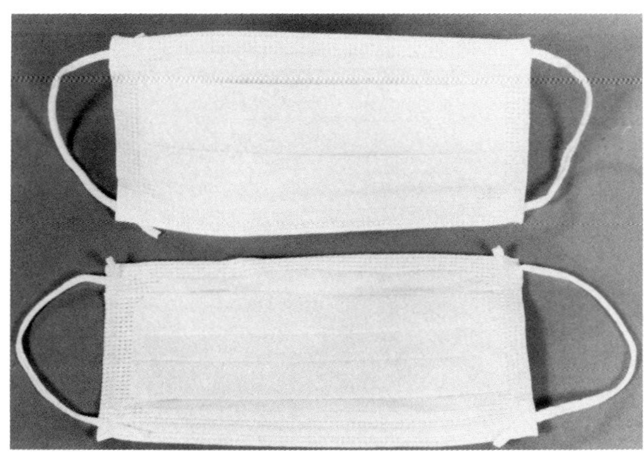

Fig. 2–30. Face masks.

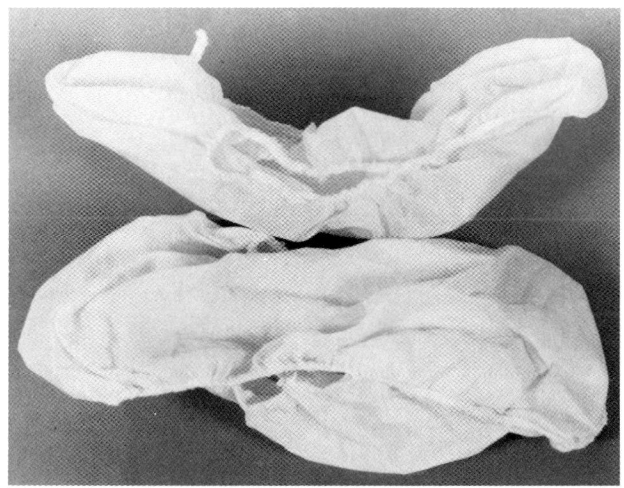

Fig. 2–31. Shoe covers.

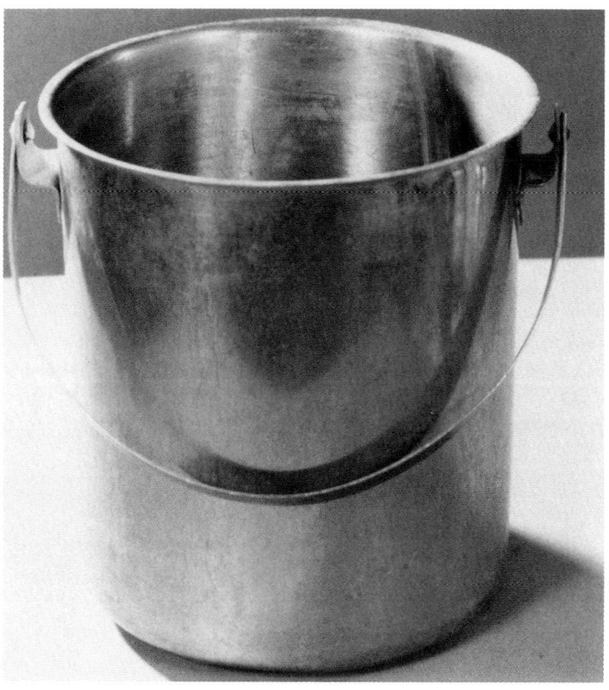

Fig. 2–32. Stainless steel bucket.

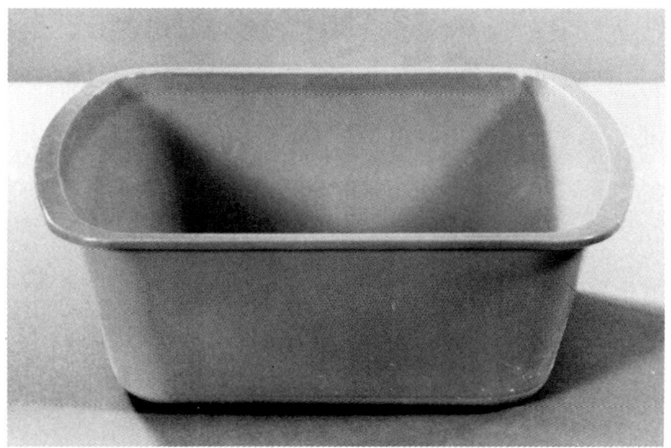

Fig. 2–33. Plastic pan.

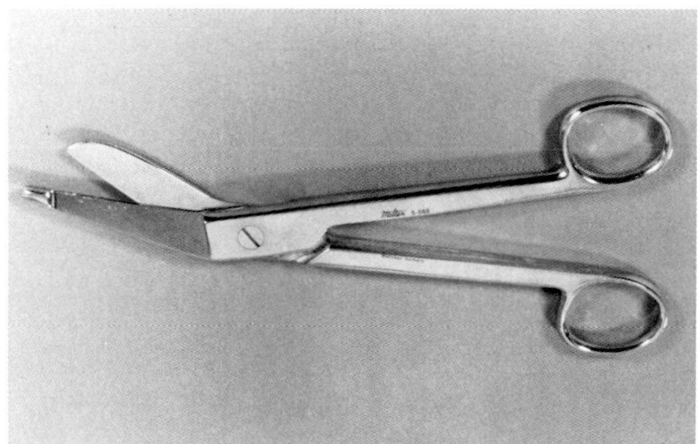

Fig. 2–34. Plaster scissors.

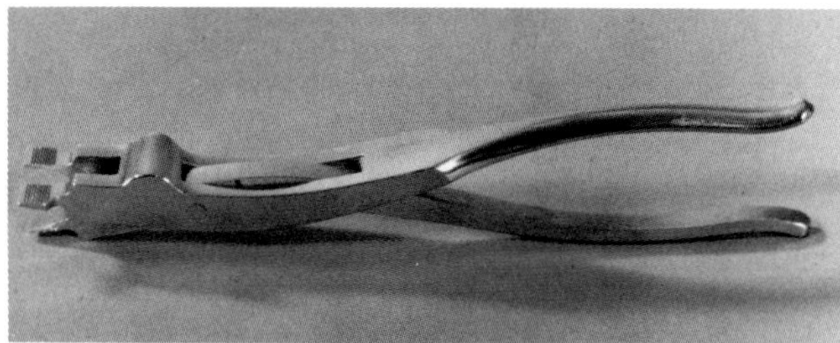

Fig. 2–35. Cast spreader.

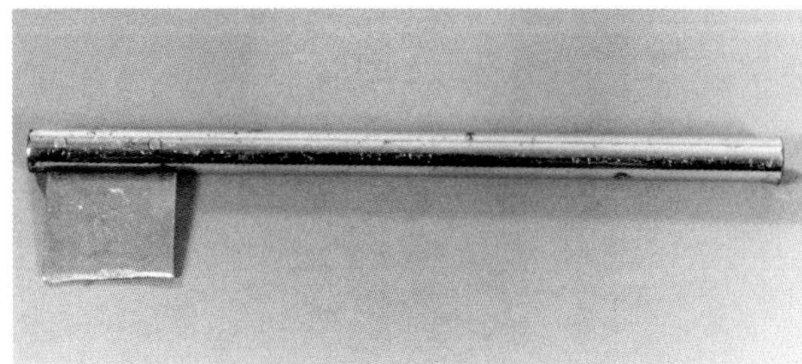

Fig. 2–36. Hatchet cast spreader.

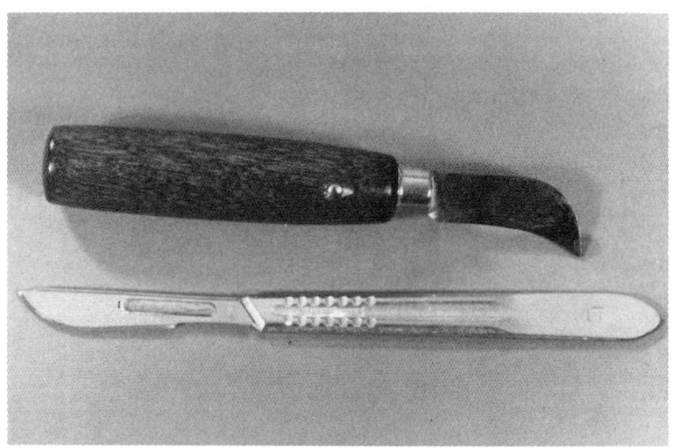

Fig. 2–37. Cast knife and scalpel.

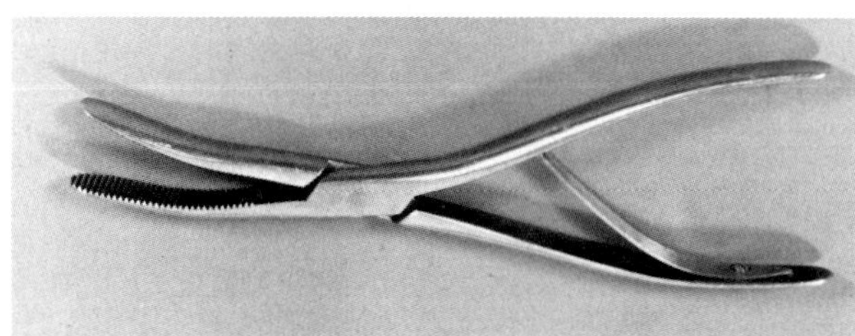

Fig. 2–38. Cast breaker.

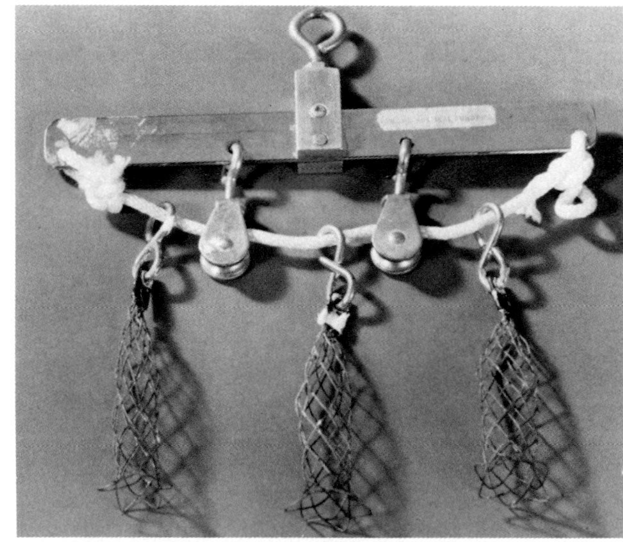

Fig. 2–39. Chinese finger traps.

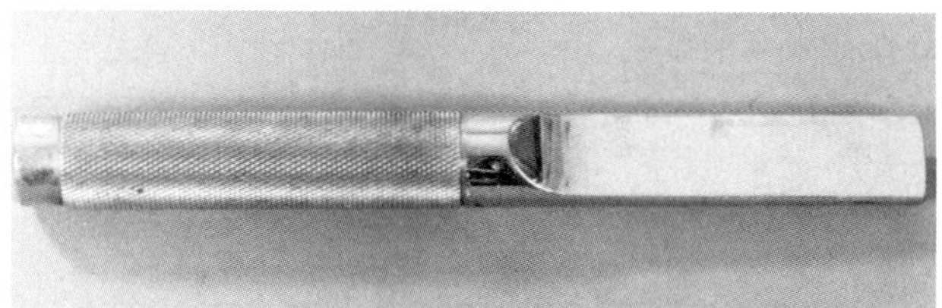

Fig. 2–40. Wedging separator.

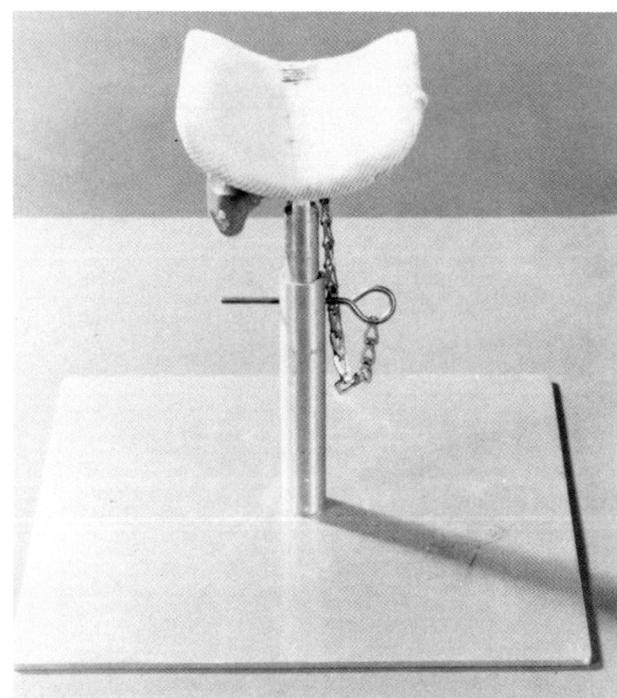

Fig. 2–41. Leg stand.

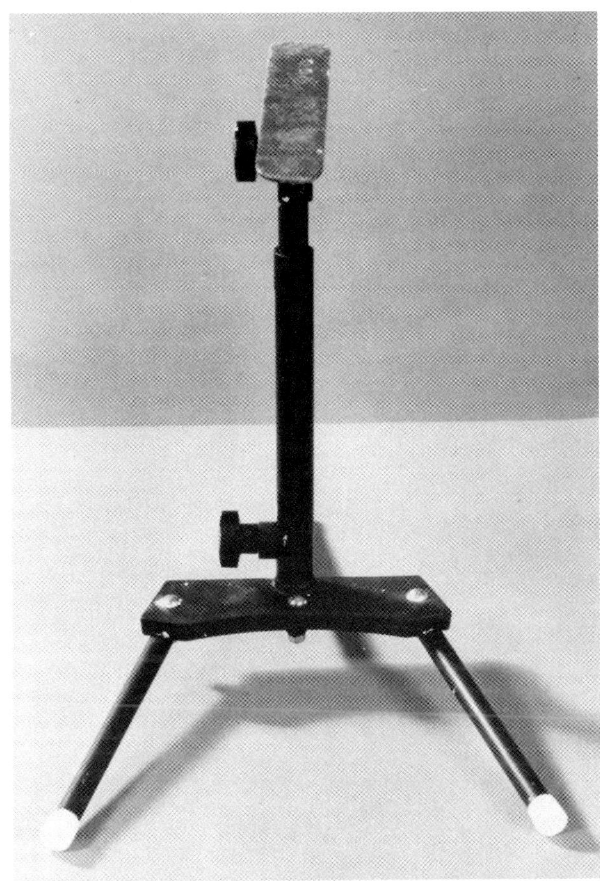

Fig. 2–42. Foot stand.

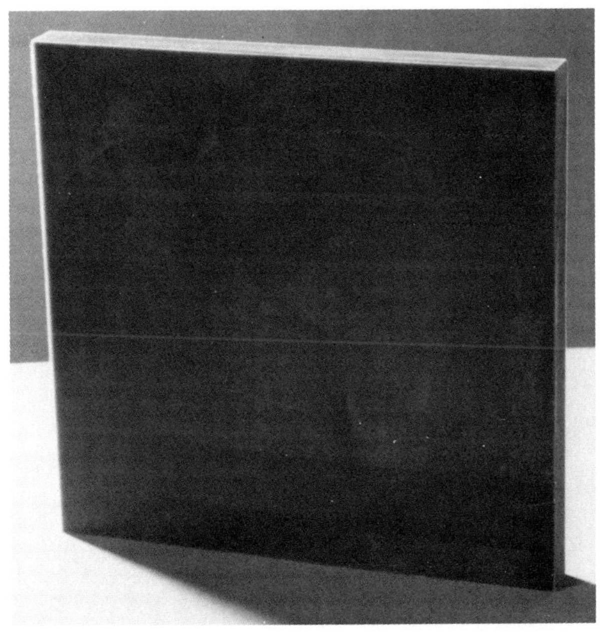

Fig. 2–43. Solid rubber block.

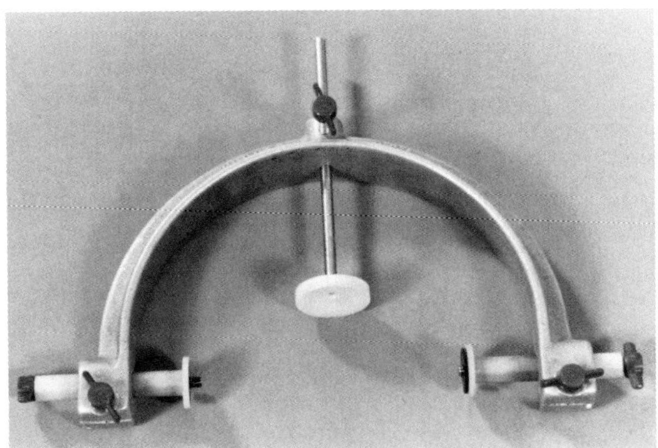

Fig. 2–44. Fracture-brace alignment fixture.

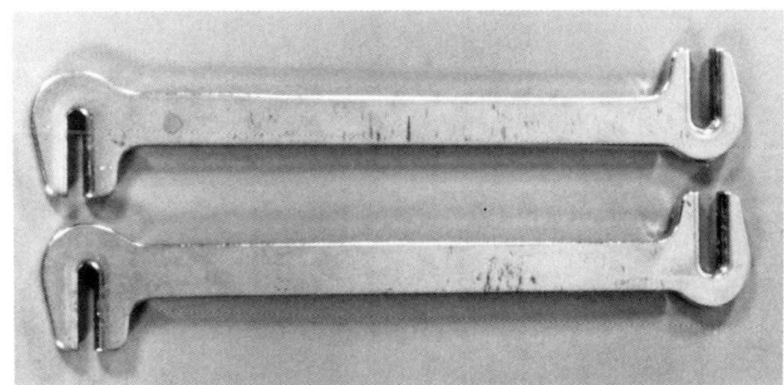

Fig. 2–45. Bending irons.

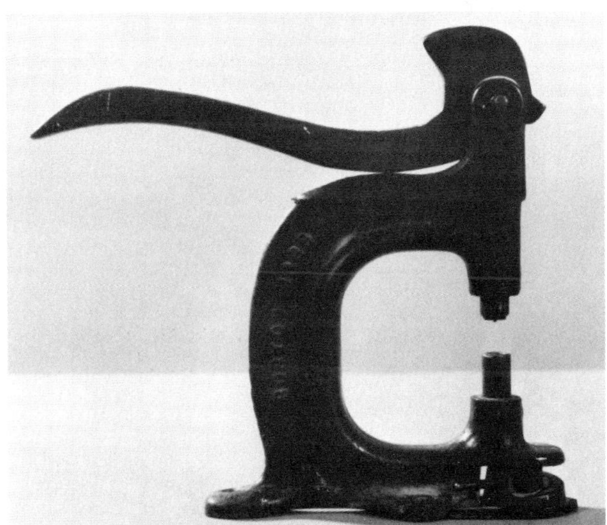

Fig. 2–46. Rivet machine.

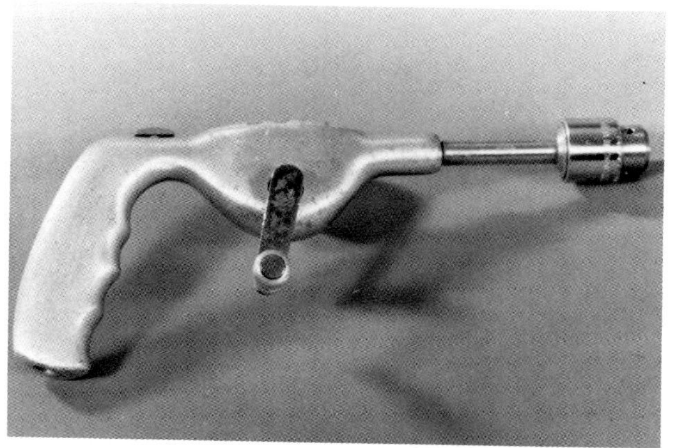

Fig. 2–47. Hand drill.

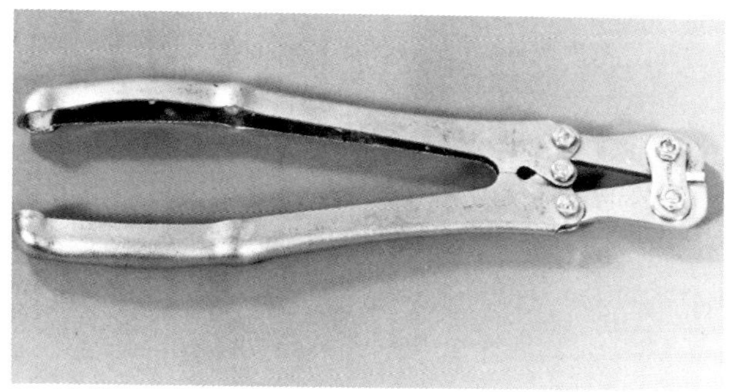

Fig. 2–48. Pin cutter.

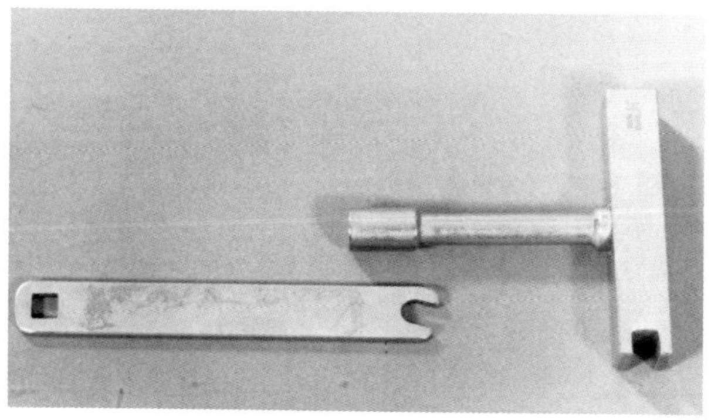

Fig. 2–49. Wrenches for Hoffmann apparatus.

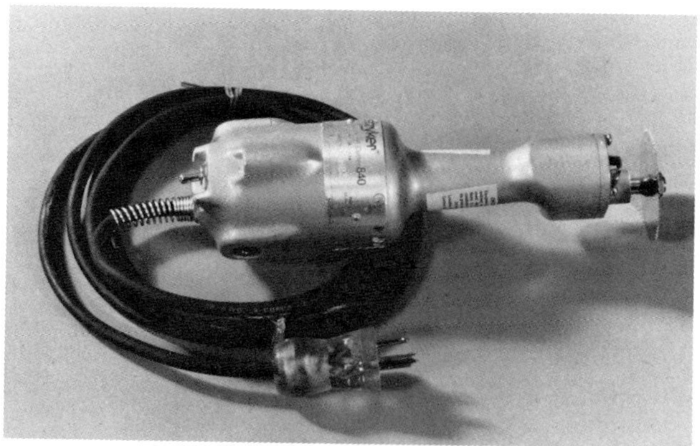

Fig. 2–50. Cast saw.

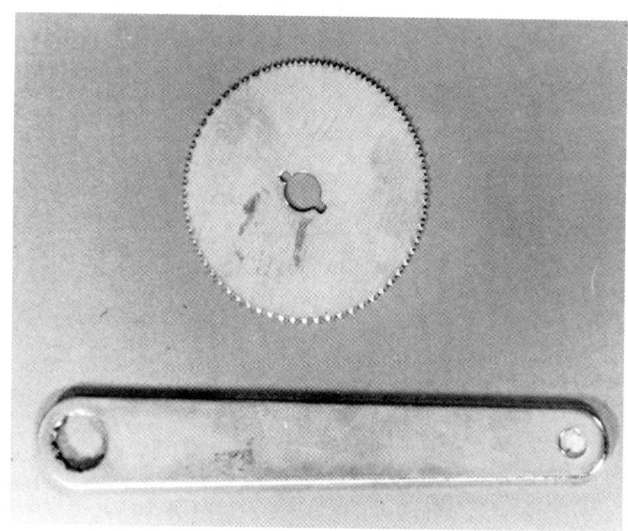

Fig. 2–51. Cast-saw blade and wrench.

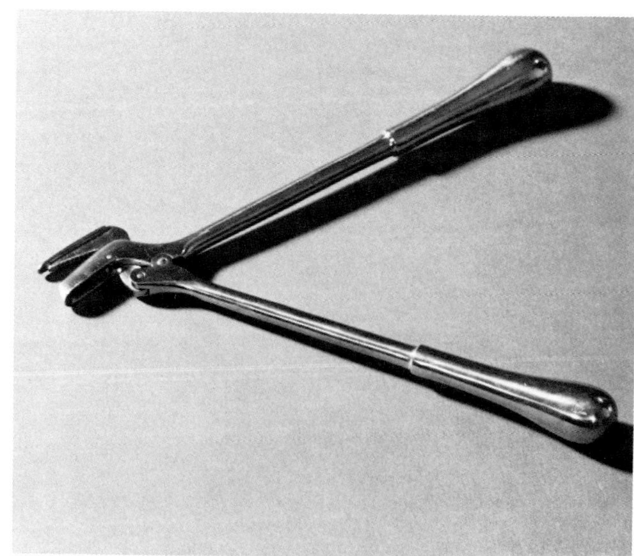

Fig. 2–52. Manual cast cutter.

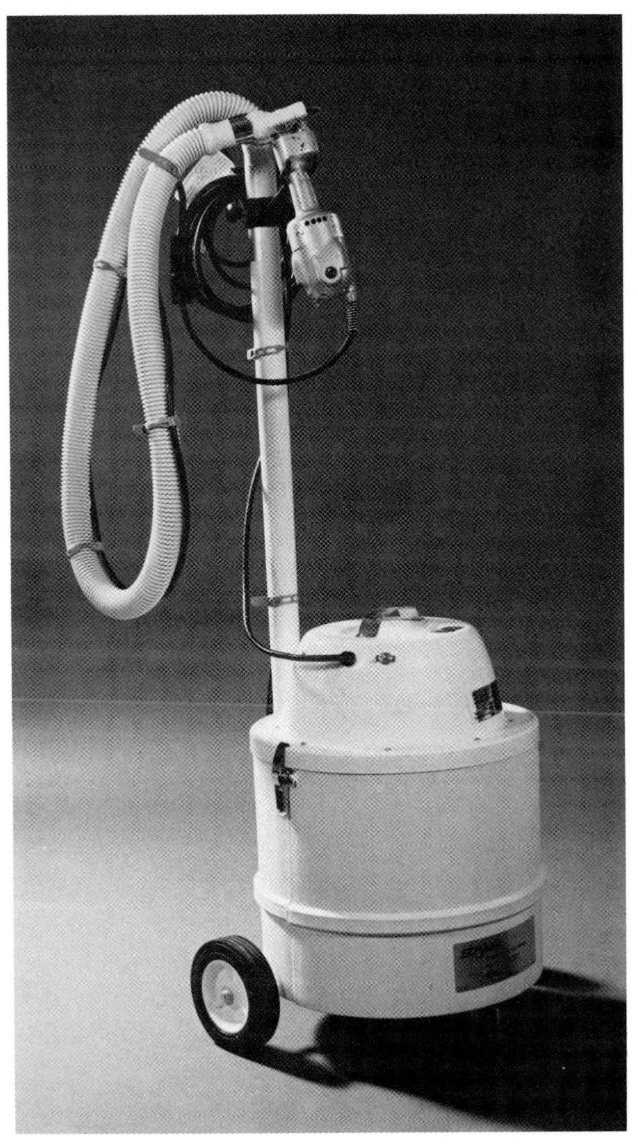

Fig. 2–53. Plaster vacuum.

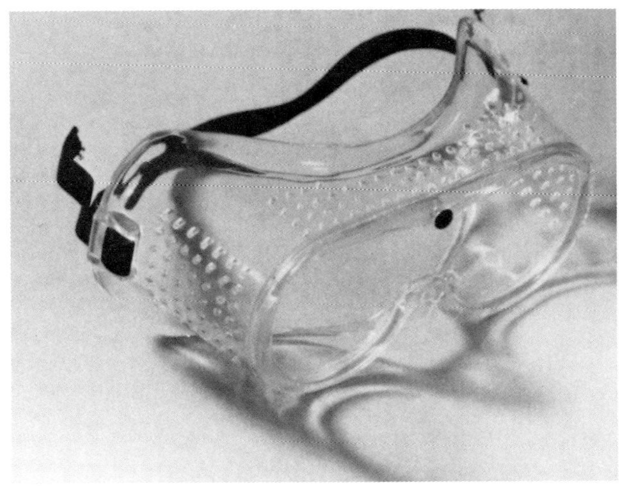

Fig. 2–54. Safety goggles.

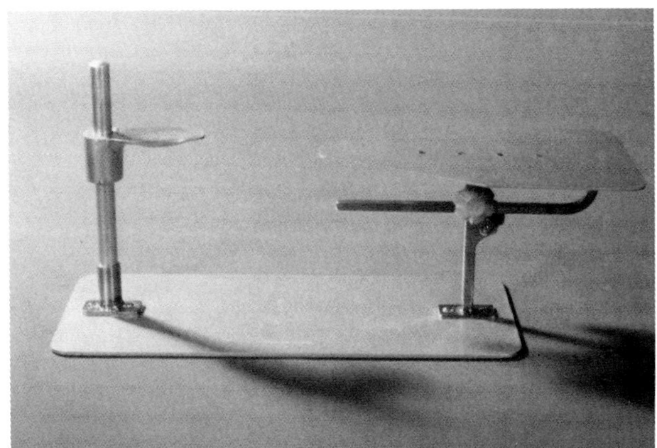

Fig. 2–55. Pediatric spica table.

CHAPTER 3. CASTING TECHNIQUES

APPLICATION OF STOCKINET

Stockinet is the first layer of padding that is in direct contact with the skin. In its application several important points should be borne in mind:

Appropriate Length and Width

As a rule, 3-inch-wide stockinet is used for arm casts, 4-inch-wide stockinet for leg casts, and 10-inch- or 12-inch-wide stockinet for body casts. Regardless of width, the stockinet should be significantly longer than the corresponding cast so that the ends of the stockinet can be folded over the ends of the cast and fixed there with a strip of plaster or fiberglass bandage to produce a neater cast and minimize skin irritation by the rough cast ends.

Removal of Transverse Wrinkles

Pressure-producing transverse wrinkles are typically present at the anterior aspect of an extremity where the joint has a 90° bend, e.g., the anterior aspects of the elbow and ankle joints. Transverse wrinkles are caused by the difference in length between the anterior and posterior aspects of the extremities and should be cut off with a pair of plaster scissors (Figs. 3-1, 3-2).

Making Smooth Transitions

In spica casts for the shoulder and hip, the extremities and the torso are enclosed in a single cast. The relatively small stockinet around the extremity thus has to become continuous with the much larger stockinet of the torso. A smooth transition can be achieved easily by splitting part of the torso stockinet at the transitional region so that the split ends can be brought down and wrapped smoothly around the stockinet of the extremity to produce smooth continuity between the two mismatched stockinets. Also, an arm or leg stockinet can be split so that it overlaps the much larger body stockinet (Figs. 3-3–3-5).

Adherence of Stockinet To Underlying Skin

Sometimes, as in a cylinder cast of the leg, an adhesive such as tincture of benzoin is applied to the stockinet to cause it to stick to the underlying skin so that the cast cannot slide up or down.

USE OF WEBRIL

Webril, which is made of soft cotton, is applied directly over the stockinet. A few points should be noted concerning its use:

Amount of Overlap

Webril may be overlapped from 25 to 50% of its width.

Thickness

It is customary to use two or three layers of Webril.

Eliminating Wrinkles

Wrinkles can be eliminated by proportionally stretching or even tearing the side of the Webril that has to go around a bigger portion of an extremity or around a torso.

Achieving Smooth Transitions

Spica Casts for Thumb and Great Toe

A 1-inch roll of Webril, obtained by equally dividing a 2-inch roll, can be used to wrap the thumb and the hand, or the great toe and the foot, before applying plaster or fiberglass bandages. When a 2-inch roll of Webril is used for the hand or foot, the Webril should be cut down to 1 inch for wrapping the thumb or the great toe.

Long-Leg and Short-Leg Casts and Long-Arm Cast

The approximately 90° bend at the ankle and elbow joints makes routine continuous Webril wrapping difficult. To avoid wrinkles, e.g., in front of the ankle, one should first apply Webril around the malleolar and midtarsal regions. The bare calcaneal region can then be covered with overlapping vertical and horizontal Webril strips until the whole heel region is adequately and uniformly padded (Figs. 3-6, 3-7).

Spica Casts For Shoulder and Hip

The Webril should be wrapped as high as possible around the extremities, and the Webril around the torso should be wrapped as close to the extremities as possible. The small gap at the junction between the extremities and the torso can then be covered easily with overlapping strips of Webril to produce a uniform padding.

USE OF FELT PADDING

Square, circular, or rectangular pieces of felt are usually used to pad the bony prominences of the body, which include the following:

Head Region

Occipital and forehead areas (Fig. 3-8) and mandibles.

Body

Clavicles and tops of the shoulders (Fig. 3-9), lateral aspects of the upper chest wall (Fig. 3-10), iliac crests (Fig. 3-11), spinous processes, and sacrum.

Upper Extremities

Olecranon, and radial and ulnar styloid processes.

Lower Extremities

Upper portion of the inner thigh, patella, fibular head, Achilles tendon and heel, and medial and lateral malleoli (Figs. 3-12–3-15).

As shown in the figures, various cuts have been made in these felt pads in order to produce a better fit for the bony prominences. For example, it is customary to make a cruciate cut in the center of a felt pad for the iliac crest (Fig. 3-11), partial diagonal cuts in a felt pad for padding in patella (Fig. 3-14), circular cut in a felt pad to pad the base of the neck (Fig. 3-9), and a circular cut through a felt pad to provide relief from a painful heel spur.

USE OF PLASTER BANDAGES

Plaster bandages are the most important and the most commonly used cast material, and familiarity with their proper use is vital in achieving optimal results.

Soaking Plaster Bandages

A roll of plaster is usually immersed in water at room temperature until air bubbles cease rising (Fig. 3-16A,B,C). Warm water shortens the setting time and is often used in applying plaster to a freshly reduced fracture.

Application of Soaked Plaster Bandages

After a roll of plaster bandage has been properly soaked, it should be removed from the water and gently squeezed to get rid of excess water. The two index fingers can be used to invaginate the centers of the two ends of the plaster roll in order to prevent telescoping of the wet plaster bandage during subsequent plaster application (Fig. 3-16D,E). During application, the plaster bandage should be snugly rolled over the limb in the same direction as the Webril and should be in constant contact with the limb. One can usually avoid wrinkles in a plaster bandage by tucking in the margin of the bandage and continuously molding the wet plaster with the palms of both hands. Each turn of the plaster bandage is usually overlapped about 50% by the succeeding turn, and 4 to 6 layers of evenly applied plaster are required to complete a cast. After all the necessary plaster bandages have been applied, and while the plaster is still wet, the whole cast should be thoroughly and evenly rubbed with the palms of both hands to convert the cast into a single smooth, strong unit. The Webril should extend $^1/_2$ to 1 inch beyond the proximal and distal margins of the plaster, so that when the ends of the stockinet are folded over the ends of the cast, the several layers of Webril will be similarly folded over the ends of the cast with the stockinet to produce smooth and well-padded cast ends. The cast is complete after the cast ends have been properly trimmed and the turned-down stockinet ends have been secured to the cast with new plaster bandages.

USE OF FIBERGLASS BANDAGES

Fiberglass bandages are applied in essentially the same manner as plaster bandages. However, the stretchability of the fiberglass bandage usually makes it unnecessary to tuck it in, and the superior strength of the fiberglass bandage makes it possible to make a strong cast with only 3 layers. When a fiberglass bandage is soaked in water before it is applied, it often sets in 2 to 3 minutes, but when the water soak is eliminated the setting time is about 7 minutes. Consequently, when a large cast such as a hip spica, shoulder spica, or body cast is being applied, the initial fiberglass bandages should be applied directly without soaking; only the later fiberglass bandages should be soaked in water. If this procedure is followed, the whole cast will be moldable to the end of the application process and a satisfactory cast will be produced.

After a fiberglass cast has hardened, small, sharp edges can often be found on its surface. These sharp edges can harm the patient and his clothing and furniture. The problem can be solved easily by removing these sharp edges with sandpaper or a fingernail file. In addition, the coarse surface of a fiberglass cast tends to produce noisy friction between the cast and the bedding, which may make it difficult for the patient to sleep. A simple way to solve this problem is to give the patient a piece of stockinet long enough to cover the entire cast for use during sleep.

USE OF PLASTER SPLINTS

Plaster splints are used to strengthen a plaster cast and tend to shorten the time required to complete it. In a long-arm cast, a 5″ × 30″ plaster splint is usually applied to the posterior surface of the arm and forearm, and only 2 or 3 layers of plaster need to be applied to the arm. Similarly, in a long-leg cast, 2 5″ × 30″ plaster splints are usually applied to the posterior aspect of the leg after the first roll of plaster bandage has been applied, and only 2 or 3 layers of plaster, applied in an overlapping circular manner, are required to finish the cast. Plaster splints are particularly indicated in providing additional strength to plaster casts worn by obese, unreliable, and young and active patients. Fiberglass splints are rarely required in fiberglass casts, because of the superior strength of the cast material.

TRIMMING OF CASTS

Trimming of a cast provides freedom of movement for the uninvolved part of the extremity beyond the cast and prevents pressure sores produced by the rough ends or openings of a cast. Casts should be trimmed, carefully and correctly, in the following places:

Distal Ends of Long-Arm and Short-Arm Casts, Shoulder Spica Casts, and Long-Arm and Short-Arm Cast-Braces. The thumbhole should be smooth and large enough for free thumb movement, and the distal end of the cast should end at the proximal palmar crease to allow free use of the fingers.

Distal Ends of Long-Leg and Short-Leg Casts, Hip Spica Casts, and Long-Leg Cast-Braces. The distal ends of these casts should be trimmed to the level of the proximal ends of the webspaces in a slightly oblique fashion. However, if a toe plate is required, the bottom portion of the cast should be allowed to extend slightly beyond the ends of all five toes.

Proximal Ends of Long-Leg Casts, Long-Leg Cast-Braces, and Cylinder Casts. A shallow semicircular piece may have to be removed from the superomedial aspect of these casts in order to provide pressure relief for the medial aspect of the upper thigh region, especially in very fat and very thin patients.

Proximal Aspect of a Shoulder Spica Cast. The proximal aspect of a shoulder spica cast should be carefully trimmed to allow complete freedom of motion of the neck without any irritation.

Perineal Region of a Hip Spica Cast. The perineal region of a hip spica cast should be smooth enough to prevent skin irritation, and the opening should be adequate for taking care of personal hygiene.

Upper Part of a Minerva Cast. The upper part of a Minerva cast should be carefully molded and smoothed off along the entire mandibular region to prevent pressure sores. The cast margins should be trimmed at least 1/3 inch from both ears to avoid irritation.

Upper Part of a Risser Cast. A Risser cast should be smoothly and carefully molded along the mandibular region; in addition, a shallow semicircular notch should be cut out of the occipital area in order to prevent pressure sore on the external occipital protuberance.

Shoulder Openings of Minerva, Risser, and Clavicular Casts. Shoulder openings should be comfortable and should provide ample room for complete use of the shoulder joints.

Lower Parts of Minerva, Risser and Body Casts. A shallow semicircular notch should be cut out of the sacrococcygeal region of Minerva, Risser, and body casts in order to prevent pressure sores.

BIBLIOGRAPHY

Bleck, E.E.: Atlas of Plaster Cast Techniques. Chicago, Year Book Publishers, 1956.

Blount, W.P.: Fractures in Children. Baltimore, Williams & Wilkins, 1955.

Connolly, J.F.: DePalma's The Management of Fractures and Dislocations. 3rd Ed. Philadelphia, W.B. Saunders, 1981.

Davis, B., and Dooley, B.: New fiberglass casting system in orthopaedic practice. Med. J. Aust., *1:* 1010, 1976.

Fleetcroft, J.: Plastering: A combination of old and new. Injury, *13:* 131, 1981.

Gartland, J.J.: Fundamentals of Orthopaedics. 3rd Ed. Philadelphia, W.B. Saunders, 1979.

Leach, R.E.: New fiberglass casting system. Clin. Orthop., *103:* 109, 1974.

Lewis, R.C.: Handbook of Traction, Casting and Splinting Techniques. Philadelphia, J.B. Lippincott, 1977.

Lovell, W.W., and Winter, R.B. (eds.): Pediatric Orthopaedics. Philadelphia, J.B. Lippincott, 1978.

Mears, D.C. (ed.): Materials in Orthopaedic Surgery. Baltimore, Williams & Wilkins, 1979.

Rockwood, C.A., Jr., and Green, D.P. (eds.): Fractures in Adults. 2nd Ed. Philadelphia, J.B. Lippincott, 1984.

Rockwood, C.A., Jr., Wilkins, K.E., and King, R.E. (eds.): Fractures in Children. Philadelphia, J.B. Lippincott, 1984.

Sarmiento, A.: Functional bracing of tibial and femoral shaft fractures. Clin. Orthop., *82:* 2, 1972.

Sarmiento, A., and Latta, L.L.: Closed functional Treatment of Fracture. Berlin, Springer-Verlag, 1981.

Sarmiento, A., et al.: Functional bracing of fractures of shaft of the humerus. J. Bone Joint Surg., *59:* 596, 1977.

Tachdjian, M.O.: Pediatric Orthopedics. Philadelphia, W.B. Saunders, 1972.

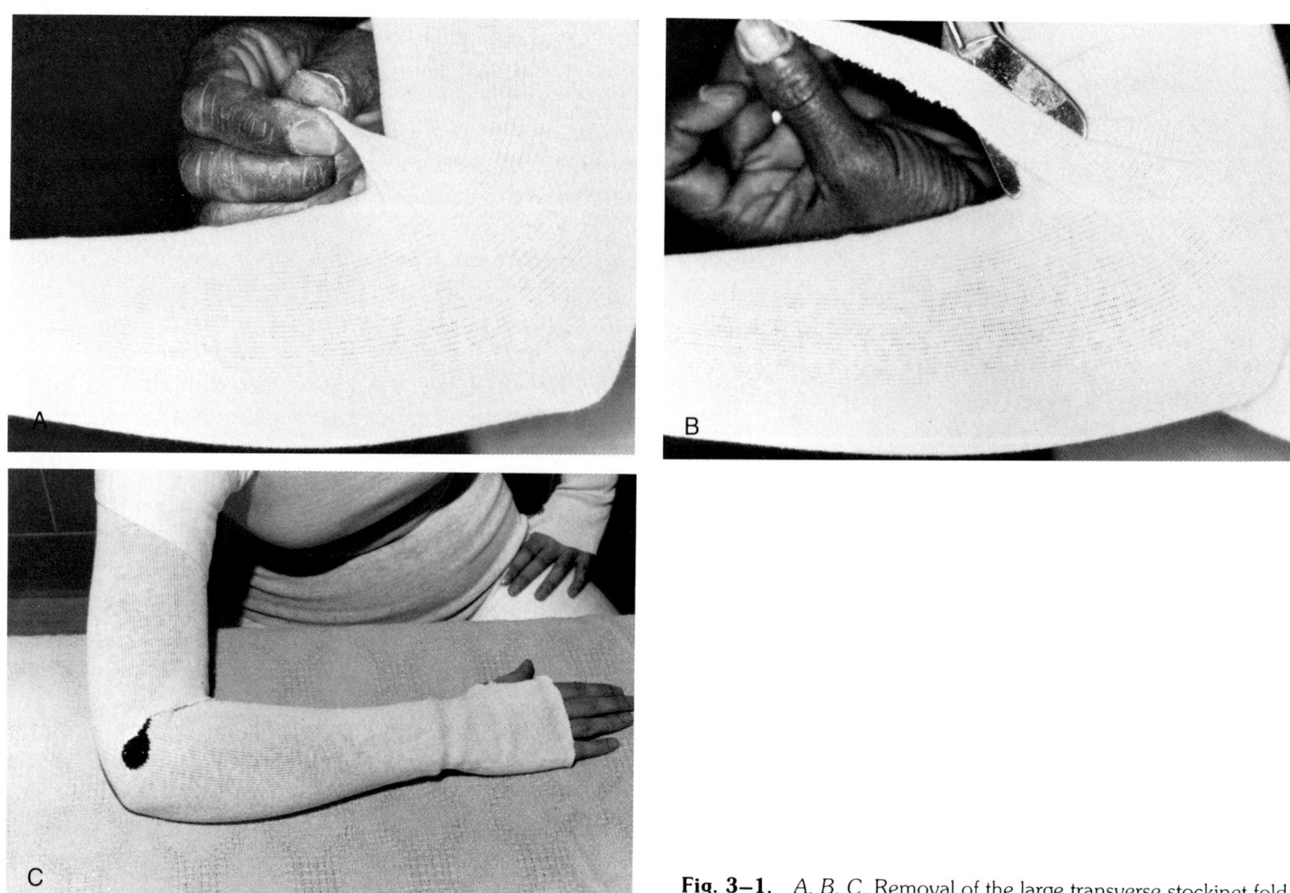

Fig. 3–1. *A, B, C,* Removal of the large transverse stockinet fold in front of the elbow.

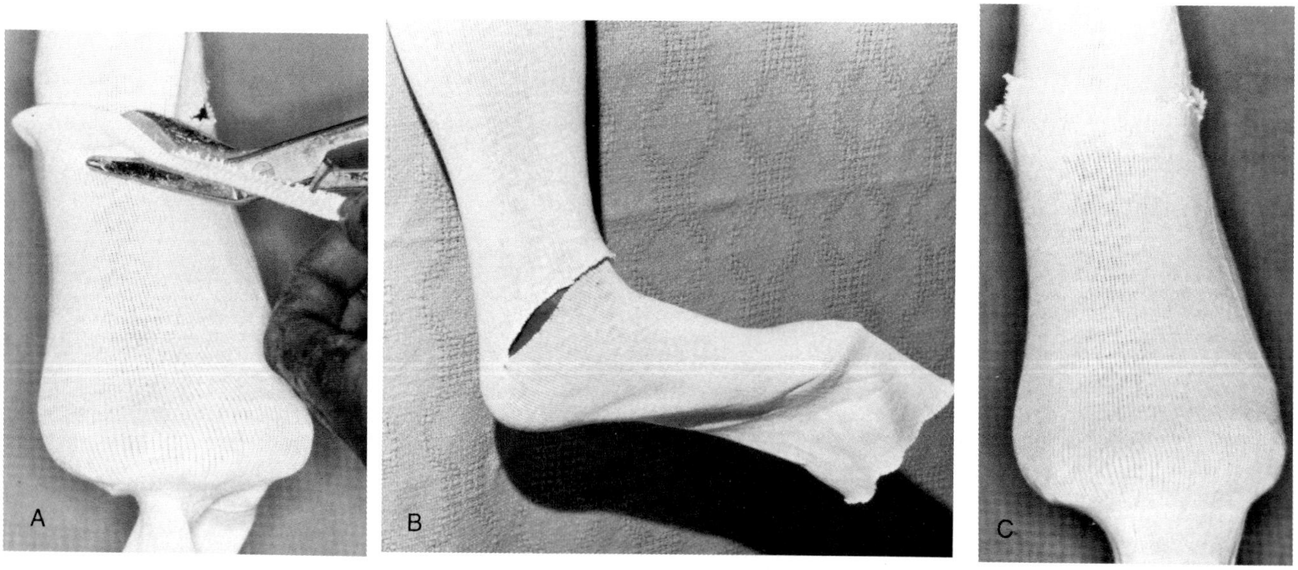

Fig. 3–2. *A, B, C,* Removal of the large transverse stockinet fold in front of the ankle joint.

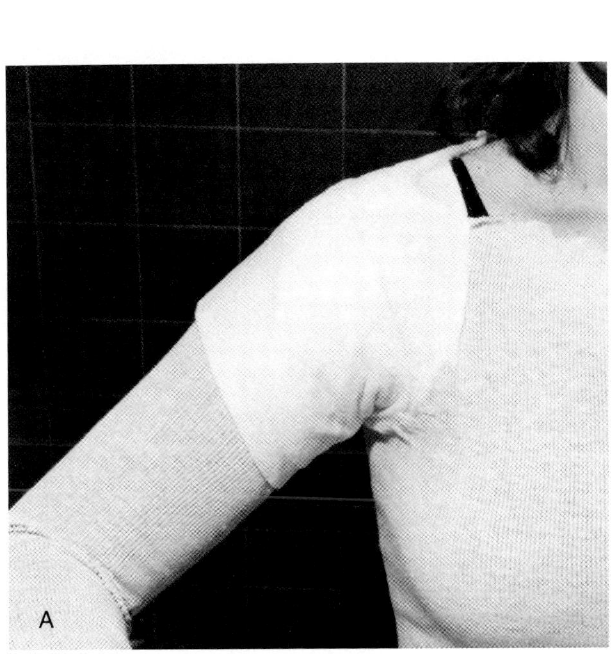

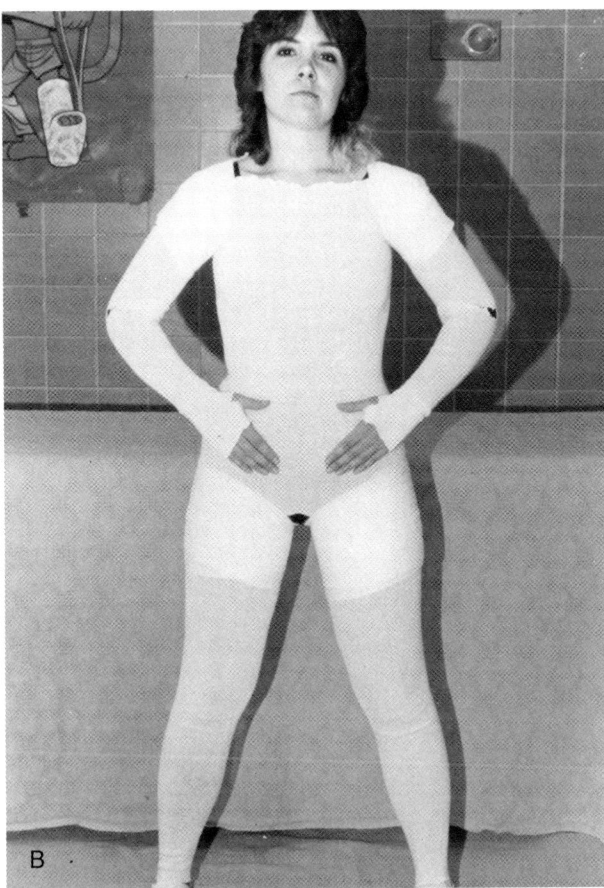

Fig. 3–3. *A, B,* To make a smooth transition of the stockinet in the shoulder region, lap the larger body stockinet over the smaller arm stockinet and then use several turns of Webril to hold the ends together.

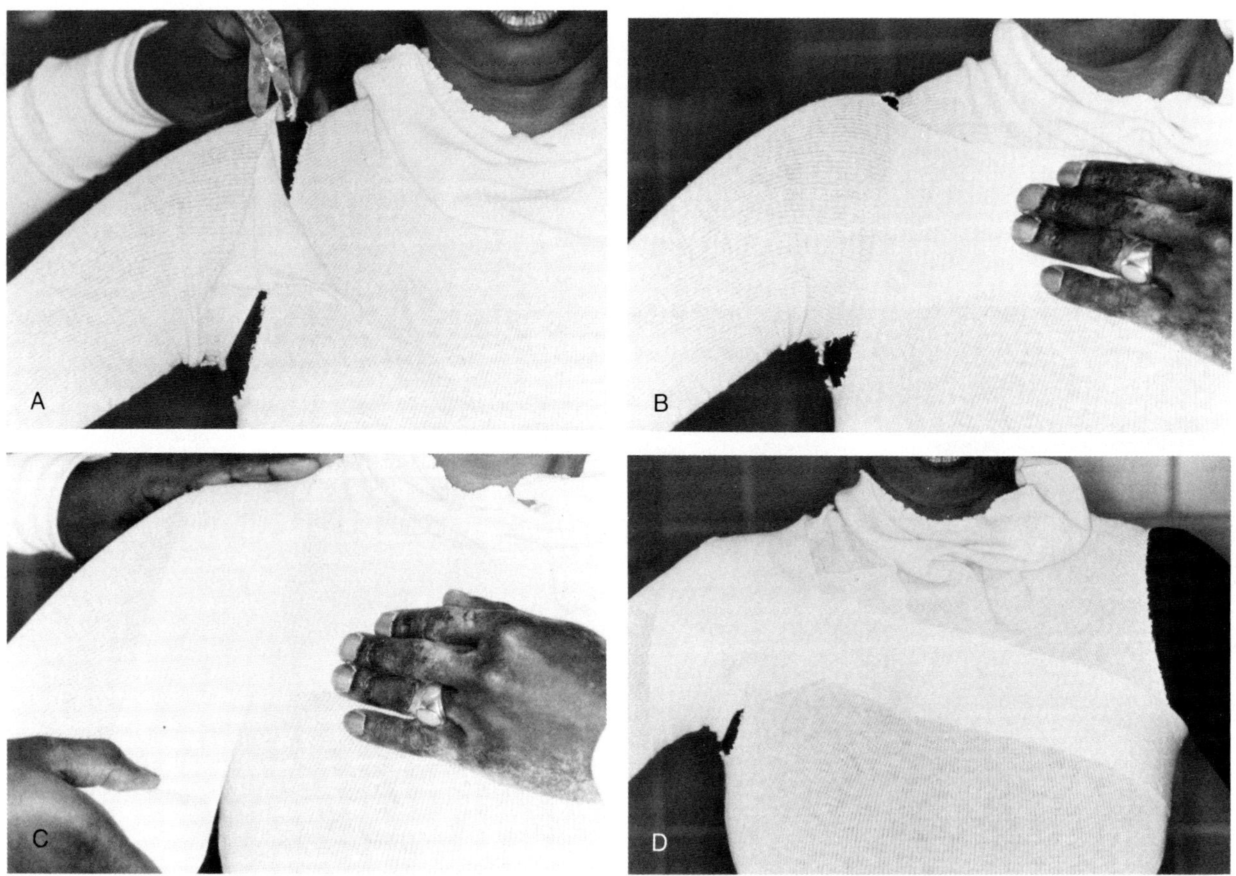

Fig. 3–4. *A–D*, An arm stockinet can be made to overlap a body stockinet by splitting it longitudinally to provide two large flaps to overlap the body stockinet. The overlapping ends can be secured with a Webril bandage.

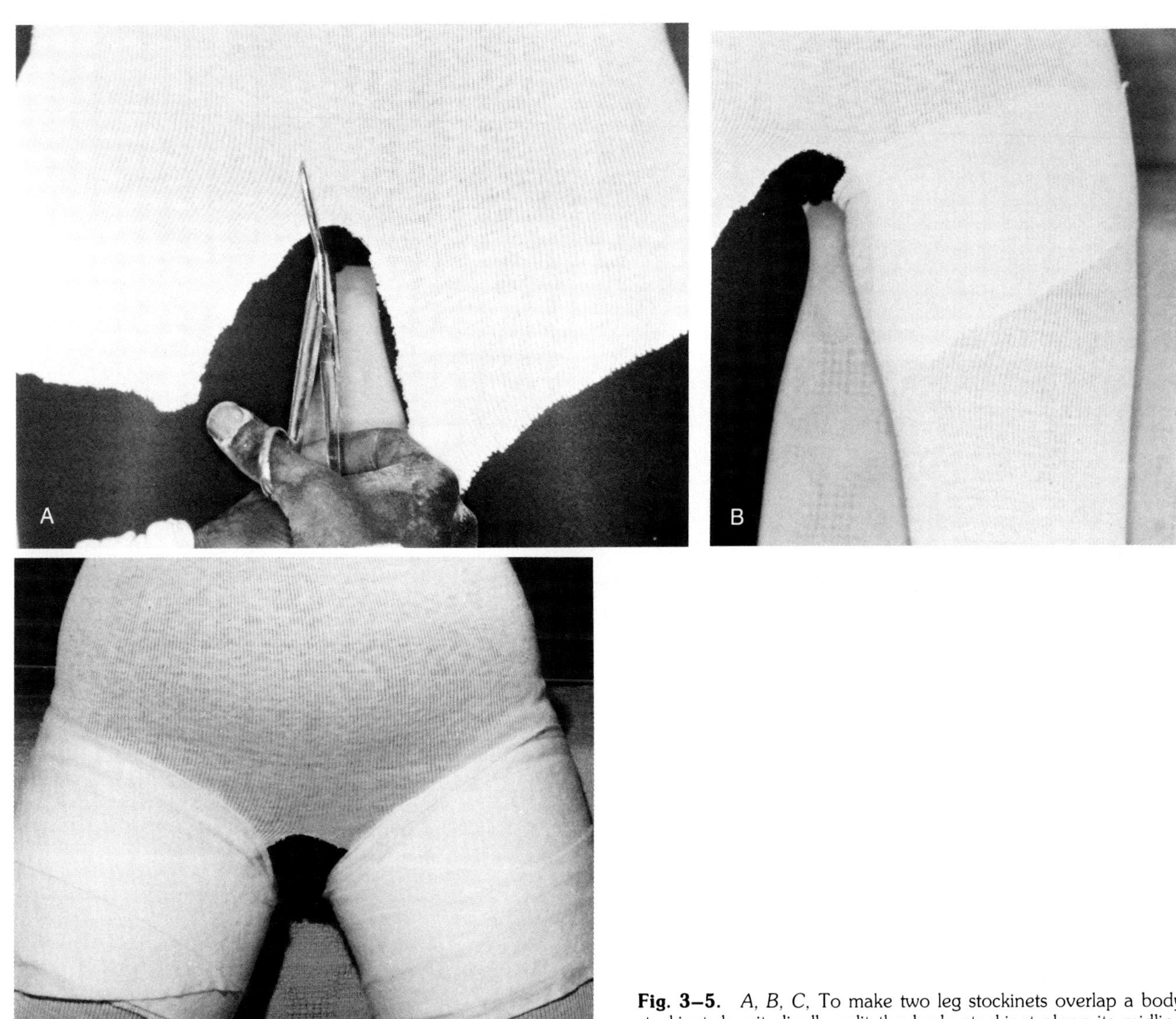

Fig. 3–5. *A, B, C,* To make two leg stockinets overlap a body stockinet, longitudinally split the body stockinet along its midline between the two upper thighs, roll the two leg stockinets up over the four cut ends of body stockinet, and hold the ends in place with Webril bandages.

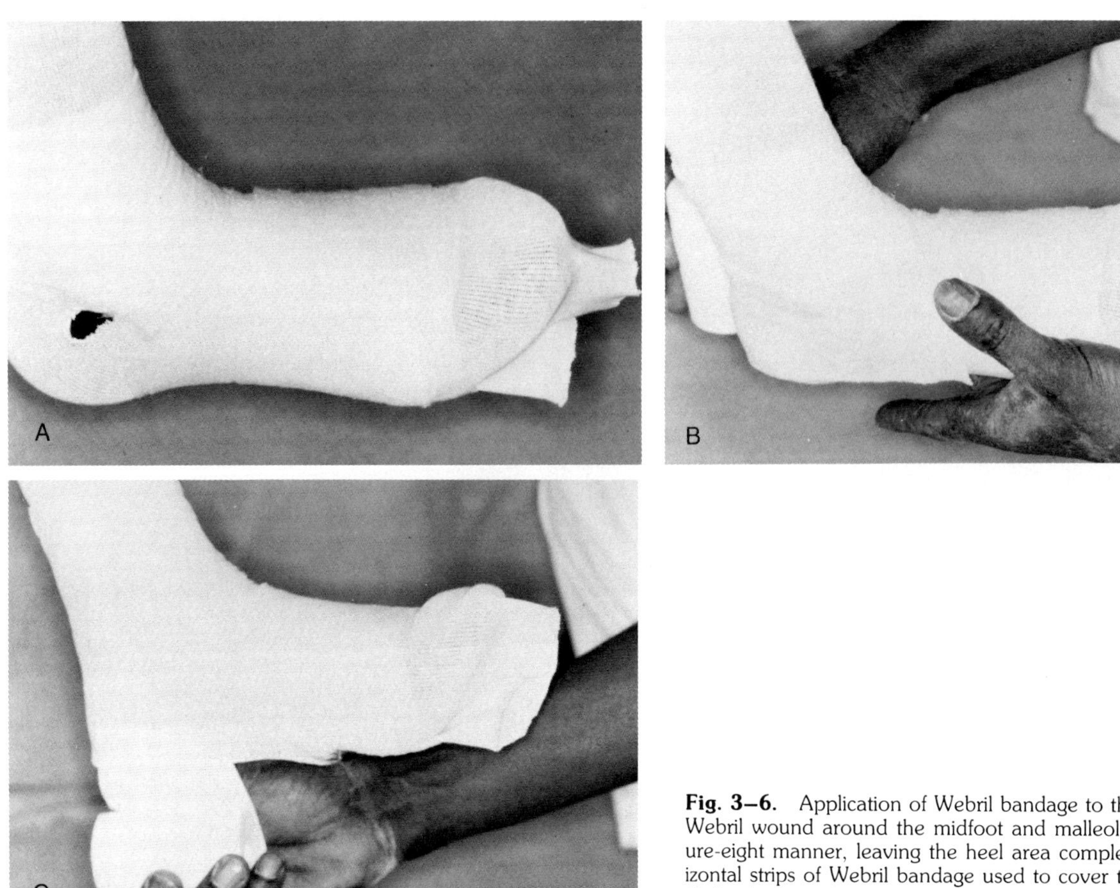

Fig. 3–6. Application of Webril bandage to the ankle region. *A*, Webril wound around the midfoot and malleolar regions in a figure-eight manner, leaving the heel area completely bare. *B*, Horizontal strips of Webril bandage used to cover the bare heel area. *C*, Application of vertical strips of Webril bandage to finish covering the heel.

Fig. 3–7. *A, B,* The supracondylar region of the humerus and the proximal radial and ulnar region are covered with Webril bandage applied in a figure-eight manner, and the bare olecranon area is covered with strips of Webril bandage.

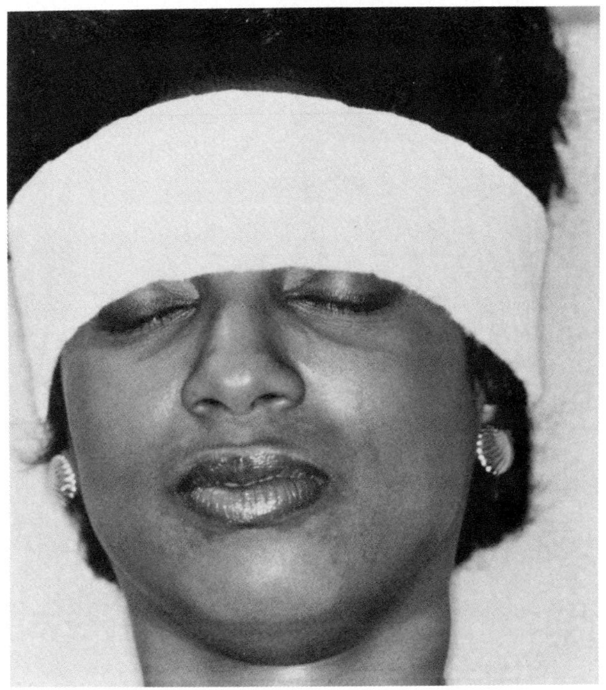

Fig. 3–8. A felt forehead band for a Minerva cast.

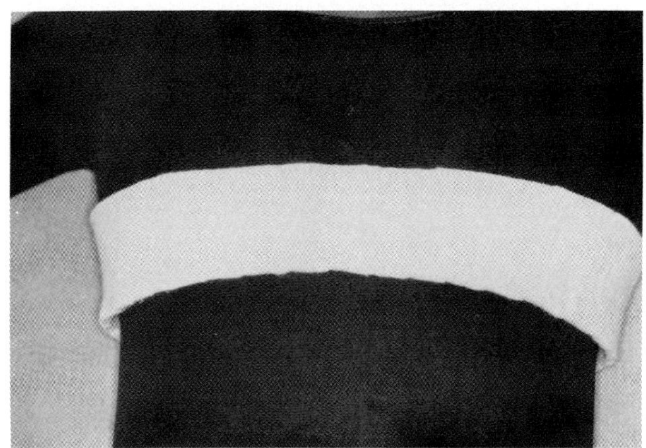

Fig. 3–10. Felt pad for upper chest wall.

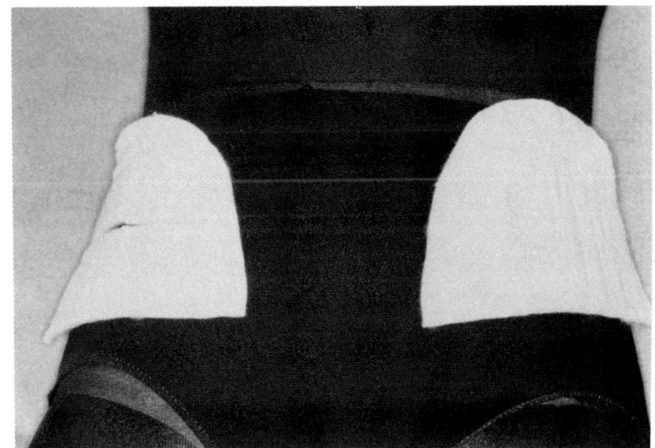

Fig. 3–11. Felt pads for anterior iliac crests.

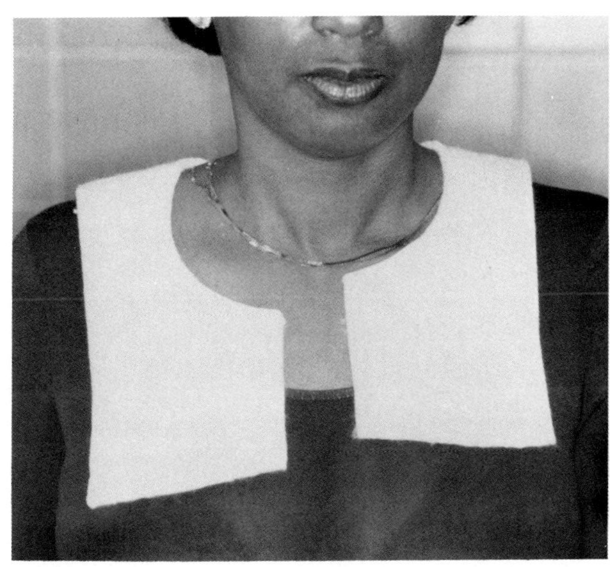

Fig. 3–9. Felt pad for shoulders and neck.

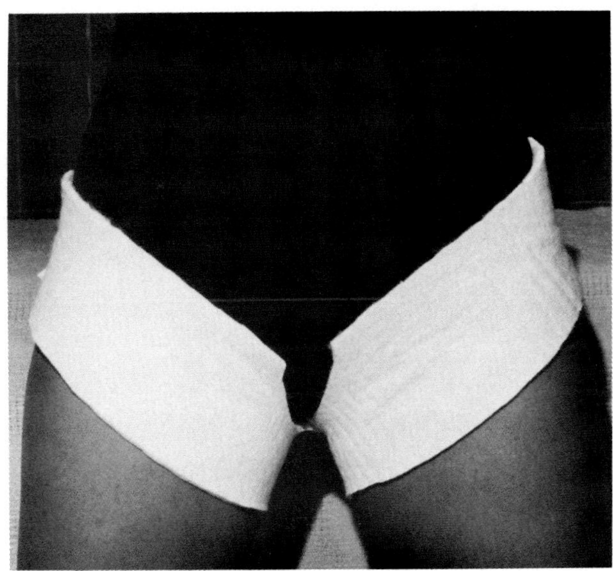

Fig. 3–12. Two felt upper medial thigh pads.

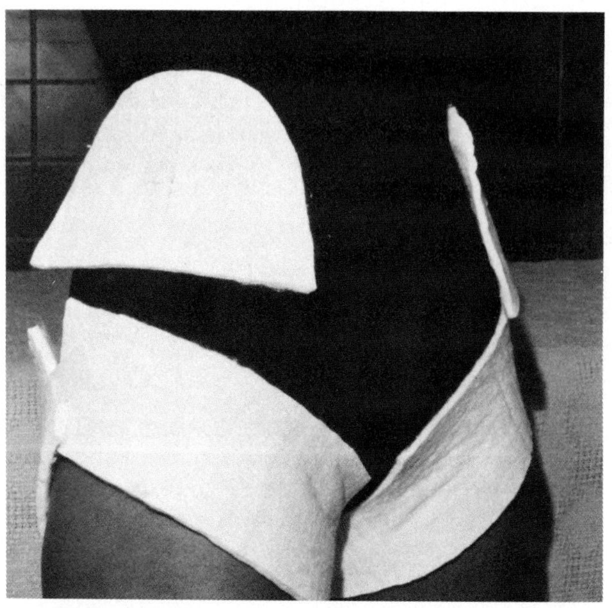

Fig. 3–13. Two felt upper medial thigh pads and two felt anterior iliac crest pads.

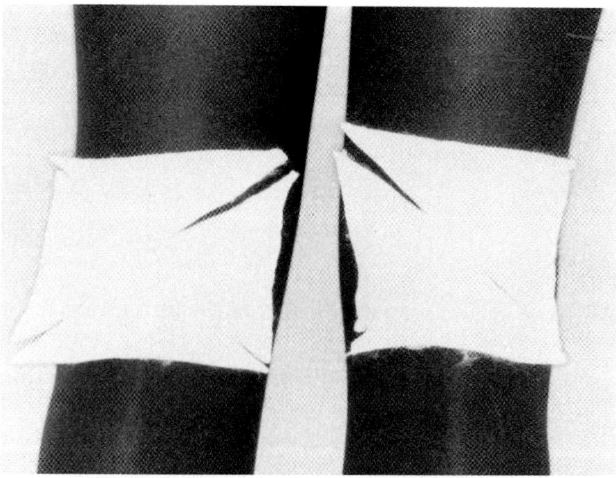

Fig. 3–14. Two felt patellar pads.

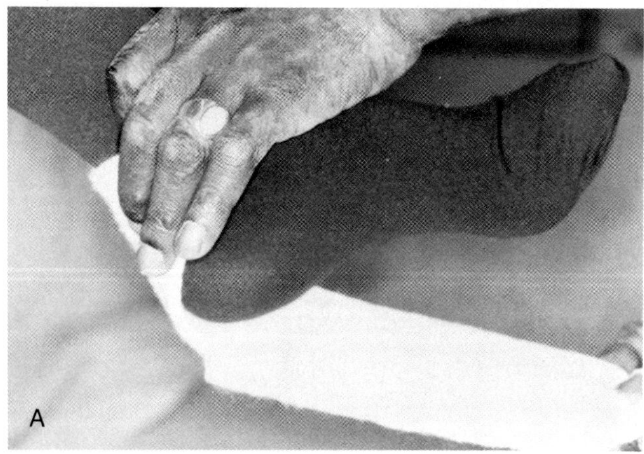

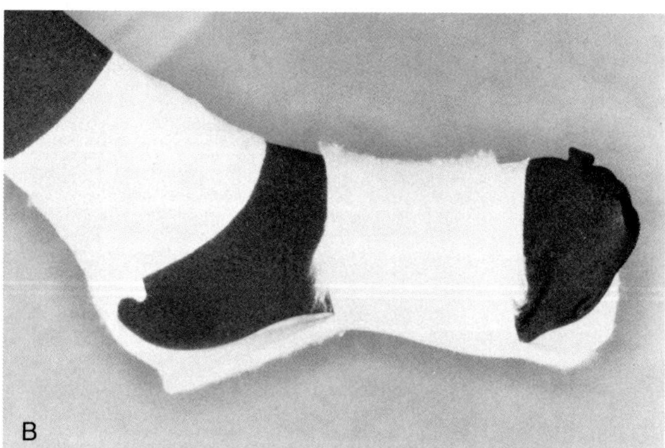

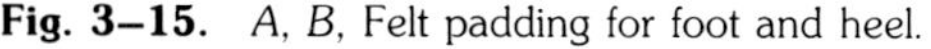

Fig. 3–15. *A*, *B*, Felt padding for foot and heel.

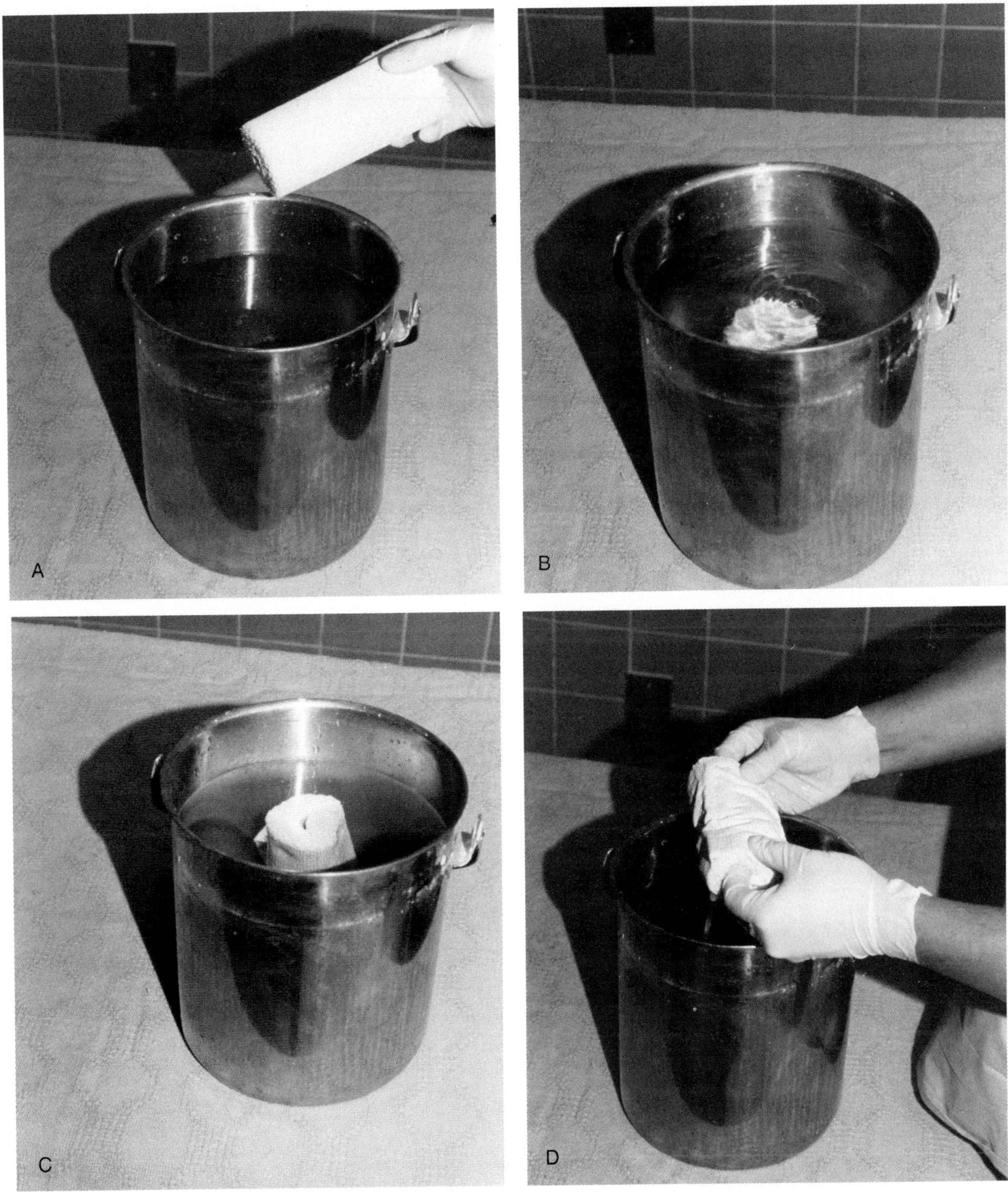

Fig. 3–16. Preparation of a plaster bandage prior to its application. *A*, A roll of plaster is ready to go into the water. *B*, Many bubbles are rising from the plaster bandage. *C*, Bubbles have ceased to rise. *D*, The central portion of the wet plaster bandage is pushed in with both index fingers to prevent telescoping of the plaster bandage during application.

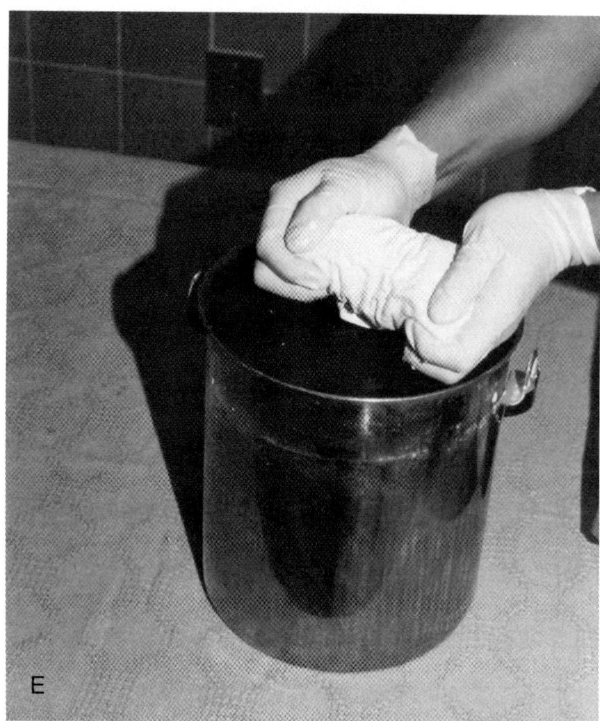

Fig. 3–16 (cont.). *E,* The wet plaster bandage is gently squeezed with both hands to get rid of excess water.

CHAPTER 4. COMPLICATIONS OF CASTS

PLASTER BURN

Third-degree burn can occasionally be produced by plaster. Severity of the burn depends on the absolute temperature and the duration of heat exposure. Plaster burns can be caused by such variables as hot dipping water, an unusually thick cast that produces too much heat, inadequate ventilation that impedes heat dissipation, fast-setting plaster that produces more heat per unit time than a slow-setting plaster, use of pillows made of highly insulating materials such as vinyl to cushion the newly applied cast, and high room temperature and humidity.

PRESSURE SORES

Pressure sores can be caused by large transverse stockinet wrinkles over the dorsum of the ankle, antecubital fossa, and popliteal fossa; irregular wadding of Webril; plaster ridges; indentations in the plaster produced by finger pressure; irregular cast ends and openings; improperly trimmed casts; and unpadded (or inadequately and incorrectly padded) bony prominences. Whenever a patient complains of a persistent pain or burning sensation under any part of a cast, the symptomatic area should be windowed and inspected immediately in order to prevent irreversible skin necrosis caused by a high-pressure point.

NERVE PALSY

Nerve palsy most commonly affects the common peroneal nerve, which, for instance, can be injured in a long-leg cast when the patient lies in bed for a prolonged period of time with his leg externally rotated. Less commonly, an ulnar nerve palsy can be caused by a constricting long-arm cast in the cubital tunnel region. In addition, the median nerve can be compressed in the carpal tunnel by various wrist and carpal fractures and dislocations, whose compressing effect is further augmented by the unyielding long-arm or short-arm cast.

ARTERIAL INJURY

Arterial injury produced by fractures or dislocations can be easily masked by reduction and cast application. Because the injured extremity is mostly covered by the cast, the cardinal signs of arterial insufficiency are obscured and tragic consequences can ensue. Arterial injury can become very difficult to deal with when the patient has multiple fractures and dislocations and is also semiconscious or unconscious.

VOLKMANN'S ISCHEMIC CONTRACTURE

Volkmann's ischemic contracture is usually caused by a fracture that produces edema and extravasation of blood into a confined space, which greatly increases intracompartmental pressure. The unyielding cast around the injured extremity further contributes to elevation of intracompartmental pressure. As a result, venous and lymphatic drainage is obstructed and the arteries and their collaterals go into severe vasospasm, producing severe ischemia of the nerves and the muscles, which subsequently become infarcted. With time, these infarcted muscles are slowly replaced by scar tissue, which also tends to involve the damaged nerves. The result is severe contracture, joint stiffness, and nerve palsy of the involved extremity.

THROMBOEMBOLIC COMPLICATIONS

Thromboembolic complications usually originate in the lower extremities (e.g., thrombophlebitis in the calf region). The presence of a cast over a fracture can make it difficult for a physician to arrive at the correct diagnosis without the aid of venography. Thrombophlebitis can lead to pulmonary embolism, which can easily cause the patient's demise. The common unpleasant sequence of thromboembolic complications is chronic venous insufficiency and recurrent thrombophlebitis.

CAST SYNDROME

Cast syndrome is caused by vascular obstruction of the duodenum by a body cast and is manifested clinically by epigastric pain and tenderness, vomiting, nausea, and symptoms and signs of electrolyte imbalance, which can cause death. The treatment consists of cutting a generous hole over the epigastrium (sometimes even complete removal of the body cast), insertion of a nasogastric tube to decompress the stomach, and careful electrolyte-replacement therapy until all symptoms subside.

CAST DERMATITIS

Cast dermatitis can be caused by poor ventilation and hygiene of the skin under the cast or by allergic reaction of the skin to chemicals in the cast.

LOOSE-CAST SYNDROME

A very loose cast can easily slide up and down an extremity to produce skin slough in areas such as the malleolar region and the dorsum of the foot.

CAST-INDUCED OPEN FRACTURE

Cast-induced open fracture can occur in a fractured extremity where the bone is very close to the skin, such as the pretibial region. The skin over a tibial fracture can be caught between the cast and the jagged broken bone and become necrotic. If neglected, an open tibial fracture can eventually lead to osteomyelitis of the tibia.

FOREIGN BODIES IN A CAST

Intentional or unintentional dropping of an object such as a hairpin, paper clip, toothpick, or coin into a cast can produce severe ulceration and infection of the skin under the cast.

CAST-INDUCED INFECTION

Fungal, parasitic, and bacterial infections sometimes follow an opening in the skin, such as a pin tract, to involve the underlying bone.

AVASCULAR NECROSIS OF THE FEMORAL HEAD

Avascular necrosis of the femoral head has been known to be caused by hip spica cast used to treat congenital dislocation of the hip in infants.

PERMANENT JOINT STIFFNESS

Permanent joint stiffness commonly occurs in the finger, shoulder, and elbow after immobilization in a cast for a prolonged period of time.

SHORTENING, ANGULATION, AND MALUNION OF FRACTURES, AND SUBLUXATION AND REDISLOCATION OF REDUCED JOINT DISLOCATIONS

All reduced fractures and dislocations should be followed closely in order to avoid such complications as shortening, angulation, and malunion of fractures, and subluxation and redislocation of reduced joint dislocations.

DISUSE OSTEOPOROSIS

Disuse osteoporosis, which is frequently associated with cast immobilization, is a reversible biological process. The lost bone can be regained gradually after full use of the injured extremity has been resumed.

CAST-ASSOCIATED HYPERTENSION

Cast-associated hypertension occasionally takes place; it is thought to be caused by stretching the sympathetic network around the blood vessels.

OBSTRUCTION OF A VENTRICULOPERITONEAL SHUNT BY A SPICA CAST

Obstruction of a ventriculoperitoneal shunt by a spica cast has been reported by Gerber (1977).

CAST-INDUCED ESOPHAGITIS

Cast-induced esophagitis, manifested clinically by epigastric pain and gastrointestinal hemorrhage and brought about by a body cast, has been described by Gryboski et al. (1978).

CAST-INDUCED HYPERCALCEMIA

Cast-induced hypercalcemia, also known as immobilization hypercalcemia, tends to be associated with polyostotic diseases such as multiple myeloma, metastases, Paget's disease of bone, malignant lymphomas, and leukemias.

BIBLIOGRAPHY

Aufranc, D.E., Jones, W.N., and Bierbaum, B.E.: Gas gangrene complicating fractures of the tibia. JAMA, *209:* 2045, 1969.

Beidler, J.G.: Skin complications following cast applications. Report of a case. Arch. Dermatol., *98:* 159, 1968.

Bisla, R.S., and Louis, H.J.: Acute vascular compression of the duodenum following cast application. Surg. Gynecol. Obstet., *140:* 563, 1975.

Brown, P.W.: The prevention of infection in open wounds. Clin. Orthop., *96:* 42, 1973.

Colwill, M.R., and Maudsley, R.H.: The management of gas gangrene with hyperbaric oxygen therapy. J. Bone Joint Surg. [Br.], *50:* 732, 1968.

Connolly, J.: Management of fractures associated with arterial injuries. Am. J. Surg., *120:* 331, 1970.

Culver, D., Crawford, J.S., Gardiner, J.H., and Wiley, A.M.: Venous thrombosis after fractures of the upper end of the femur. A study of incidence and site. J. Bone Joint Surg. [Br.], *52:* 61, 1970.

Doporto, J.M., and Rafique, M.: Vascular insufficiency complicating trauma to the lower limb. J. Bone Joint Surg. [Br.], *51:* 680, 1969.

Evarts, C.M.: The cast syndrome. Report of a case after spinal fusion for scoliosis. Clin. Orthop., *75:* 164, 1971.

Evarts, C.M., Winter, R.B., and Hall, J.E.: Vascular compression of the duodenum associated with the treatment of scoliosis. Review of the literature and report of eighteen cases. J. Bone Joint Surg. [Am.], *53:* 431, 1971.

Foisie, P.S.: Volkmann's ischemic contracture: An analysis of its proximate mechanism. N. Engl. J. Med., *226:* 671, 1942.

Gannaway, J.K., and Hunter, J.R.: Thermal effects of casting materials. Clin. Orthop., *181:* 191, 1983.

Gerber, A.M.: Iatrogenic failure of a ventriculoperitoneal shunt. Case report. J. Neurosurg., *46:* 830, 1977.

Gilbert, J.A., and Phillips, H.O.: The effects of steam sterilization on plaster casting materials. Clin. Orthop., *190:* 241, 1984.

Gordon, S.L., and Dunn, E.J.: Peroneal nerve palsy as a complication of clubfoot treatment. Clin. Orthop., *101:* 229, 1974.

Gore, D.R.: Iatrogenic avascular necrosis of the hip in young children. A review of six cases. J. Bone Joint Surg. [Am.], *56:* 493, 1974.

Greenberg, L.: A bacteriological analysis of plaster of paris bandages. Can. Med. Assoc. J., *60:* 4, 1949.

Griffiths, D.L.: Hazard of closed reduction of fractures. Tex. Med., *64:* 46, 1968.

Gryboski, J.D., et al. "Body-brace" oesophagitis, a complication of kyphoscoliosis therapy. Lancet, *2:* 449, 1978.

Hankin, F.M., Gragg, A.J., and Kaufer, H.: Bleeding beneath postoperative plaster casts. Orthop. Nurs., *2:* 27, 1983.

Harandi, B.A., and Zahir, A.: Severe hypertension following correction of flexion contracture of the knee. A report of two cases. J. Bone Joint Surg. [Am.], *56:* 1733, 1974.

Hearin, J.B.: Duodenal ileus with special reference to superior mesenteric artery compression. Radiology, *86:* 305, 1966.

Hicks, J.H.: External splintage as a cause of movement of fractures. Lancet, *1:* 667, 1960.

Hughes, C.W., Lineberger, E.C., and Bowers, W.F.: Anterior tibial compartment syndrome: A plea for early surgical treatment. Milit. Med., *126:* 124, 1961.

Hughes, J.P., McEntire, J.E., and Setze, T.K.: Cast syndrome: Duodenal dilatation or obstruction in a patient in a body cast, with review of the literature. Arch. Surg., *108:* 230, 1974.

Kaplan, S.S.: Burns following application of plaster splint dressings. Report of two cases. J. Bone Joint Surg. [Am.], *63:* 670, 1981.

Kozinn, H.A.: Clostridium Welchii infection due to plaster of paris after a shelf procedure of the hip. N. Engl. J. Med., *267:* 348, 1962.

Lavalette, R., Pope, M.H., and Dickstein, H.: Setting temperatures of plaster casts. The influence of technical variables. J. Bone Joint Surg. [Am.], *64:* 907, 1982.

Lawrence, G.D., Loeffler, R.G., Martin, L.G., and Connor, T.B.: Immobilization hypercalcemia. Some new aspects of diagnosis and treatment. J. Bone Joint Surg. [Am.], *55:* 87, 1973.

Leach, R.E., Hammond, G., and Stryker, W.S.: Anterior tibial compartment syndrome—acute and chronic. J. Bone Joint Surg. [Am.], *49:* 451, 1967.

Linson, M.A., Lewinnek, G., and White, A.A.: Ischemic complications of femoral cast-bracing: Report of two cases. Clin. Orthop., *162:* 189, 1982.

Lipscomb, P.R.: The etiology and prevention of Volkmann's ischemic contracture. Surg. Gynecol. Obstet., *103:* 353, 1956.

Logan, W.S., and Perry, H.O.: Cast dermatitis due to formaldehyde sensitivity. Arch. Dermatol., *106:* 717, 1972.

Logan, W.S., and Perry, H.O.: Contact dermatitis to resin-containing casts. Clin. Orthop., *90:* 150, 1973.
Lovell, C.R., and Staniforth, P.: Contact allergy to benzalkonium chloride in plaster of paris. Contact Dermatitis, *7:* 343, 1981.
Marks, M.I., Guruswamy, A., and Gross, R.H.: Ringworm resulting from swimming with polyurethane cast. J. Pediatr. Orthop., *3:* 511, 1983.
Matsen, F.A., III.: Compartmental syndrome: An unified concept. Clin. Orthop., *113:* 8, 1975.
Matsen, F.A., III., and Clawson, K.: The deep posterior compartment syndrome of the leg. J. Bone Joint Surg. [Am.], *57:* 34, 1975.
Micheli, L.J.: Thromboembolic complications of cast immobilization for injuries of the lower extremities. Clin. Orthop., *108:* 191, 1975.
Mubarak, S.J., and Owen, C.A.: Double-incision fasciotomy of the leg for decompression in compartment syndromes. J. Bone Joint Surg. [Am.], *59:* 184, 1977.
Murray, E.G.D., and Denton, G.D.: Plaster of paris as a source of infection in tetanus and gas gangrene. Can. Med. Assoc. J., *60:* 1, 1949.
Nelson, J.P., Ferris, D.O., and Ivins, J.C.: The cast syndrome: Case report. Postgrad. Med., *42:* 457, 1967.
Pichler, B.A., and Snyder, M.: Contact dematitis caused by plaster casting material. J. Am. Podiatr. Med. Assoc., *75:* 108, 1985.
Pope, M.H., Callahan, G., and Lavalette, R.: Setting temperature of synthetic casts. J. Bone Joint Surg. [Am.], *67:* 262, 1985.
Rabinou, K., and Paulin, S.: Roentgen diagnosis of venous thrombosis in the leg. Arch. Surg., *104:* 134, 1972.
Reid, R.L., and Gamon, R.S., Jr.: The cast syndrome. Clin. Orthop., *29:* 164, 1971.
Ritmann, W.W., Schibili, M., Matter, P., and Allgower, M.: Open fractures—long-term results in 200 consecutive cases. Clin. Orthop., *138:* 132, 1979.
Rutala, W.A., Sauiteer, S.M., Thomann, C.A., and Wilson, M.B.: Plaster-associated bacillus cereus wound infection. A case report. Orthopedics, *9:* 575, 1986.
Salter, R.B., Kostuik, J., and Dallas, S.: Avascular necrosis of femoral head as a complication of treatment for congenital dislocation of the hip in young children: A clinical and experimental investigation. Can. J. Surg., *12:* 44, 1969.
Seddon, H.J.: Volkmann's ischemia in the lower limb. J. Bone Joint Surg. [Br.], *48:* 627, 1966.
Seligson, D., and Harman, K.: Negative experiences with pins and plaster for femoral fractures. Clin. Orthop., *138:* 243, 1979.
Silverman, B.J., and Graham, J.J.: Cast syndrome and scoliosis. Bull. Hosp. Joint Dis., *31:* 97, 1970.
Staniforth, P.: Allergy to benzalkonium chloride in plaster of paris after sensitization to cetrimide. A case report. J. Bone Joint Surg. [Br.], *62:* 500, 1980.
Thompson, S.A., and Majoney, L.S.: Volkmann's ischemic contracture and its relationship to fracture of the femur. J. Bone Joint Surg. [Br.], *33:* 336, 1951.
Turner, M.C., Ruley, E.J., Buckley, K.M., and Strife, C.F.: Blood pressure elevation in children with orthopaedic immobilization. J. Pediatr., *95:* 989, 1979.
Volkmann, R. von: Die ischamischen Muskellahmungen und Kontrakturen. Zentralbl. Chir., *8:* 801, 1881.
Waldvogel, F.A., and Vasey, H.: Osteomyelitis: The past decade. N. Engl. J. Med., *303:* 360, 1980.
Wehbe, M.A.: Plaster uses and misuses. Clin. Orthop., *167:* 242, 1982.
Weitz, E.M., and Carson, G.: The anterior tibial compartment syndrome in a twenty month old infant (a complication of the use of a bow leg brace). Bull. Hosp. Joint Dis., *30:* 16, 1969.
Whitehouse, G.H., and Griffiths, G.J.: The phlebographic demonstration of venous thrombosis occurring during the treatment of scoliosis. Clin. Radiol., *29:* 579, 1978.

CHAPTER 5. SHORT–ARM CASTS, CAST–BRACES, AND SPLINTS

SHORT–ARM CAST

Indications

A short-arm cast (Fig. 5-1) is used for stable fractures of the distal radius and ulna, dislocations of the wrist joint, and fractures and dislocations of carpal bones.

Cast Materials Needed

Plaster Short-Arm Cast

3″ stockinet

2 rolls of 3″ Webril

2 rolls of 4″ plaster bandage

Fiberglass Short-Arm Cast

3″ stockinet

2 rolls of 3″ Webril

2 rolls of 3″ fiberglass bandage

Patient's Position

A short-arm cast is best applied with the patient in a supine position with the shoulder joint abducted 90° and the elbow flexed 90°. Chinese finger traps can then be applied to the thumb and fingers to provide traction, and counter-traction can be applied to the arm by means of weights attached to a wide sling around the upper arm.

Technique for Applying a Plaster Short-Arm Cast

Stockinet

A half-moon-shaped thumbhold about $1^1/_2$″ in diameter is cut out of the stockinet about 4″ from one end of the stockinet with a pair of plaster scissors. The stockinet is placed over the forearm and the hand with the thumb sticking out through the thumbhole (Fig. 5-2A).

Webril

Webril bandage is wrapped from the proximal ends of the fingers to the elbow joint. To make the Webril go around the thumb webspace in a smooth manner, a transverse cut or tear of about 75% of the width of the Webril should be made before the Webril is wrapped around the thumb webspace so that the base of the thumb is covered with several smooth layers of Webril (Fig. 5-2B,C,D)

Plaster Bandage

The plaster bandage should extend from the proximal palmar crease to about 1″ below the flexion crease of the elbow. After a thin layer of plaster has been applied around the forearm, the first layer of the plaster for the palm area is given a twist of 180° along its longitudinal axis to produce a small plaster rope, which is wrapped around the first webspace and crosses the palm along the proximal palmar crease to provide added strength for the palmar portion of the cast (Fig. 5-2E). A transverse cut of about 75% of the width of the plaster bandage should then be made before the second layer of plaster bandage is wrapped around the thumb webspace. The ends of stockinet and Webril are folded down over the cast end and are secured to the cast by applying a new roll of plaster bandage over the entire cast (Fig. 5-2F,G). The cast is thoroughly and evenly rubbed to fuse the layers of plaster into a single strong unit (Fig. 5-2H,I). The thumbhole is carefully trimmed to allow full use of the thumb (Fig. 5-2J,K).

Technique for Applying a Fiberglass Short-Arm Cast

Stockinet and Webril

The stockinet and the Webril are applied exactly as for the short-arm plaster cast (Fig. 5-3A,B).

Fiberglass Bandage

In order to shorten the setting time of the fiberglass bandage, the bandage is soaked briefly in water and then removed from the water and gently squeezed (Fig. 5-3C,D,E). The first roll of bandage is rolled onto the entire forearm. Then 2 or 3 turns of fiberglass bandage are made across the thumb webspace and around the hand, with a cut of about 75% of the width of the bandage for each pass across the webspace (Fig. 5-3F,G). The ends of the stockinet are then folded down over the cast ends, and a new roll of fiberglass bandage is used to finish the cast (Fig. 5-3H).

SHORT–ARM THUMB SPICA CAST

Indications

A short-arm thumb spica cast (Fig. 5-4) is used for fractures and dislocations of the navicular, trapezium, first metatarsal, and their articulations.

Cast Materials Needed

Plaster Short-Arm Thumb Spica Cast

3″ stockinet

1 roll of 3″ Webril

1 roll of 2″ Webril

2 rolls of 4″ plaster bandage

1 roll of 2″ plaster bandage

Fiberglass Short-Arm Thumb Spica Cast

3″ stockinet

1 roll of 3″ Webril

1 roll of 2″ Webril

2 rolls of 3″ fiberglass bandage

1 roll of 2″ fiberglass bandage

Patient's Position

The position of the patient should be the same as for a short-arm cast.

Technique for Applying a Short-Arm Thumb Spica Cast

Stockinet

A $1^1/_2$″ half-moon-shaped thumbhole is made about $2^1/_2$″ from one end of the stockinet, and a cut is made between the thumbhole and the end of the stockinet. The split ends of the stockinet can then be wrapped around the thumb and the thumb webspace. An alternative method is to apply a stockinet as for a short-arm cast, leaving the thumb bare (Fig. 5-5A).

Webril

The 3″ Webril is used mainly to wrap around the forearm, and the 2″ Webril is used around the thumb and hand (Fig. 5-5B,C,D).

Application of Plaster or Fiberglass Bandage

The 4″ plaster bandage or the 3″ fiberglass bandage is applied mainly to the forearm, and the 2″ plaster or fiberglass bandage to the thumb and the hand. The distal end of the cast should end at the proximal palmar crease, and the proximal end should end about 1″ distal to the flexion crease of the elbow (Figs. 5-E,F,G, 5-6). Before the cast has hardened, the palmar aspect of the cast should be molded carefully with the thumbs to conform to the thenar and hypothenar eminences and the midpalmar concavity in order to minimize the motion of the wrist.

SUPRACONDYLAR CAST

Indications

A supracondylar cast (Fig. 5-7) is used for unstable fractures and dislocations of the wrist and for fractures of the radius and ulna. Because a supracondylar cast allows elbow motion but severely restricts supination and pronation of the forearm, it can be used to replace a long-arm cast in many instances.

Cast Materials Needed

Plaster Supracondylar Cast

3″ stockinet

3 rolls of 3″ Webril

4 rolls of 4″ plaster bandage

Fiberglass Supracondylar Cast

3″ stockinet

3 rolls of 3″ Webril

2 rolls of 3″ fiberglass bandage

1 roll of 4″ fiberglass bandage

Patient's Position

A supracondylar cast is best applied with the patient in a recumbent position with the elbow bent 90° and the forearm in neutral rotation.

Technique for Applying a Supracondylar Cast

Stockinet

A 3″ stockinet with a thumbhole is applied to the whole arm from the bases of the fingers to the upper arm (Fig. 5-8A).

Webril

Webril is applied from the distal palmar crease to the middle of the upper arm. To eliminate wrinkles over the antecubital fossa, Webril should first be applied in overlapping figure-eights immediately above and below the elbow joint, and the bare olecranon region can then be covered with overlapping Webril strips until the whole elbow region is evenly and adequately padded (Fig. 5-8B).

Application of Fiberglass Bandage

Two rolls of 3″ fiberglass bandage are applied to the arm from the proximal palmar crease to the mid-portion of the upper arm. Four layers of fiberglass bandage should be wrapped around the supracondylar region to provide the required strength for the supracondylar flanges. These layers should be molded carefully around the medial and lateral humeral condyles. Similarly, the stockinet end should be folded over the distal end of the cast, which should be molded closely to fit the thenar and hypothenar eminences and the mid-palmar concavity (Fig. 5-8C,D). After the cast has hardened, cutting lines for 2 supracondylar flanges (which prevent rotation of the forearm) and 2 U-shaped notches are marked on it with a wax pencil. The anterior notch, which allows elbow flexion, should be $1^{1}/_{2}''$ to 2″ distal to the elbow flexion crease, and the posterior notch, which allows elbow extension, should extend 3″ distal to the tip of the olecranon (Fig. 5-8E,F). An oscillating saw is then used to cut the cast along the marked line (Fig. 5-8G,H,I). A longitudinal cut through the redundant portion of the cast allows it to be removed with ease (Fig. 5-8J,K). The Webril is trimmed about $^{1}/_{4}''$ above the upper margin of the cast in order to provide additional padding for the upper cast end after the stockinet has been turned down (Fig. 5-8L,M). Flexion and extension of the elbow should be checked at this point (Fig. 5-8N,O). After the proximal stockinet end has been split longitudinally along its anterior and posterior aspects, plastic adhesive is liberally applied to the two supracondylar flanges and the adjacent upper portion of the cast (Fig. 5-8P,Q). The stockinet is folded down over the upper margin of the cast and is allowed to stick to the cast (Fig. 5-8R). A roll of 4″ fiberglass bandage is applied over the entire cast to the bases of the 2 supracondylar flanges (Fig. 5-8S,T). The finished cast should be checked to confirm free motion of thumb and fingers, complete elbow flexion and extension, and virtual absence of rotation of the forearm (Fig. 5-8U,V,W).

OLD–FASHIONED SUPRACONDYLAR CAST

An old-fashioned supracondylar cast (Fig. 5-9) is made in the same manner as a standard supracondylar cast except that the medial and lateral supracondylar flanges and the infra-olecranon U-shaped notch are replaced by a posterior supracondylar extension above the humeral olecranon fossa to hug the triceps tendon. Disadvantages of the old-fashioned supracondylar cast include limitation of extension of the elbow joint and potential irritation of the skin over the triceps tendon by the cast extension.

SUPRACONDYLAR CAST–BRACE WITH DORSAL WRIST HINGE

Indications

A supracondylar cast-brace with dorsal wrist hinge (Fig. 5-10), which allows motion in both elbow and wrist joints, is used mainly in treating fractures of the radius and ulna.

Cast Materials Needed

Plaster Supracondylar Cast-Brace with Dorsal Wrist Hinge

3″ stockinet

3 rolls of 3″ Webril

4 rolls of 4″ plaster bandage

1 roll of 2″ plaster bandage

1 small gate hinge

Fiberglass Supracondylar Cast-Brace with Dorsal Wrist Hinge

3″ stockinet

3 rolls of 3″ Webril

2 rolls of 3″ fiberglass bandage

1 roll of 4″ fiberglass bandage

1 roll of 2″ fiberglass bandage

1 small gate hinge

Patient's Position

The position of the patient is the same as for a supracondylar cast.

Technique for Applying a Supracondylar Cast-Brace with Dorsal Wrist Hinge

The initial application of stockinet, Webril, and plaster or fiberglass bandages is the same as for a supracondylar cast. After the supracondylar cast is finished, an oscillating cast saw is used to make 2 cuts on the dorsal aspect of the cast, 1 proximal and 1 distal to the wrist joint. The distal cut should be along a line extending from the proximal end of the thumb webspace to the base of fifth metacarpal, and the proximal cut should be approximately 1 inch proximal to the tips of the radial and ulnar styloid processes. These 2 cuts are made prior to installation of the hinge in order to avoid the difficulty of cutting the cast material under the hinge. The small gate hinge is placed over the dorsal aspect of the cast, care being taken to make sure that the hinge is directly on top of the wrist joint before the ends of the hinge are fixed to the cast with 2″ plaster or fiberglass bandage. The plaster or fiberglass between the two cuts is removed from the dorsal and volar aspects of the wrist with an oscillating cast saw. The underlying Webril and stockinet are cut transversely and secured to the proximal and distal portions of the cast-brace with narrow strips of plaster or fiberglass bandage (Fig. 5-11Q).

OLD–FASHIONED SUPRACONDYLAR CAST–BRACE WITH DORSAL WRIST HINGE

An old-fashioned supracondylar cast-brace with a dorsal wrist hinge (Fig. 5-12) is made by first applying an old-fashioned supracondylar cast and then installing a dorsal wrist hinge.

BIVALVING OF SHORT–ARM CAST, SHORT–ARM THUMB SPICA CAST, AND SUPRACONDYLAR CAST

Casts are often bivalved in order to provide additional room for postoperative or posttraumatic swelling of the extremities, to facilitate inspection and treatment of open wounds, and to allow unobstructed physiotherapy and occupational therapy.

Bivalving of a Short-Arm Cast

A short-arm cast can be bivalved easily along its radial and ulnar borders. A cast spreader can then be used to pry the cast open. The underlying Webril should be cut before splitting the stockinet in order to avoid skin damage. The margins of the bivalved cast can be lined with moleskin, and the two halves of the bivalved cast can be reapplied to the injured extremity and held together with Velcro straps or webbings with attached buckles (Figs. 5-13, 5-14). An alternative method for bivalving a short-arm cast is to make a longitudinal cut along the midline of the volar and dorsal surfaces of the cast (Fig. 5-15).

Bivalving of a Short-Arm Thumb Spica Cast

A short-arm thumb spica cast can be bivalved by making one longitudinal cut along the radial border to the thumb webspace and another longitudinal cut along the ulnar border of the cast (Figs. 5-16, 5-17). The bivalved cast can be lined with moleskin and then put together with Velcro straps or webbings and buckles.

Bivalving of a Supracondylar Cast

A supracondylar cast can be bivalved by splitting the cast longitudinally along the midline of its volar and dorsal surfaces (Fig. 5-18). An alternative method is to make two oblique cuts, one from the first webspace to the middle of the anterior notch of the cast immediately distal to the antecubital fossa, and the other from the ulnar border of the distal end of the cast to the middle of the infra-olecranon notch of the cast (Figs. 5-19, 5-20).

SHORT–ARM SPLINTS

Sugar-Tong Short-Arm Splint

A sugar-tong short-arm splint (Fig. 5-21) can be made of plaster or fiberglass splints and bandages, which should be padded with felt, foam rubber sheet, or several layers of Webril. This splint is used mainly to treat fractures and dislocations of the wrist and forearm. The sugar-tong splint should be applied to the injured forearm or wrist when the cast material is still soft, and an Ace bandage is usually wrapped around the splint. A shoulder immobilizer or a forearm sling is commonly used to support the weight of the forearm and splint.

Finger Splint

Finger splints are used in the treatment of fractures and dislocations of the phalanges and metacarpals. An adjacent normal finger is commonly immobilized with the injured finger to provide added support and to prevent development of malalignment of the injured finger. Ready-made plaster or fiberglass splints, or splints made of folded plaster or fiberglass bandages, should be tailored to fit the involved fingers and the corresponding portions of hand and forearm. These tailored splints should be padded with felt, foam rubber sheet, or multiple layers of Webril before they are applied to the volar aspects of the fingers, hand, and forearm, and Ace bandages should be used to hold the splints in place (Figs. 5-22, 5-23).

Thumb Splint

Thumb splints are used to treat injuries of the thumb and can be made of ready-made plaster or fiberglass splints, or folded plaster or fiberglass bandages. These splints should be padded with felt, foam rubber sheet, or multiple layers of Webril before they are applied to the thumb and radial aspect of the forearm (Fig. 5-24) and should be held in place with Ace bandages.

Wrist Splint

Wrist splints are frequently used for injuries of the wrist and are almost always placed on the volar aspect of the wrist. They are made of plaster or fiberglass splints or bandages and are padded with felt, foam rubber sheet, and multiple layers of Webril. Ace bandage is routinely used to hold a wrist splint to the volar aspect of the hand, wrist, and forearm (Fig. 5-25H).

The Author's Preferred Wrist Splints

A nicely fitted ulnar gutter wrist splint (Fig. 5-26) can be made by applying a short-arm cast, then longitudinally splitting the cast along the midline of its volar and dorsal surfaces, cutting the underlying Webril and stockinet, discarding the top half of the cast, lining the margins of the bottom half of the cast with moleskin, reapplying the bottom half of the cast to the ulnar aspect of the wrist and forearm, and binding it to the wrist and forearm with an Ace bandage. Similarly, a nicely fitting volar wrist splint (Fig. 5-27) can be obtained by cutting a short-arm cast along its radial and ulnar borders, cutting the underlying Webril and stockinet, discarding the top half of the cast, lining the margins of the bottom half of the cast with moleskin, reapplying the bottom half of the cast to the volar aspect of the wrist and forearm, and holding it to the wrist and forearm with an Ace bandage.

SHORT–ARM CAST WITH BIPOLAR K–WIRES THROUGH THE METACARPALS AND OLECRANON

A short-arm cast with bipolar K-wires through the metacarpals and olecranon (Fig. 5-28) is most commonly used in treating unstable, comminuted, and transarticular fractures of the distal radius and fractures of the radius and ulna. The rigidity of the cast keeps the distance between the two K-wires constant and thus maintains the reduced fractures for healing to take place. The materials used in this cast are virtually identical to those used in a standard short-arm cast. The cast can be applied under general anesthesia or under axillary nerve block. Before the cast is applied, a K-wire is driven through the second and third metacarpals, and another K-wire through the olecranon. Traction is then applied to the fingers by means of Chinese finger traps, and counter-traction is applied to the upper arm by means of a padded sling around the arm with weights attached to it. The reduction of fracture is checked with x-ray photography or an image intensifier, and if the reduction is satisfactory, a short-arm cast incorporating the bipolar K-wires can be applied in the regular manner. The K-wires are trimmed with a pin cutter, and a small strip of plaster is wrapped around the ends of the wires to prevent damage to clothes, bedding, or furniture. The palmar portion of the cast can be removed (Fig. 5-29) to improve finger and thumb function and to reduce the chance of skin irritation of the hand by the distal portion of the cast.

BIBLIOGRAPHY

Abouna, J.M., and Brown, H.: The treatment of mallet finger. The results in a series of 148 consecutive cases and review of the literature. Br. J. Surg., *55*:658, 1968.

Adler, G.A., and Light, T.R.: Simultaneous complex dislocation of the metacarpophalangeal joints of the long and index fingers. A case report. J. Bone Joint Surg. [Am.], *63*:1007, 1968.
Adler, J.B., and Shaftan, G.W.: Fractures of the capitate. J. Bone Joint Surg. [Am.], *44*:1537, 1962.
Armstrong, G.W.D.: Rotational subluxation of the scaphoid. Canad. J. Surg., *11*:306, 1968.
Bach, J., Draslov, B., and Jergensen, B.: Positioning, splinting and pressure management of the burned hand: A method. Scand. J. Plast. Reconstr. Surg., *18*:145, 1984.
Baldwin, L.W., Miller, D.L., Lockhart, L.D., and Evans, E.B.: Metacarpophalangeal joint dislocations of the fingers. A comparison of the pathological anatomy of index and little finger dislocations. J. Bone Joint Surg. [Am.], *49*:1587, 1967.
Barton, N.J.: Fractures of the shafts of the phalanges of the hand. Hand, *11*:119, 1979.
Bartone, N.F., and Grieco, R.V.: Fractures of the triquetrum. J. Bone Joint Surg. [Am.], *38*:353, 1956.
Bennett, E.H.: Fractures of the metacarpal bones. Dublin, J. Med. Sci., *73*:72, 1882.
Bilos, Z.J., and Hui, P.W.T.: Dorsal dislocation of the lunate with carpal collapse. J. Bone Joint Surg. [Am.], *63*:1484, 1981.
Bilos, Z.J., Pankovich, A.M., and Yelda, S.: Fracture-dislocation of the radiocarpal joint: A clinical study of five cases. J. Bone Joint Surg. [Am.], *59*:198, 1977.
Boe, S.: Dislocation of the trapezium (multangulum majus): A case report. Acta Orthop. Scand., *50*:85, 1979.
Bora, F.W., Jr., and Didizian, N.H.: The treatment of injuries to the carpometacarpal joint of the little finger. J. Bone Joint Surg. [Am.], *56*:1459, 1974.
Bowen, T.L.: Injuries of the hamate bone. Hand, *5*:235, 1973.
Bowers, W.H., and Horst, L.C.: Gamekeeper's thumb. J. Bone Joint Surg., [Am.], *59*:519, 1977.
Brady, L.P.: Double pin fixation of severely comminuted fractures of the distal radius and ulna. South. Med. J., *56*:307, 1963.
Brooks, D.: Splint for mallet fingers. Br. Med. J., *2*:1238, 1964.
Bryan, R.S., and Dobyns, J.H.: Fractures of the carpal bones other than lunate and navicular. Clin. Orthop., *149*:107, 1980.
Bunger, C., Slund, K., and Rasmussen, P.: Early results after Colles' fracture: Functional bracing in supination vs. dorsal plaster immobilization. Arch. Orthop. Trauma Surg., *103*:25, 1984.
Burnham, P.J.: Physiological treatment for fractures of the metacarpals and phalanges. JAMA, *169*:663, 1959.
Buzby, B.F.: Isolated radial dislocation of carpal scaphoid. Ann. Surg., *100*:553, 1934.
Camp, R.A., Weatherwax, R.J., and Miller, E.B.: Chronic post-traumatic radial instability of the thumb metacarpophalangeal joint. J. Hand Surg., *5*:221, 1980.
Campbell, R.D., Jr., Lance, E.M., and Yeoh, C.B.: Lunate and perilunar dislocations. J. Bone Joint Surg., [Br.], *46*:55, 1964.
Cannon, N.M. (ed.): Manual of Hand Splinting. New York, Churchill Livingstone, 1985.
Cole, J.M., and Obletz, B.E.: Comminuted fracture of the distal end of the radius treated by skeletal transfixation in plaster cast. An end-result study of thirty-three cases. J. Bone Joint Surg. [Am.], *48*:931, 1966.
Cooney, W.P., III., Dobyns, J.H., and Linscheid, R.L.: Fractures of the scaphoid. A rational approach to management. Clin. Orthop., *149*:90, 1980.
Cordrey, L.J., and Ferrer-Torells, M.: Management of fractures of the greater multangular: Report of five cases. J. Bone Joint Surg. [Am.], *42*:1111, 1960.
Duke, R.: Dislocation of the hamate bone: Report of a case. J. Bone Joint Surg. [Br.], *45*:744, 1963.
Dutton, R.O., and Meals, R.A.: Complex dorsal dislocation of the thumb metacarpophalangeal joint. Clin. Orthop., *164*:160, 1982.
Elliott, R.A.: Splints for mallet and boutonnier deformities. Plast. Reconstr. Surg., *52*:282, 1973.
Fess, E.E., Gettle, K.S., and Strickland, J.W.: Hand Splinting. Principles and Methods. St. Louis, C.V. Mosby, 1981.
Hall, R.F., Jr., Gleason, T.F., and Kasa, R.F.: Simultaneous closed dislocations of the metacarpophalangeal joints of the index, long, and ring fingers: A case report. J. Hand Surg., *10*:81, 1985.
Hartwig, R.H., and Louis, D.S.: Multiple carpometacarpal dislocations. J. Bone Joint Surg. [Am.], *61*:906, 1979.
Harvey, F.J., and Bye, W.D.: Bennett's fracture. Hand, *8*:48, 1976.
Harwin, S.F., Fox, J.M., and Sedlin, E.D.: Volar dislocation of the bases of the second and third metacarpals. J. Bone Joint Surg. [Am.], *57*:849, 1975.
Howes, D.S., and Kaufman, J.J.: Plaster splints: Techniques and indications. Am. Fam. Physician, *30*:215, 1984.
Immermann, E.W.: Dislocation of the pisiform. J. Bone Joint Surg. [Am.], *30*:489, 1948.
Jensen, J.S.: Operative treatment of chronic subluxation of the first carpometacarpal joint. Hand, *7*:269, 1975.

Lamb, D.W., Abernathy, P.J., and Fragiadakis, E.: Injuries of the metacarpophalangeal joint of the thumb. Hand, *3*:164, 1971.

Latta, L., Sarmiento, A., and Tarr, R.R.: The rationale of functional bracing of fractures. Research experiences. Clin. Orthop., *146*:28, 1980.

Leslie, I.J., and Dickson, R.A.: The fractured carpal scaphoid: Natural history and factors influencing outcome. J. Bone Joint Surg. [Br.], *63*:225, 1981.

Lewis, H.H.: Dislocation of the lesser multangular: Report of a case. J. Bone Joint Surg. [Am.], *44*:1412, 1962.

London, P.S.: Observations on the treatment of some fractures of the forearm by splintage that does not include the elbow. Injury, *2*:252, 1971.

Malick, M.H.: Manual on Static Hand Splinting. 4th Ed. Pittsburgh, Harmarville Rehabilitation Center, 1980.

Mayfield, J.K.: Mechanism of carpal injuries. Clin. Orthop., *149*:45, 1980.

Mazet, R., Jr.: A Manual of Closed Reduction of Closed Fractures and Dislocations. Springfield, Charles C Thomas, 1967.

Moneim, M.S., Bolger, J.T., and Omer, G.E.: Radiocarpal dislocation—classification and rationale for management. Clin. Orthop., *192*:199, 1985.

Nicholas, J.J., et al.: Splinting in rheumatoid arthritis: II. Evaluation of light cast fiberglass polymer splints. Arch. Phys. Med. Rehabil., *63*:95, 1982.

Niehuss, J.E.: An improved method to attach straps to plaster splints. Phys. Ther., *45*:1059, 1965.

O'Brien, E.T.: Fractures of the metacarpals and phalanges. *In* Operative Hand Surgery. Edited by D.P. Green. New York, Churchill Livingstone, 1982.

Pagalidis, T., Kuczynski, K., and Lamb, D.W.: Ligamentous stability of the base of the thumb. Hand, *13*:29, 1981.

Pollen, A.G.: The conservative treatment of Bennett's fracture—subluxation of the thumb metacarpal. J. Bone Joint Surg. [Br.], *50*:91, 1968.

Pollen, A.G.: Fractures and Dislocations in Children. Baltimore, Williams and Wilkins, 1973.

Robertson, R.C., Cawley, J.J., Jr., and Faris, A.M.: Treatment of fracture-dislocation of the interphalangeal joints of the hand. J. Bone Joint Surg., *28*:68, 1946.

Robins, R.H.C.: Injuries of the metacarpophalangeal joints. Hand, *3*:159, 1971.

Sarmiento, A., Cooper, J.S., and Sinclair, W.F.: Forearm fractures: Early functional bracing—preliminary report. J. Bone Joint Surg. [Am.], *57*:297, 1975.

Sarmiento, H., Kinman, P.B., Murphy, R.B., and Phillips, J.G.: Treatment of ulnar fractures by functional bracing. J. Bone Joint Surg. [Am.], *58*:1104, 1976.

Sarmiento, A., Pratt, G.W., Berry, N.D., and Sinclair, W.F.: Colles' fractures—functional bracing in supination. J. Bone Joint Surg. [Am.], *57*:311, 1975.

Sarmiento, A., Zagorski, J.B., and Sinclair, W.F.: Functional bracing of Colles' fractures: A prospective study of immobilization versus pronation. Clin. Orthop., *146*:175, 1980.

Saunier, J., and Chamay, A.: Volar perilunar dislocation of the wrist. Clin. Orthop., *157*:139, 1981.

Schick, M.: Long term follow-up of treatment of comminuted fractures of the distal end of the radius by transfixation with Kirschner wires and cast. J. Bone Joint Surg. [Am.], *44*:337, 1962.

Shepherd, E., and Solomon, D.J.: Carpo-metacarpal dislocation. J. Bone Joint Surg. [Br.], *42*:772, 1960.

Smith, R.J.: Posttraumatic instability of the metacarpophalangeal joint of the thumb. J. Bone Joint Surg. [Am.], *59*:14, 1977.

Solgaard, S.: Classification of distal radius fractures. Acta Orthop. Scand., *56*:249, 1985.

Souter, W.A.: The boutonniere deformity. A review of 101 patients with division of the central slip of the extensor expansion of the fingers. J. Bone Joint Surg. [Br.], *49*:710, 1967.

Sprague, B.L.: Proximal interphalangeal joint injuries and their initial treatment. J. Trauma, *15*:380, 1975.

Stark, H.H., Jobe, F.W., Boyes, J.H., and Ashworth, C.R.: Fracture of the hook of the hamate in athletes. J. Bone Joint Surg. [Am.], *59*:575, 1977.

Stein, A.H., Jr.: Dorsal dislocation of the lesser multangular bone. J. Bone Joint Surg. [Am.], *53*:377, 1971.

Stein, A.H., Jr., and Katz, S.F.: Stabilization of comminuted fracture of the distal inch of radius: Percutaneous pinning. Clin. Orthop., *108*:174, 1975.

Stener, B.: Hyperextension injuries to the metacarpophalangeal joint of the thumb—rupture of ligaments, fracture of sesamoid bones, rupture of flexor pollicis brevis. An anatomical and clinical study. Acta Chir. Scand., *125*:275, 1963.

Stewart, H.D., Innes, A.R., and Burke, F.D.: Functional cast-bracing for Colles' fractures. A comparison between cast-bracing and conventional plaster casts. J. Bone Joint Surg. [Br.], *66*:749, 1984.

Strong, M.L.: A new method of extension-block splinting for the proximal interphalangeal joint—preliminary report. J. Hand Surg., *5*:606, 1980.

Surman, R.K.: Unstable fractures of the distal end of the radius (transfixation pins and a cast). Injury, *15*:206, 1983.

Trojan, E.: Fracture dislocation of the bases of the proximal and middle phalanges of the fingers. Hand, *4*:60, 1972.

Van-Straten, O., and Mahler, D.: Four new hand splints. Br. J. Plast. Surg., *34*:345, 1981.

Varian, J.P.: The ridged plaster volar slab. Hand, *7*:78, 1975.

Zide, B.M., Bevin, A.G., and Hollis, L.I.: Examples of simply fabricated, custom-made splints for the hand. J. Hand Surg., *6*:35, 1981.

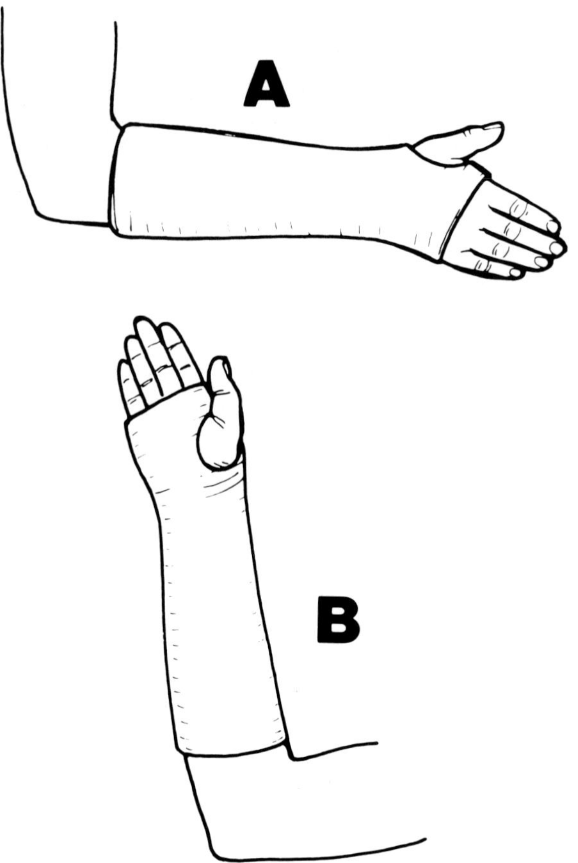

Fig. 5–1. Dorsal (*A*) and volar (*B*) views of a short-arm cast.

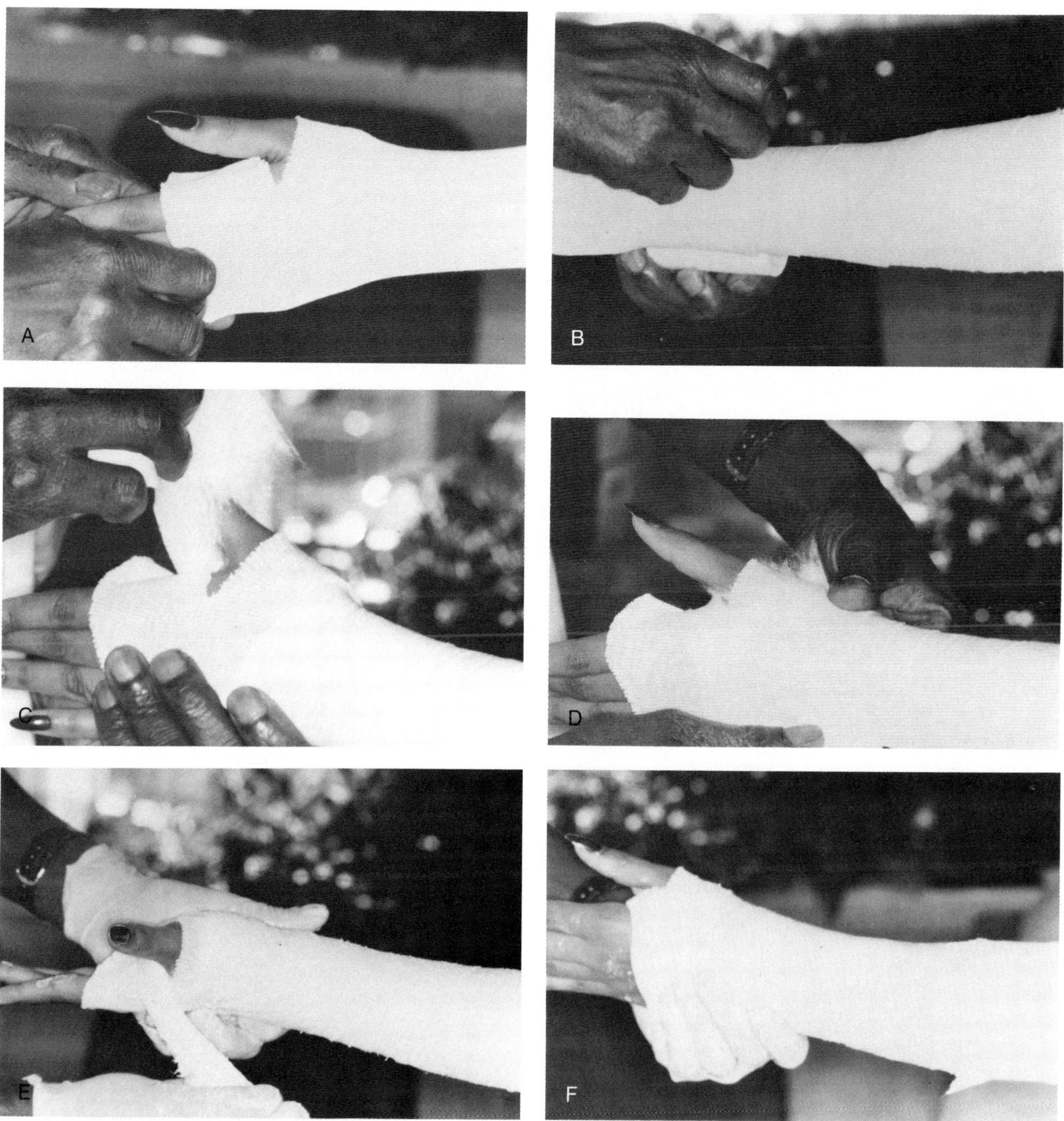

Fig. 5–2. The making of a plaster short-arm cast. *A*, 3″ stockinet has been placed over the forearm and the hand, with the thumb sticking out through the small half-moon-shaped thumbhole. *B*, 3″ Webril has been wrapped around the forearm. *C*, A transverse tear of about 75% of the width of the Webril has been made in order to wrap the Webril around the first webspace and the base of the thumb in a smooth manner. *D*, All the Webril necessary for a short-arm cast has been applied. *E*, The plaster bandage has been twisted along its longitudinal axis to produce a small plaster rope, which is used to wrap around the palm region to provide added strength for the distal end of the cast. *F*, The ends of the stockinet are folded down over the cast ends after first roll of plaster has been applied.

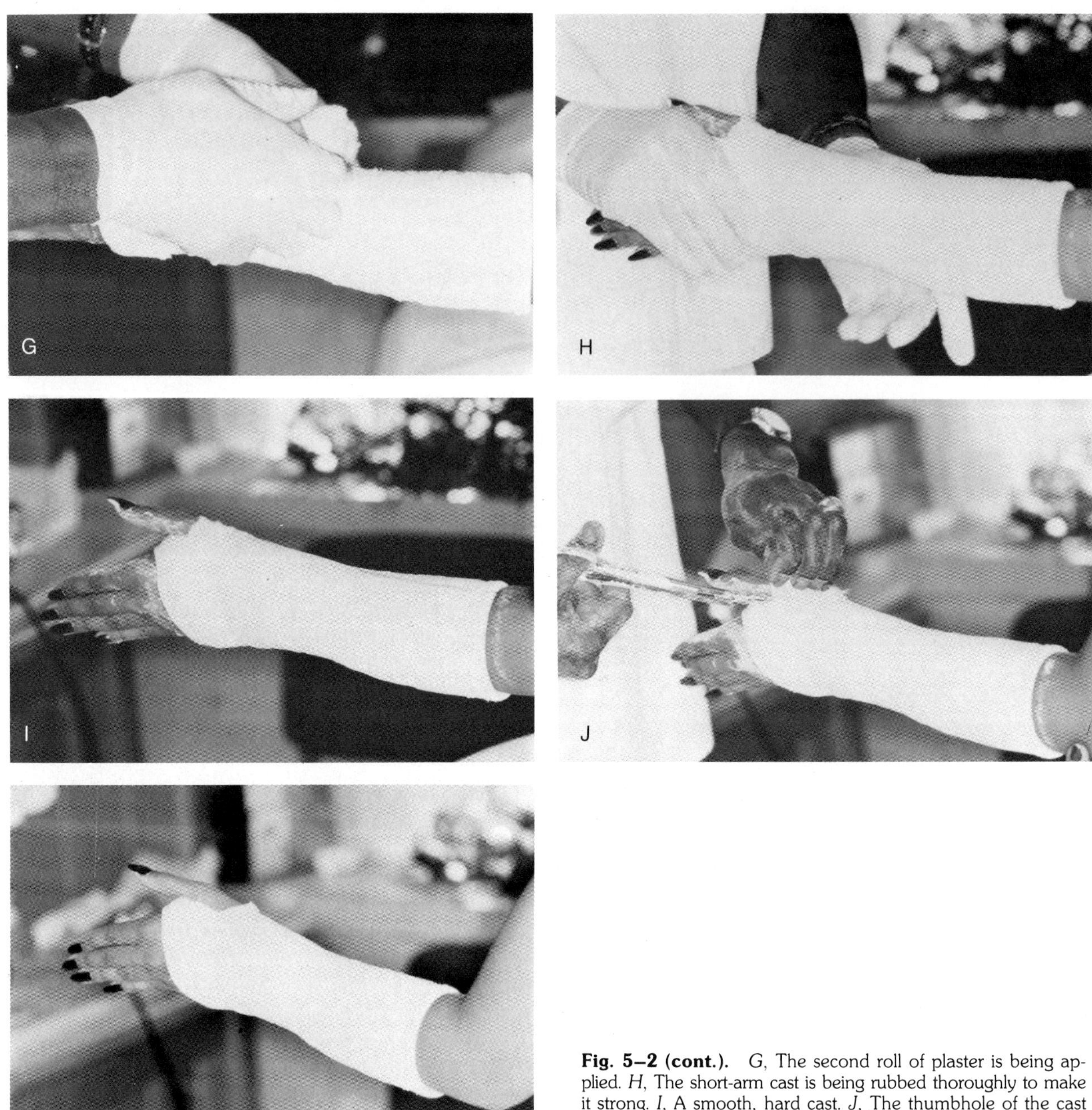

Fig. 5–2 (cont.). *G*, The second roll of plaster is being applied. *H*, The short-arm cast is being rubbed thoroughly to make it strong. *I*, A smooth, hard cast. *J*, The thumbhole of the cast is carefully trimmed to allow full use of the thumb. *K*, A completely finished short-arm cast.

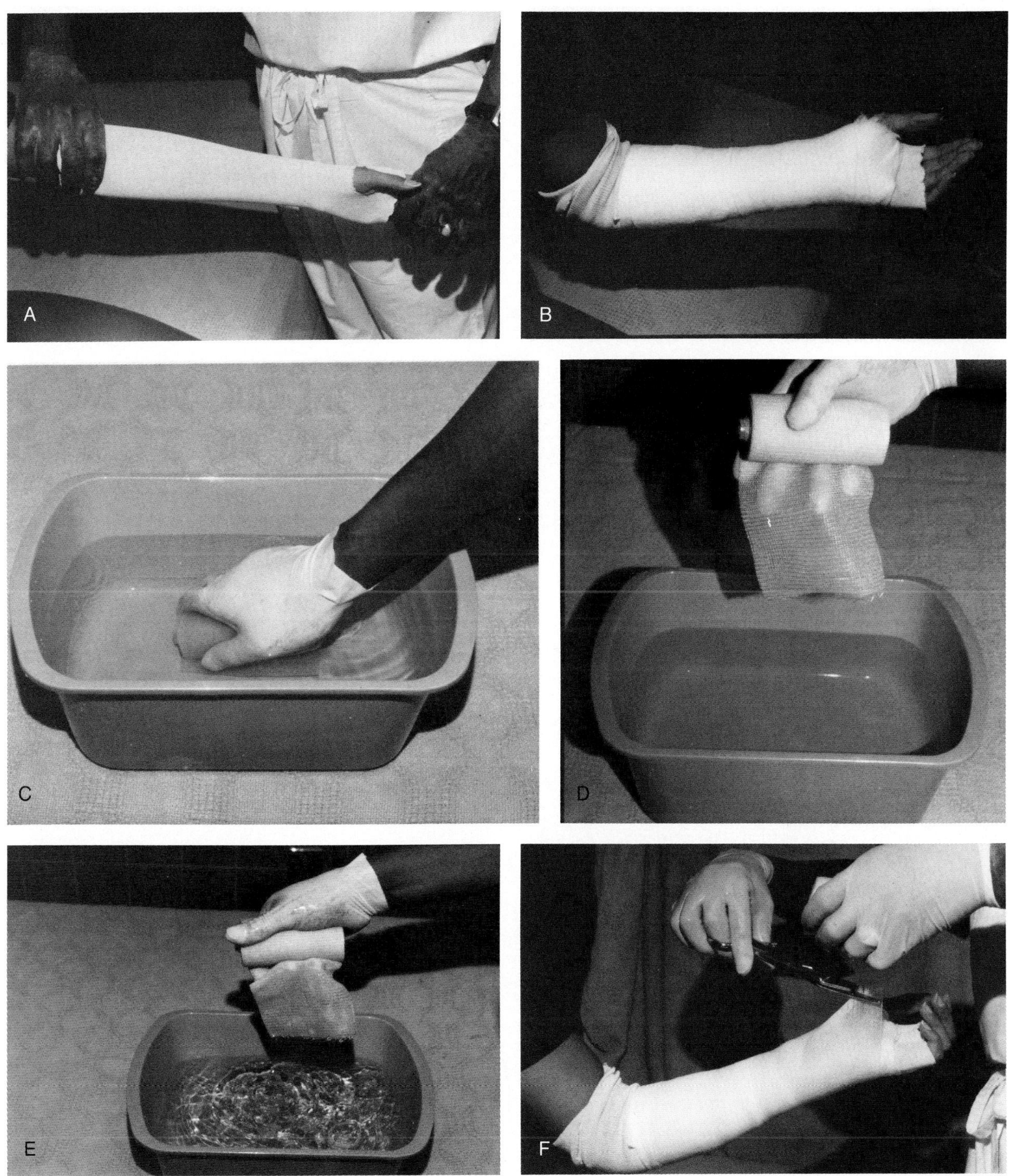

Fig. 5–3. The making of a fiberglass short-arm cast. *A*, A 3″ stockinet has been applied to the forearm and hand. *B*, Two rolls of 3″ Webril have been wrapped around the forearm and hand. *C*, A 3″ fiberglass bandage is being soaked in water. *D*, The fiberglass bandage is removed from the water. *E*, The bandage is gently squeezed to get rid of excess water. *F*, The first roll of fiberglass bandage has been wrapped around the forearm, and a pair of plaster scissors is being used to make a transverse cut through about 75% of the width of the fiberglass bandage.

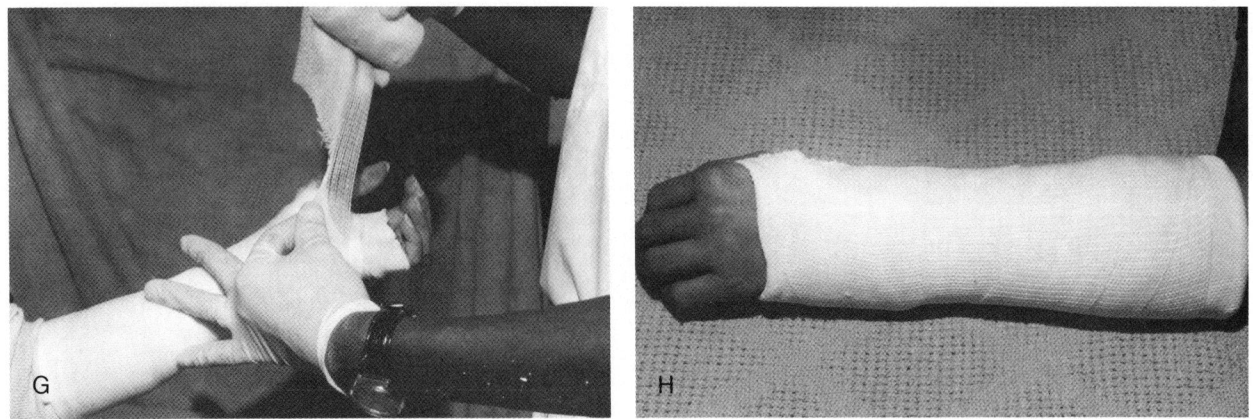

Fig. 5–3 (cont.). *G*, The cut portion of the fiberglass bandage is now ready to go over the first webspace and around the proximal part of the hand in a smooth manner. *H*, The finished cast. The two stockinet ends have been turned down over the cast ends, and a new roll of fiberglass bandage has been placed over the entire cast.

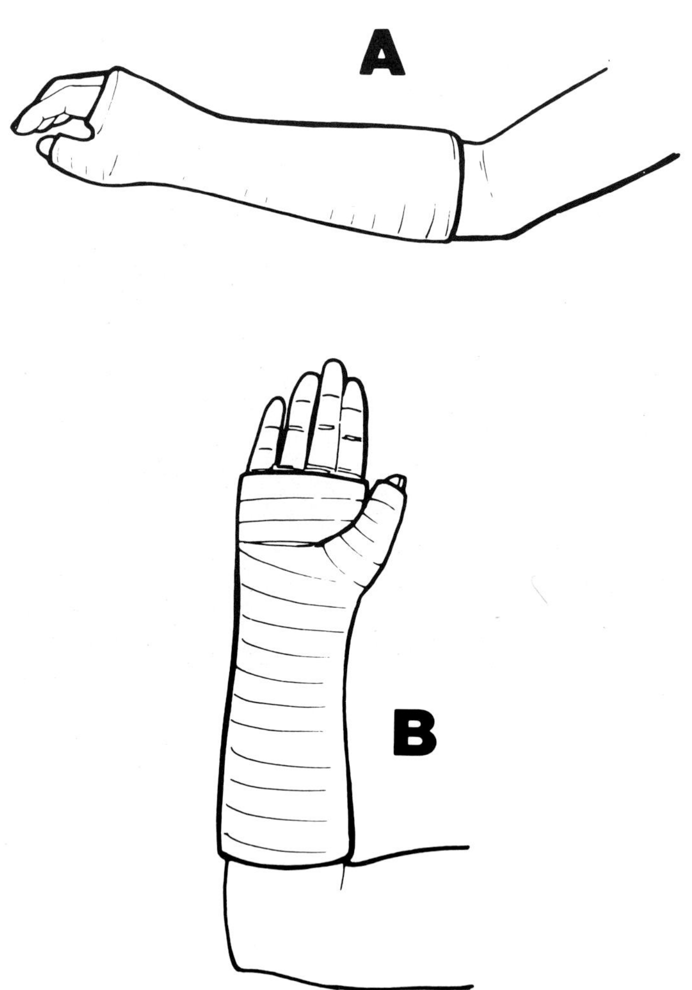

Fig. 5–4. Anterior (*A*) and medial (*B*) views of a short-arm thumb spica cast.

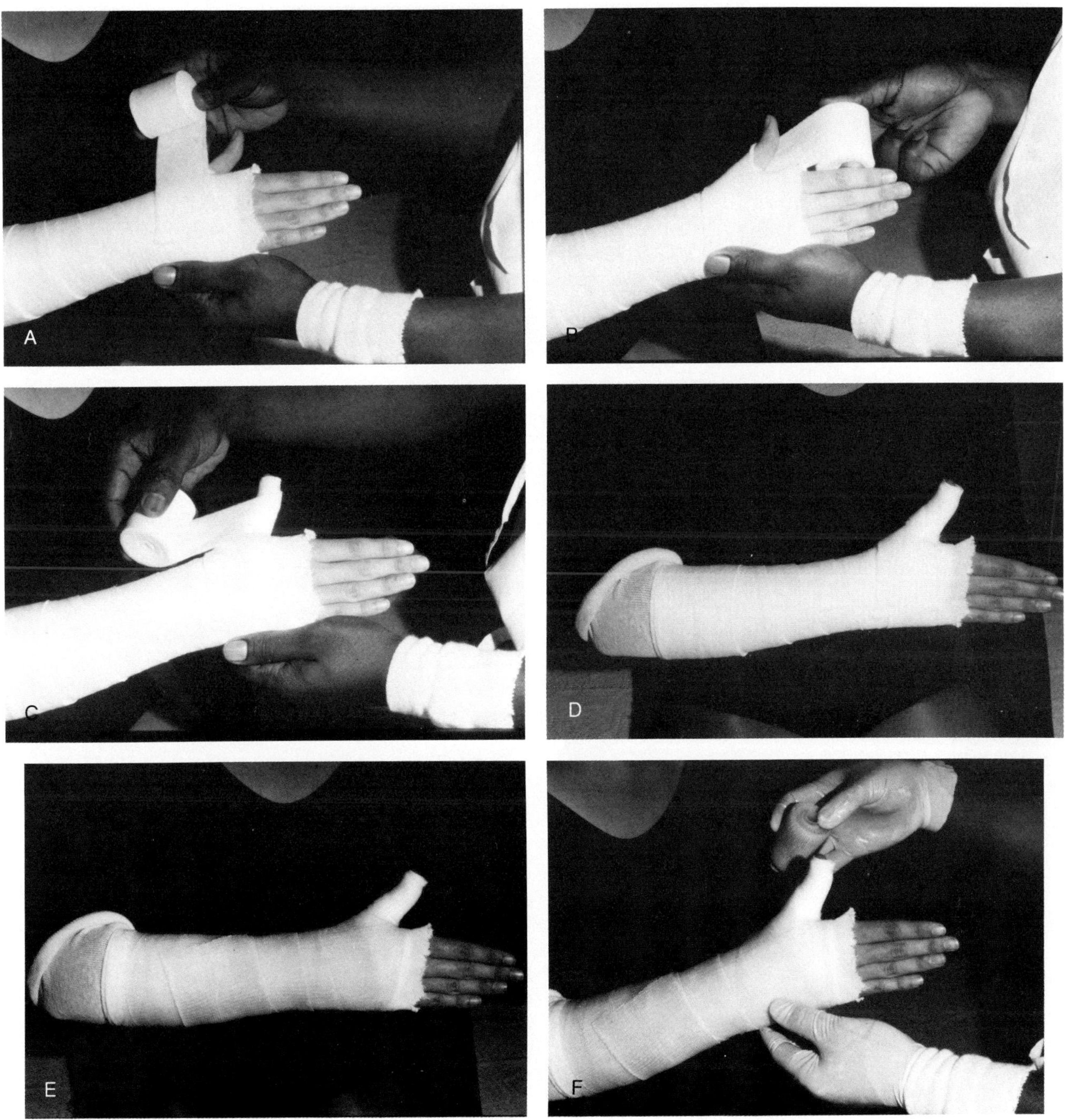

Fig. 5–5. The making of a short-arm thumb spica cast. A stockinet identical to the one used in a short-arm cast is used in making this cast. *A*, *B*, A roll of 3″ Webril has been wrapped around the forearm and hand. *C*, *D*, A roll of 2″ Webril is used to cover the thumb and the proximal portion of the hand. *E*, A roll of 3″ fiberglass bandage has been applied to the forearm and hand. *F*, A roll of 2″ fiberglass bandage is being used to cover the thumb and the proximal portion of the hand and wrist.

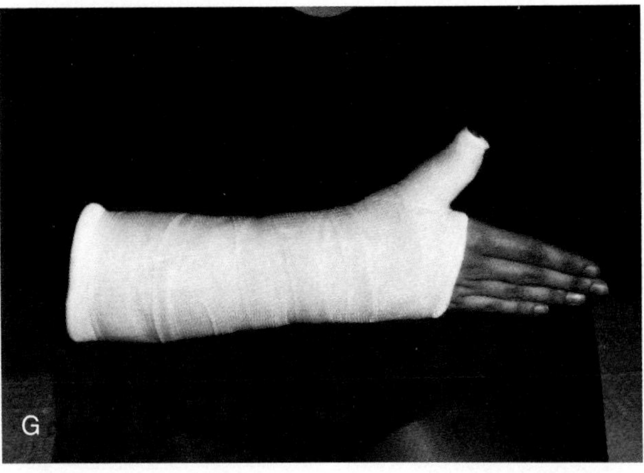

Fig. 5–5 (cont.). *G*, After the two stockinet ends are folded over the proximal and distal ends of the cast, a second roll of 3″ fiberglass bandage is used to finish the cast.

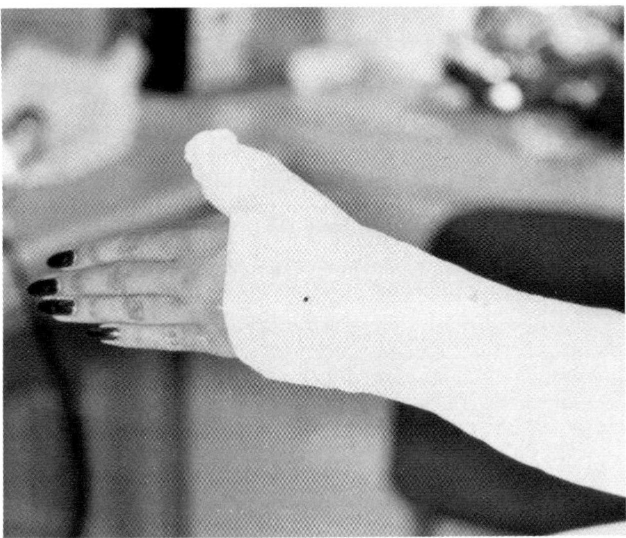

Fig. 5–6. A completed plaster short-arm thumb spica cast.

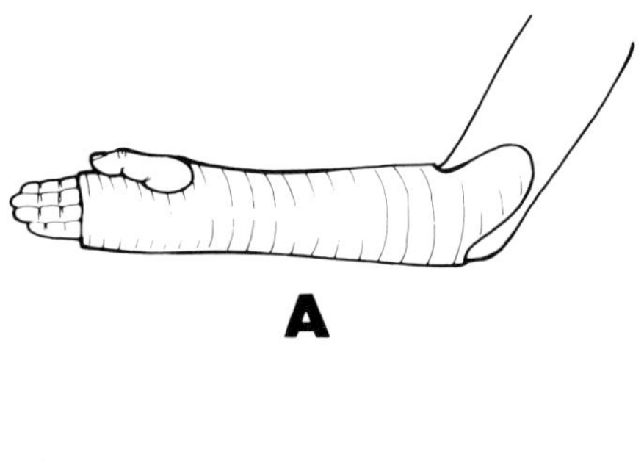

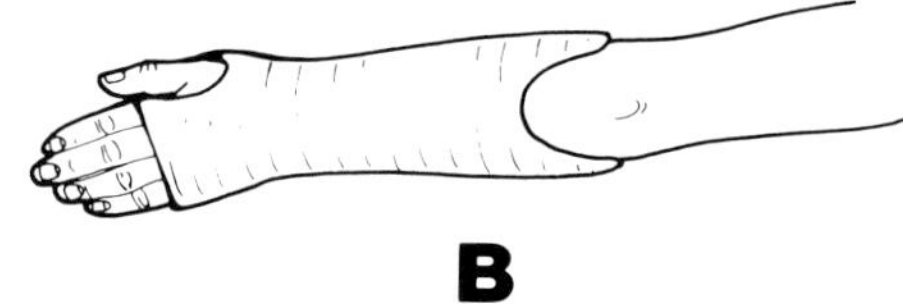

Fig. 5–7. Medial (*A*) and posterior (*B*) views of a supracondylar cast.

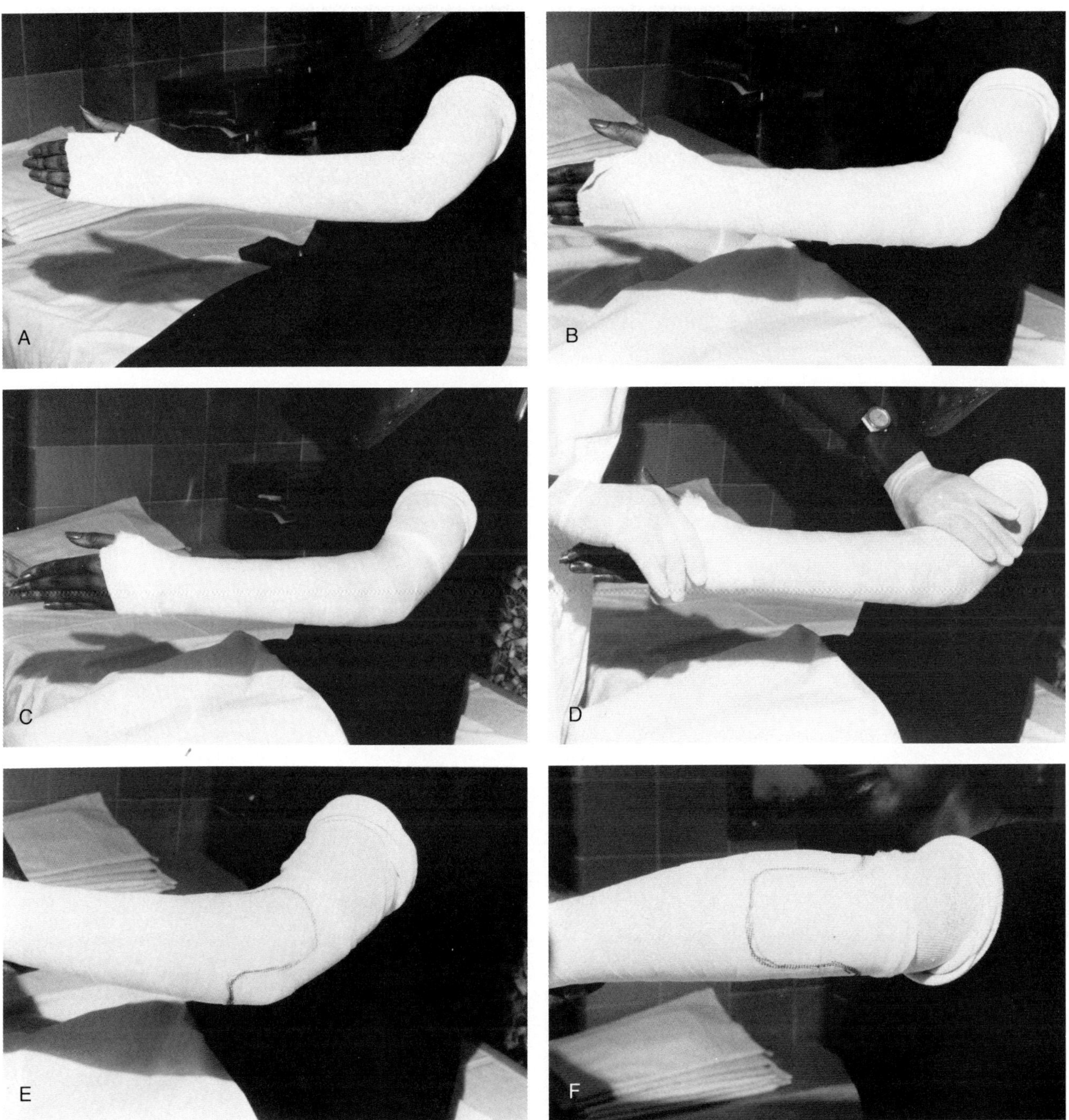

Fig. 5–8. The making of a fiberglass supracondylar cast. *A*, 3″ stockinet with a thumbhole has been applied to the arm from the bases of the fingers to the upper arm. *B*, 3″ Webril has been wrapped around the arm from the distal palmar crease to the mid-arm level. *C*, Two rolls of 3″ fiberglass bandage have been applied to the arm from the proximal palmar crease to the middle of the upper arm, and the distal stockinet end has been folded over the distal end of the cast. *D*, While the cast is setting, it should be molded carefully to the medial and lateral humeral condyles proximally, and the thenar and hypothenar eminences and the mid-palmar concavity distally. *E*, *F*, The supracondylar flanges and the two U-shaped notches below the elbow flexion crease and the olecranon have been marked on the cast with a wax pencil.

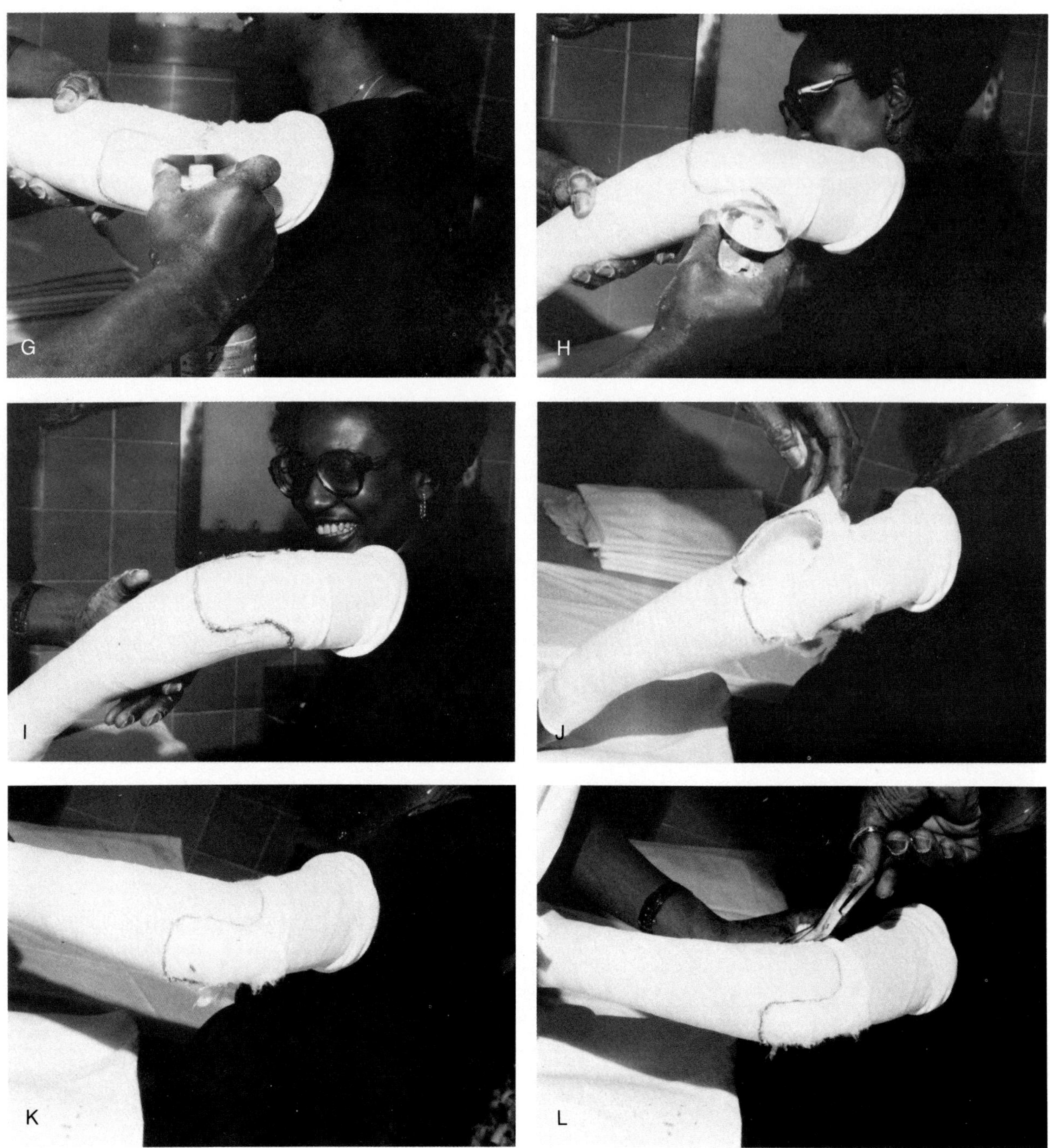

Fig. 5–8 (cont.). *G, H, I,* An oscillating saw is used to cut completely around the cast along the wax pencil line. *J, K,* The upper, redundant portion of the cast is removed by splitting it longitudinally along its anterior aspect. *L,* The cast material is cut along the trimming line.

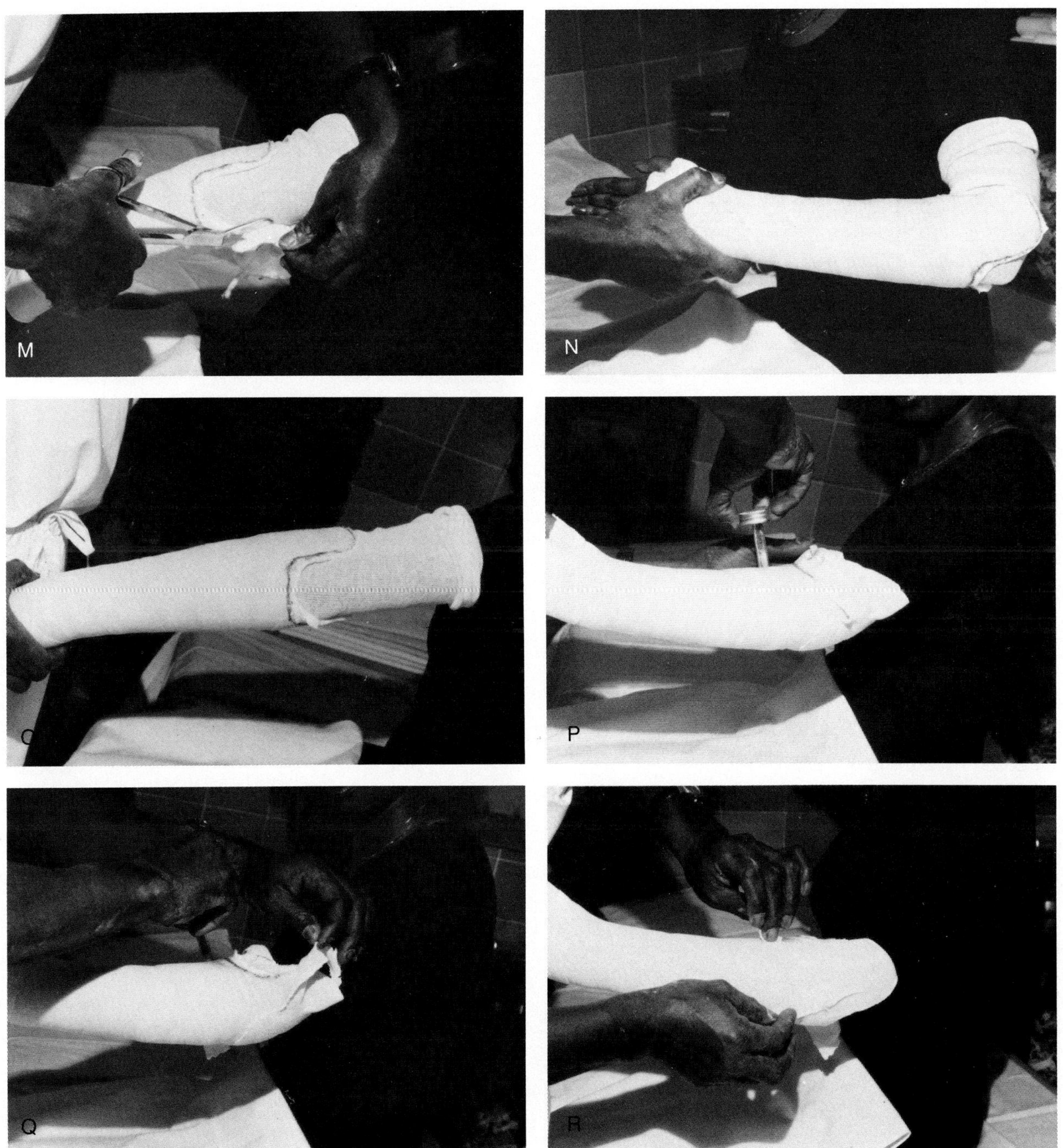

Fig. 5–8 (cont.). *M*, The Webril is trimmed about 1/4" above the upper end of the cast so that it can provide additional padding for the cast end when the stockinet has been folded down over the upper end of the cast. *N*, *O*, Flexion and extension of the elbow are checked carefully and are found to be satisfactory. *P*, *Q*, The upper stockinet end has been split longitudinally along its anterior and posterior aspects, and plastic adhesive is applied generously to the adjacent upper portion of the cast. *R*, The split upper stockinet end is pulled down tightly over the upper end of the cast and is allowed to stick to the adjacent upper portion of the cast.

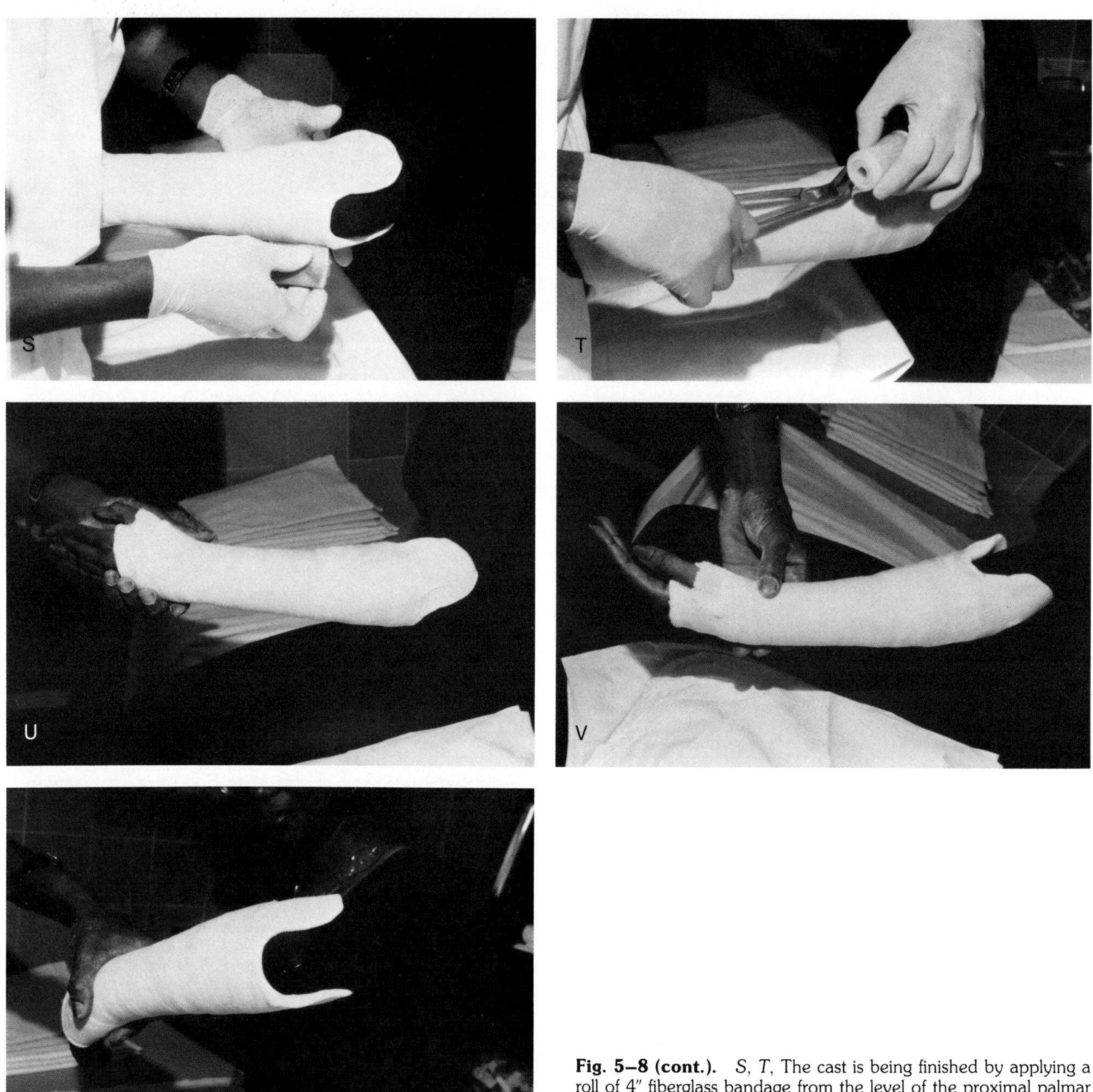

Fig. 5–8 (cont.). *S, T,* The cast is being finished by applying a roll of 4″ fiberglass bandage from the level of the proximal palmar crease to the level of the bases of the two supracondylar flanges. *U, V, W,* Lateral, oblique, and posterior views of a finished supracondylar cast show that it has proper fit and excellent function.

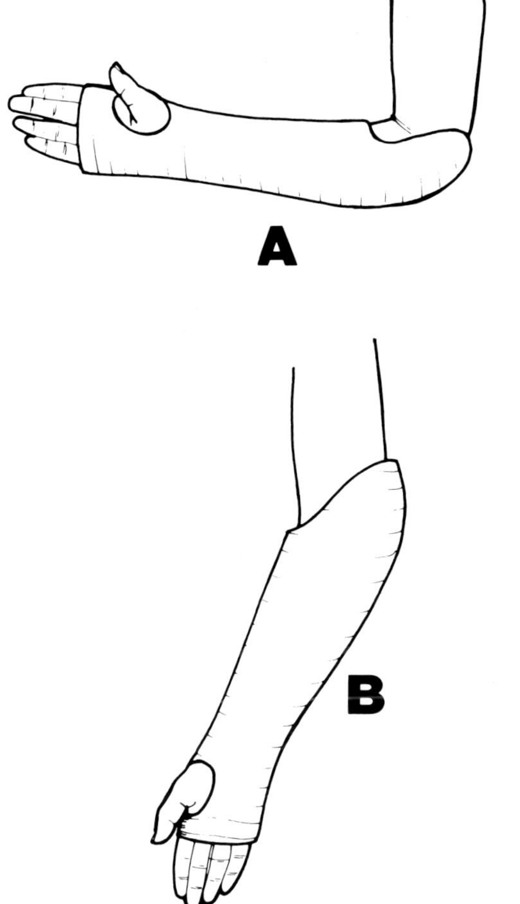

Fig. 5–9. Medial views of an old-fashioned supracondylar cast with the elbow in flexion (*A*) and extension (*B*).

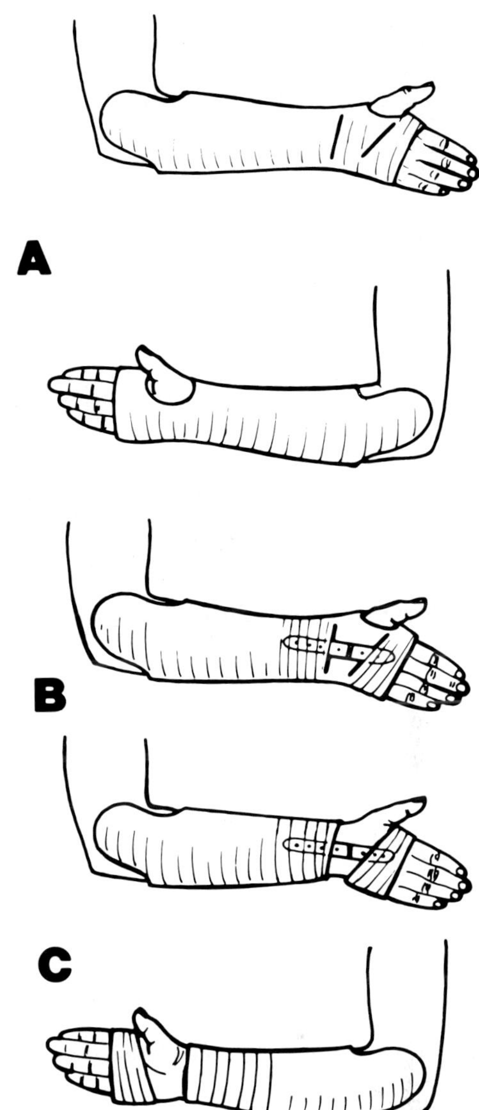

Fig. 5–10. Making of a supracondylar cast-brace with a dorsal wrist hinge. *A*, Dorsal and volar views of a supracondylar cast showing the two cuts, proximal and distal to the wrist joint, on the dorsal aspect of the cast. *B*, A small gate hinge has been attached to the dorsal aspect of the wrist region of the cast. *C*, The cast materials between the two cuts have been completely removed, and the wrist joint can now be extended and flexed.

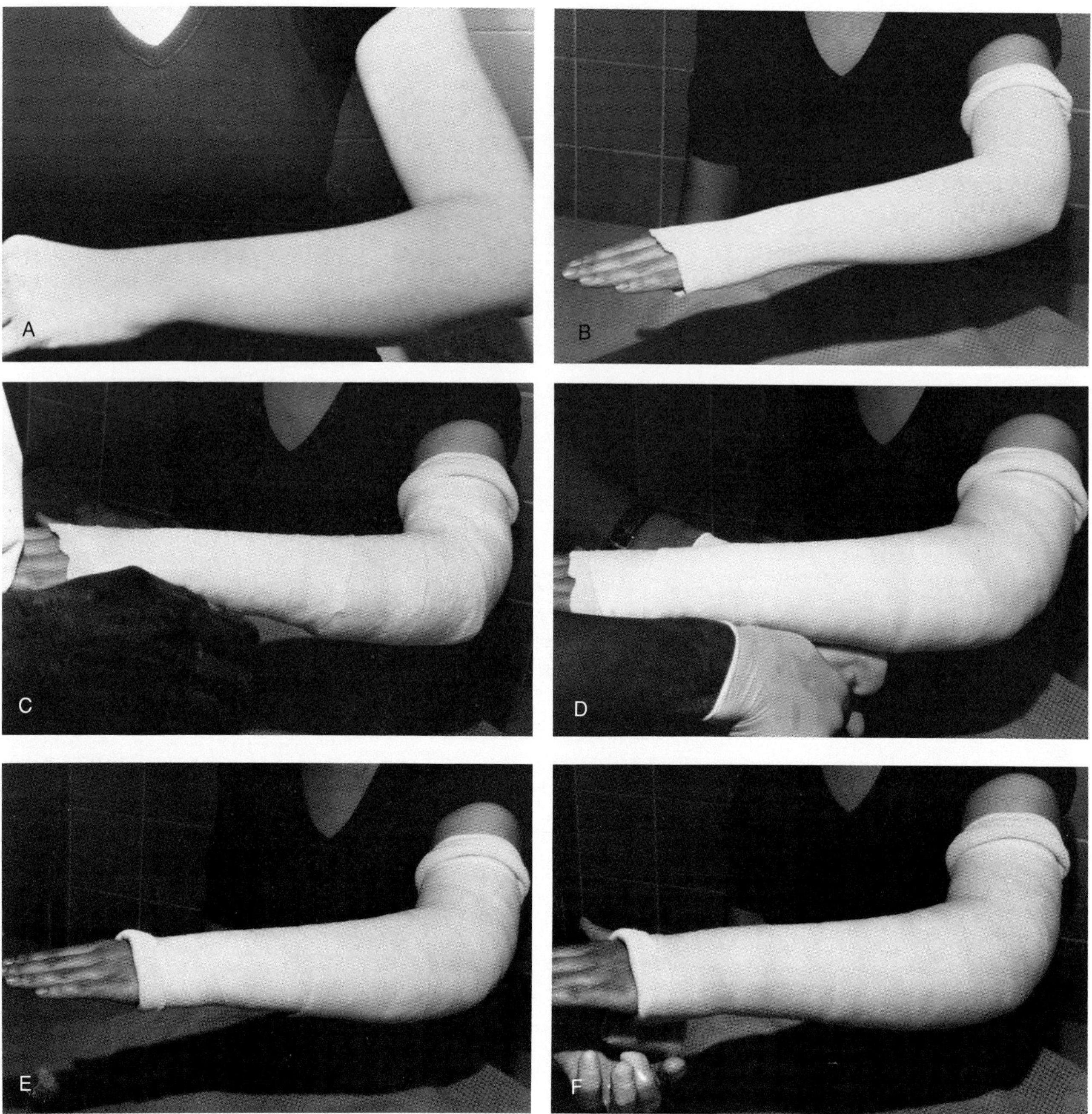

Fig. 5–11. *A*, A supracondylar cast-brace with dorsal wrist hinge should be applied with the elbow flexed 90° and the forearm in a neutral position. *B*, A 3″ stockinet is applied from the bases of the fingers to the upper arm. *C*, Webril bandages are applied from the distal palmar crease to the mid-arm level. *D*, *E*, Fiberglass bandages are applied from the mid-arm level to the proximal palmar crease, and the distal end of the stockinet is folded down over the distal end of the cast. *F*, The distal end of the cast is finished by fixing the stockinet end to the distal end of the cast with a fiberglass bandage.

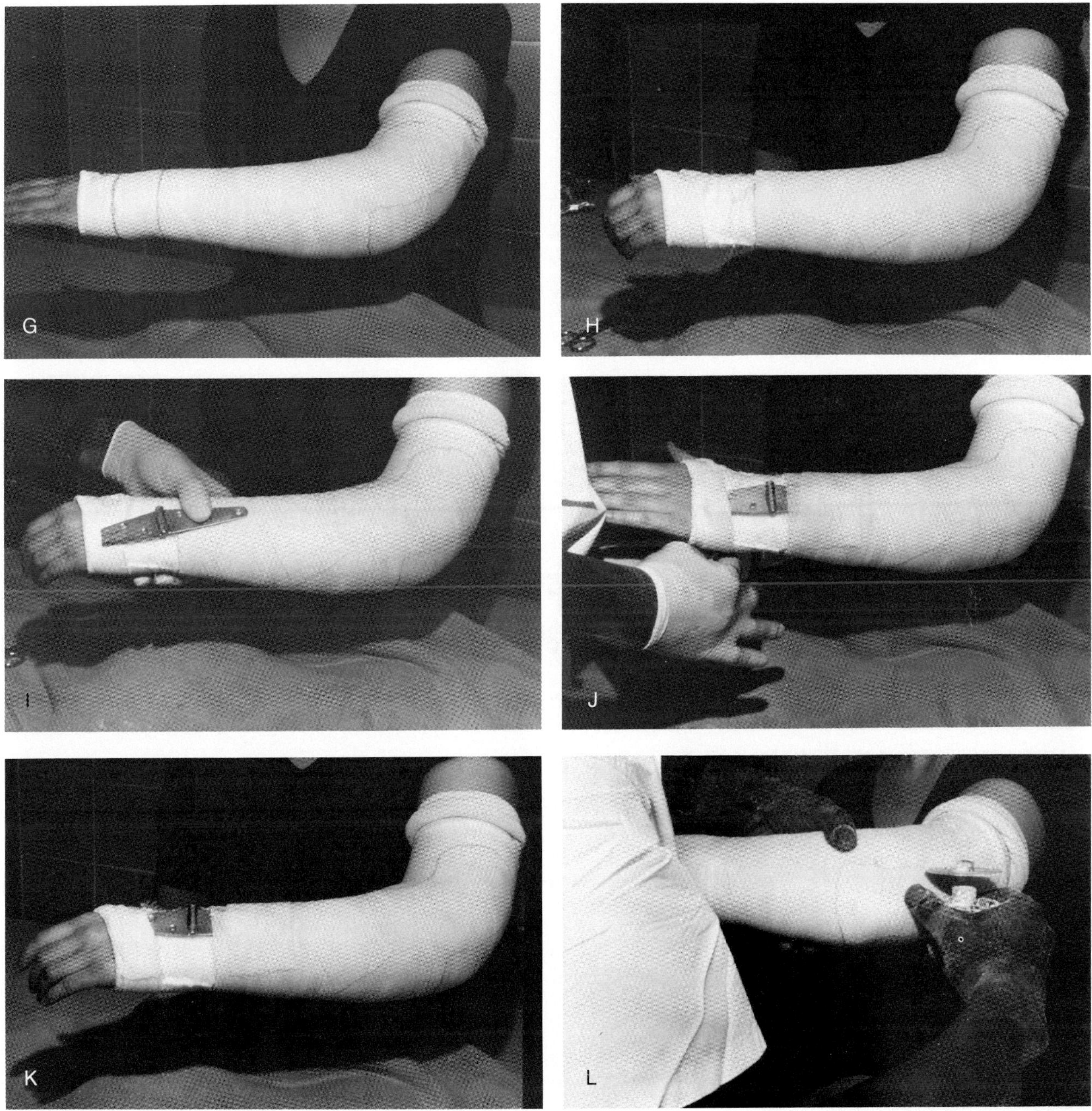

Fig. 5–11 (cont.). *G, H,* The section of the cast over the dorsal aspect of the wrist joint is marked with a wax pencil and then removed with a cast saw. *I, J,* The small gate hinge is placed over the dorsal aspect of the wrist joint and fixed to the distal end of the cast with fiberglass bandages. *K,* The two supracondylar flanges have been marked on the supracondylar portion of the cast with a wax pencil. *L,* A cast saw is used to cut the cast materials along the lines marked with wax pencil.

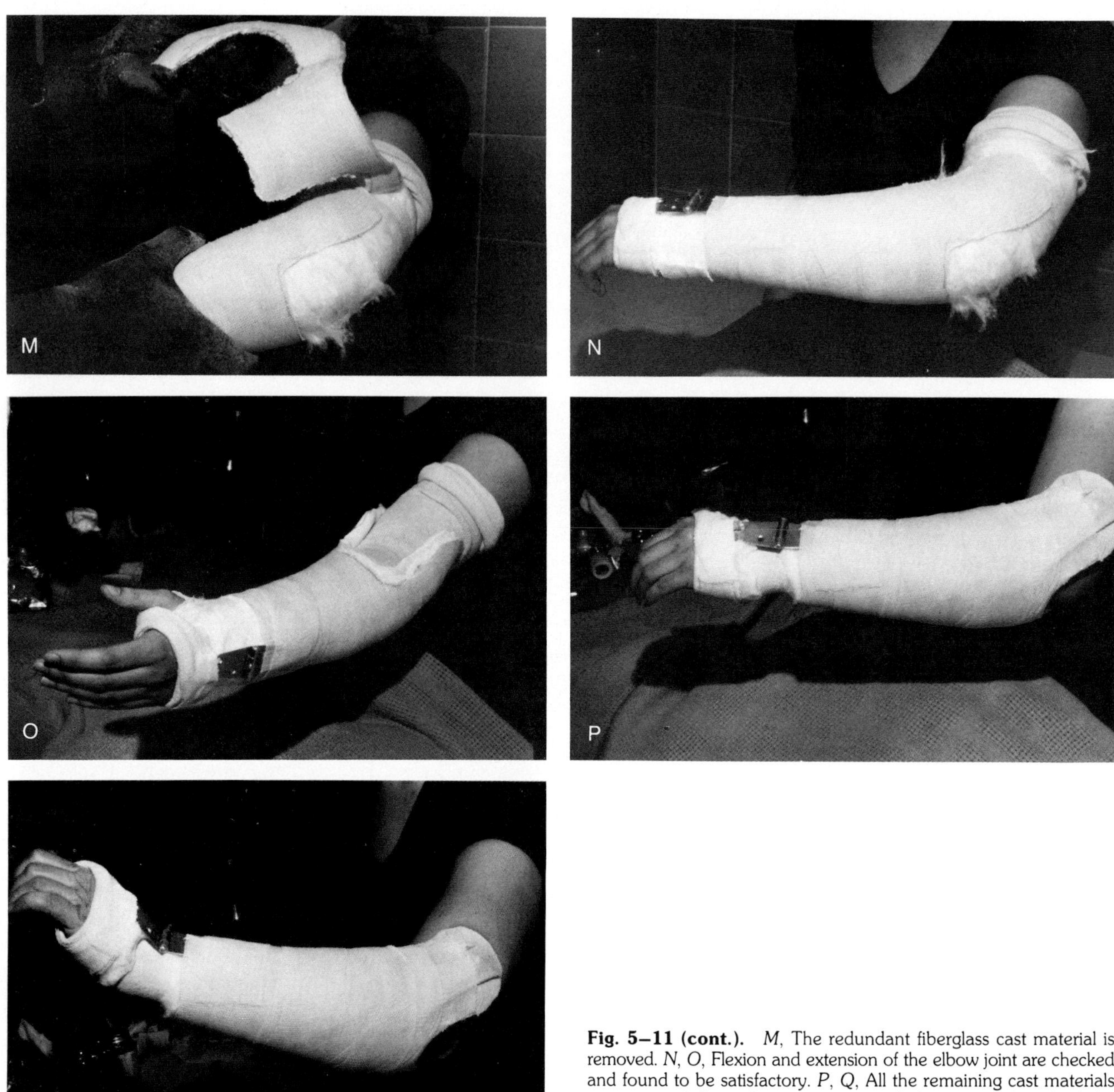

Fig. 5–11 (cont.). *M*, The redundant fiberglass cast material is removed. *N*, *O*, Flexion and extension of the elbow joint are checked and found to be satisfactory. *P*, *Q*, All the remaining cast materials are removed from the wrist joint, and the proximal end of the stockinet is turned down over the two supracondylar flanges and fixed to the cast with a new roll of fiberglass bandage.

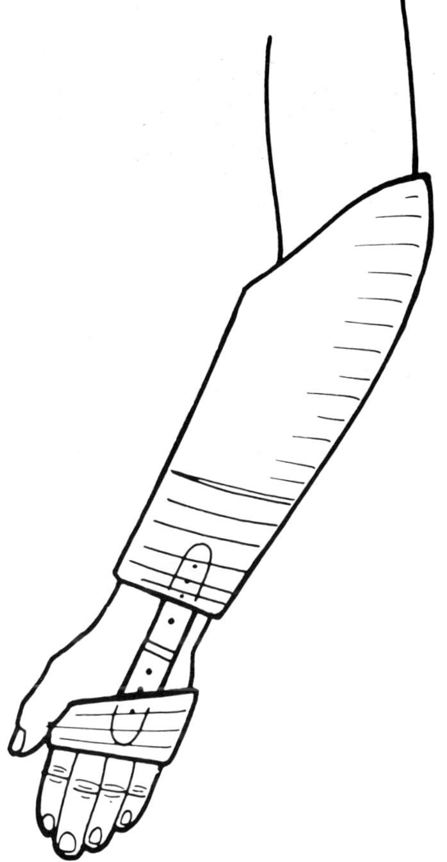

Fig. 5–12. An old-fashioned supracondylar cast-brace with a dorsal wrist hinge.

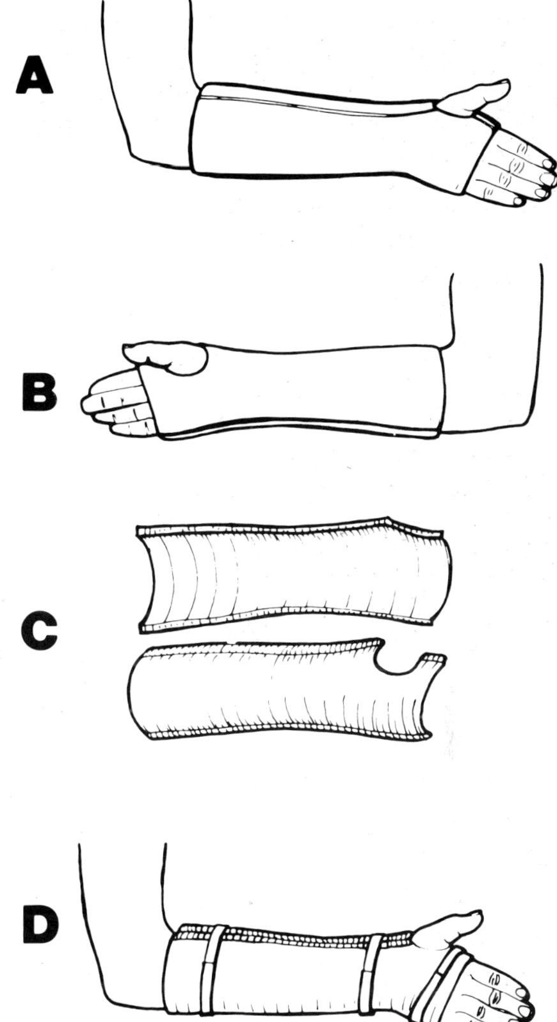

Fig. 5–13. Bivalving of a short-arm cast. *A*, Radial cut of the cast. *B*, Ulnar cut of the cast. *C*, The margins of the two halves of the bivalved cast have been lined with moleskin. *D*, The two halves of the bivalved cast have been reapplied to the injured extremity and are held together with three Velcro straps.

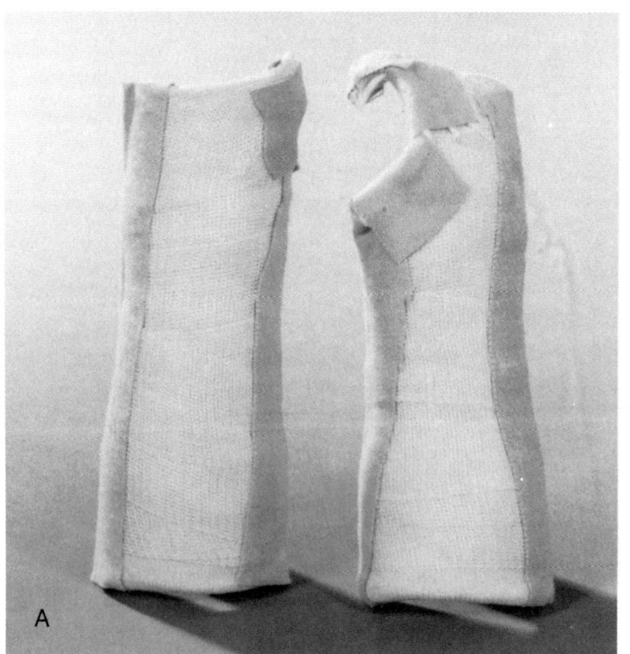

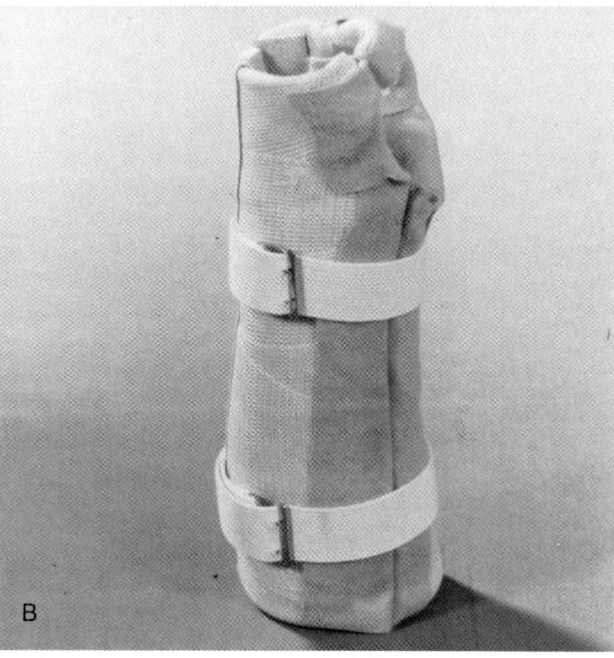

Fig. 5–14. *A*, A bivalved short-arm cast whose margins have been fully lined with moleskin. *B*, The two halves of a fully lined bivalved cast have been assembled and are held together with webbings and buckles.

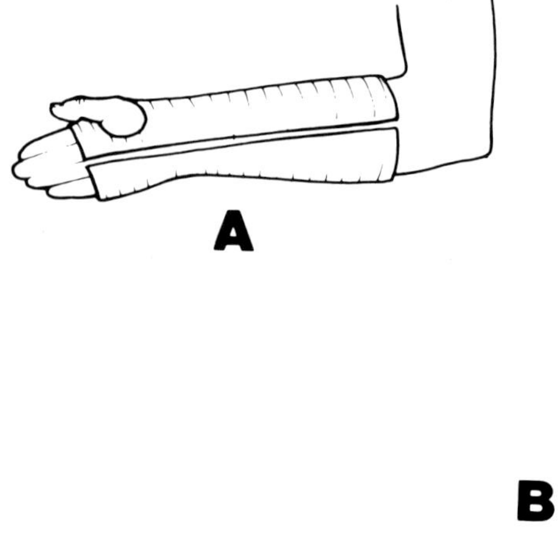

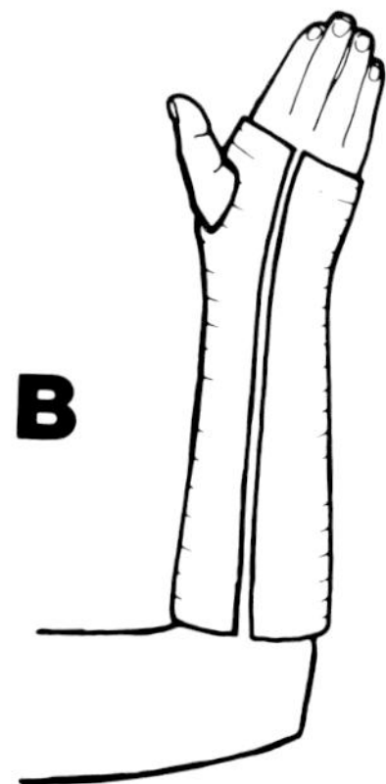

Fig. 5–15. A short-arm cast has been bivalved along the midline of its volar (*A*) and dorsal (*B*) surfaces.

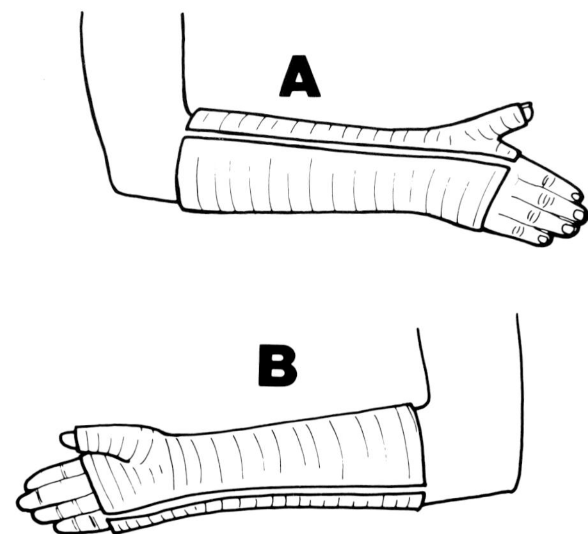

Fig. 5–16. A short-arm thumb spica cast has been bivalved along its radial (*A*) and ulnar (*B*) borders.

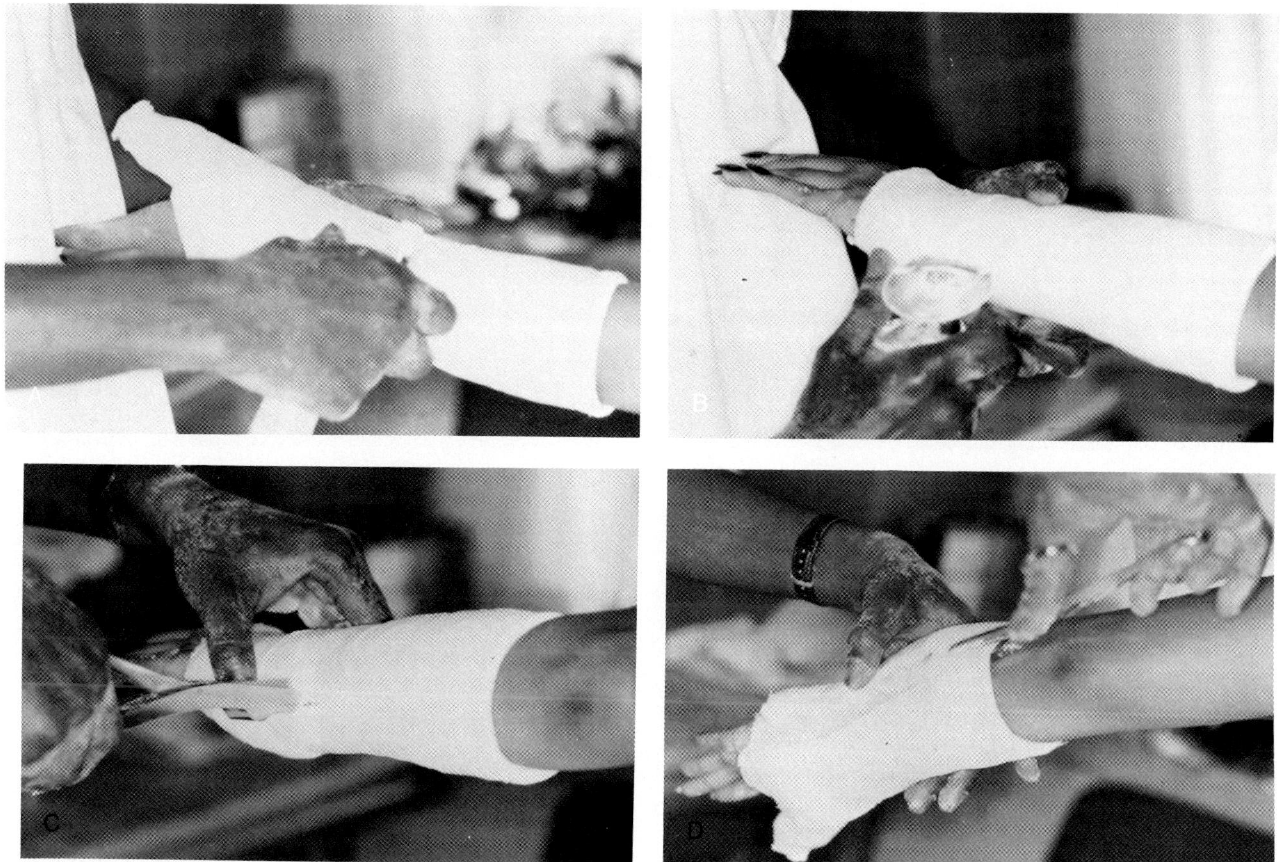

Fig. 5–17. Bivalving of a short-arm thumb spica cast. *A*, Cutting a short-arm thumb spica cast along its radial border. *B*, Cutting the cast along its ulnar border. *C*, Separating the two halves of the bivalved cast with a cast spreader. *D*, The Webril and stockinet are being cut with a pair of plaster scissors.

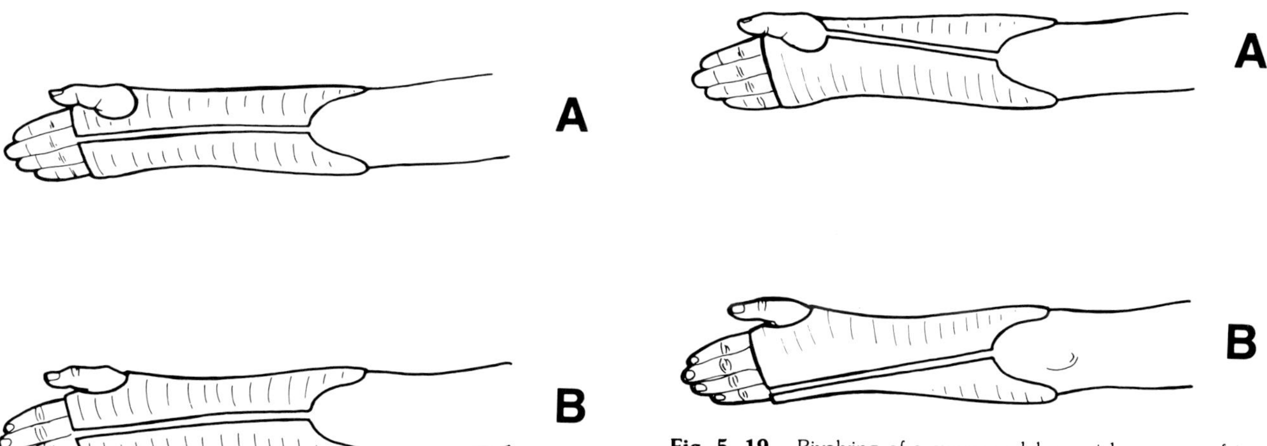

Fig. 5–18. A supracondylar cast has been bivalved along the midlines of its volar (*A*) and dorsal (*B*) surfaces.

Fig. 5–19. Bivalving of a supracondylar cast by means of two oblique cuts: from the first webspace to the middle of the anterior notch of the cast immediately distal to the antecubital fossa (*A*) and from the ulnar border of the distal end of the cast to the middle of the posterior notch immediately distal to the olecranon (*B*).

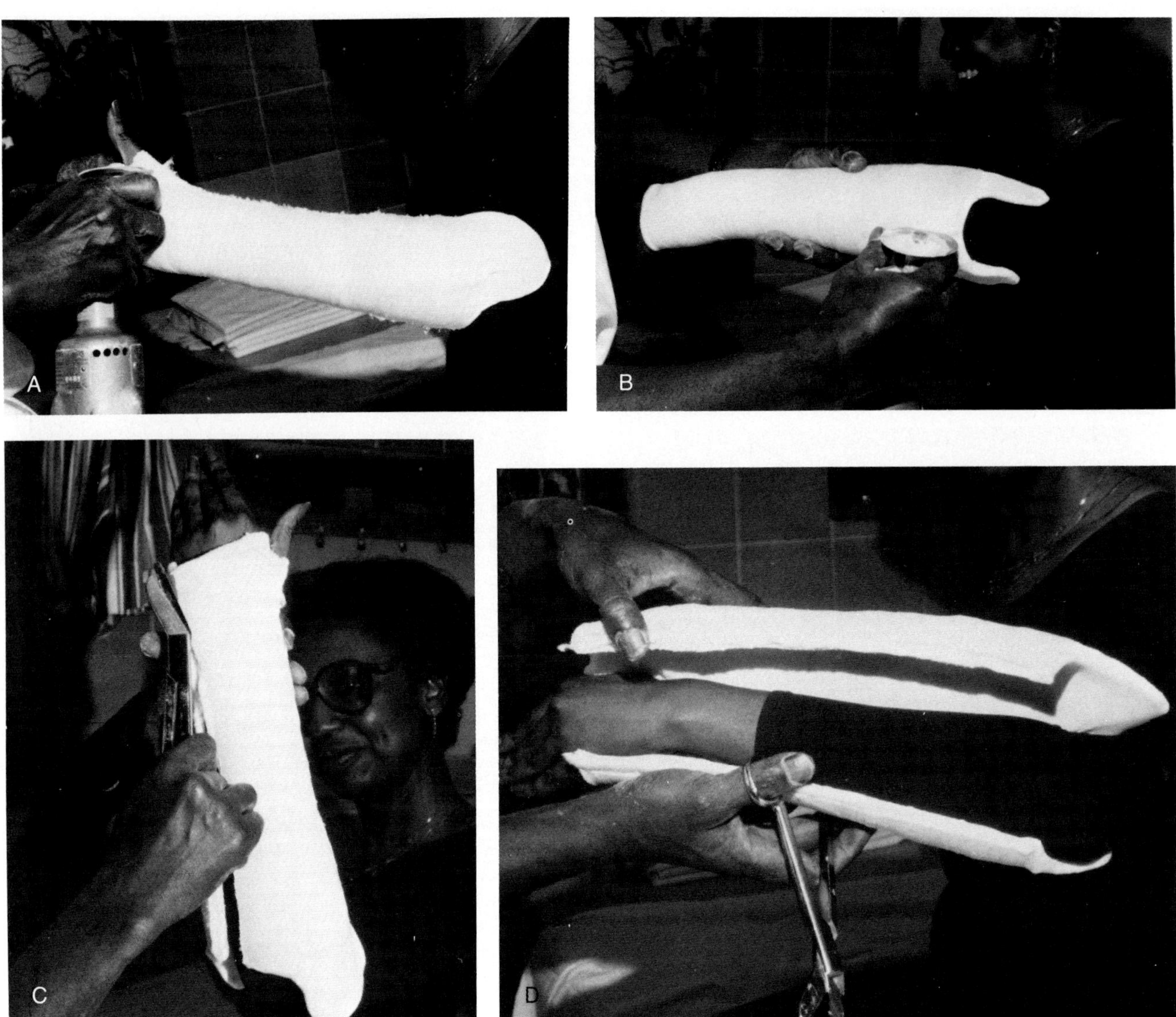

Fig. 5–20. Bivalving of a supracondylar cast. *A*, An oblique cut is made from the first webspace to the anterior notch of the cast immediately distal to the antecubital fossa. *B*, *C*, Another oblique cut is made from the ulnar border of the distal end of the cast to the middle of the infra-olecranon notch. *D*, The two halves of the supracondylar cast can now be separated after the underlying Webril and stockinet have been split longitudinally.

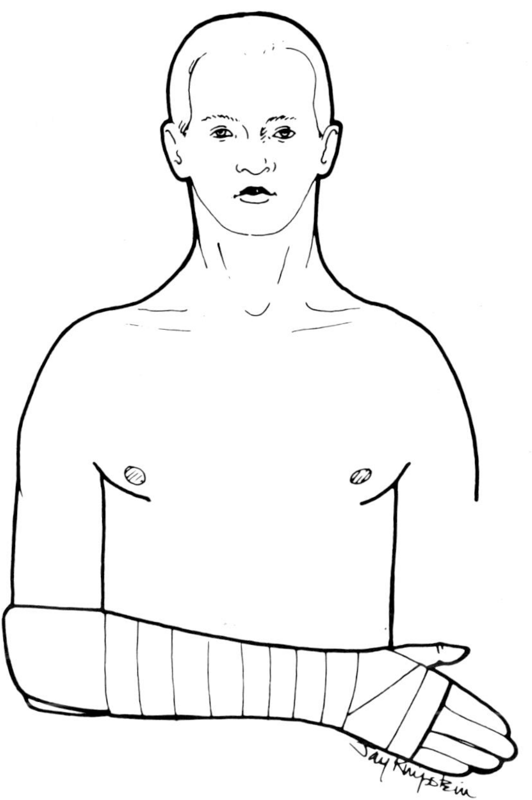

Fig. 5–21. A sugar-tong forearm splint.

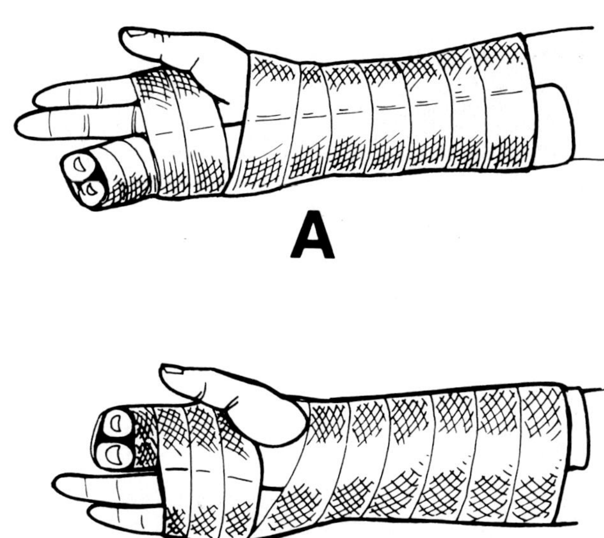

Fig. 5–22. Volar finger splints. *A*, An ulnar volar finger splint for injuries of the little and ring fingers. *B*, A radial volar finger splint for injuries of the index and long fingers.

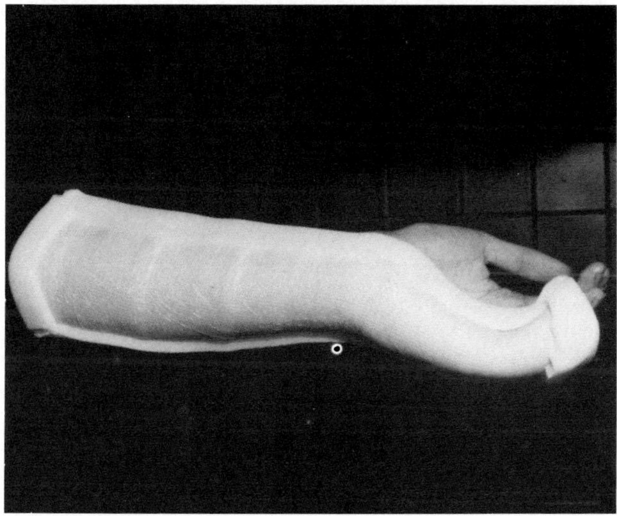

Fig. 5–23. An ulnar volar finger splint made of a tailored fiberglass splint and padded with a foam rubber sheet has been applied to the ulnar aspect of the hand and forearm.

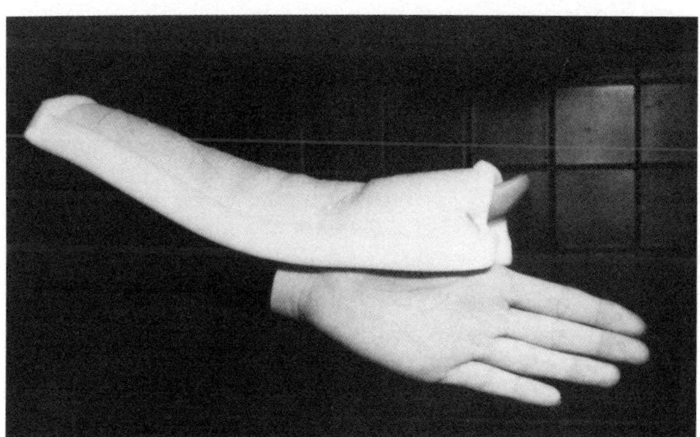

Fig. 5–24. A thumb splint made of a tailored fiberglass splint that has been padded with a piece of foam rubber sheet.

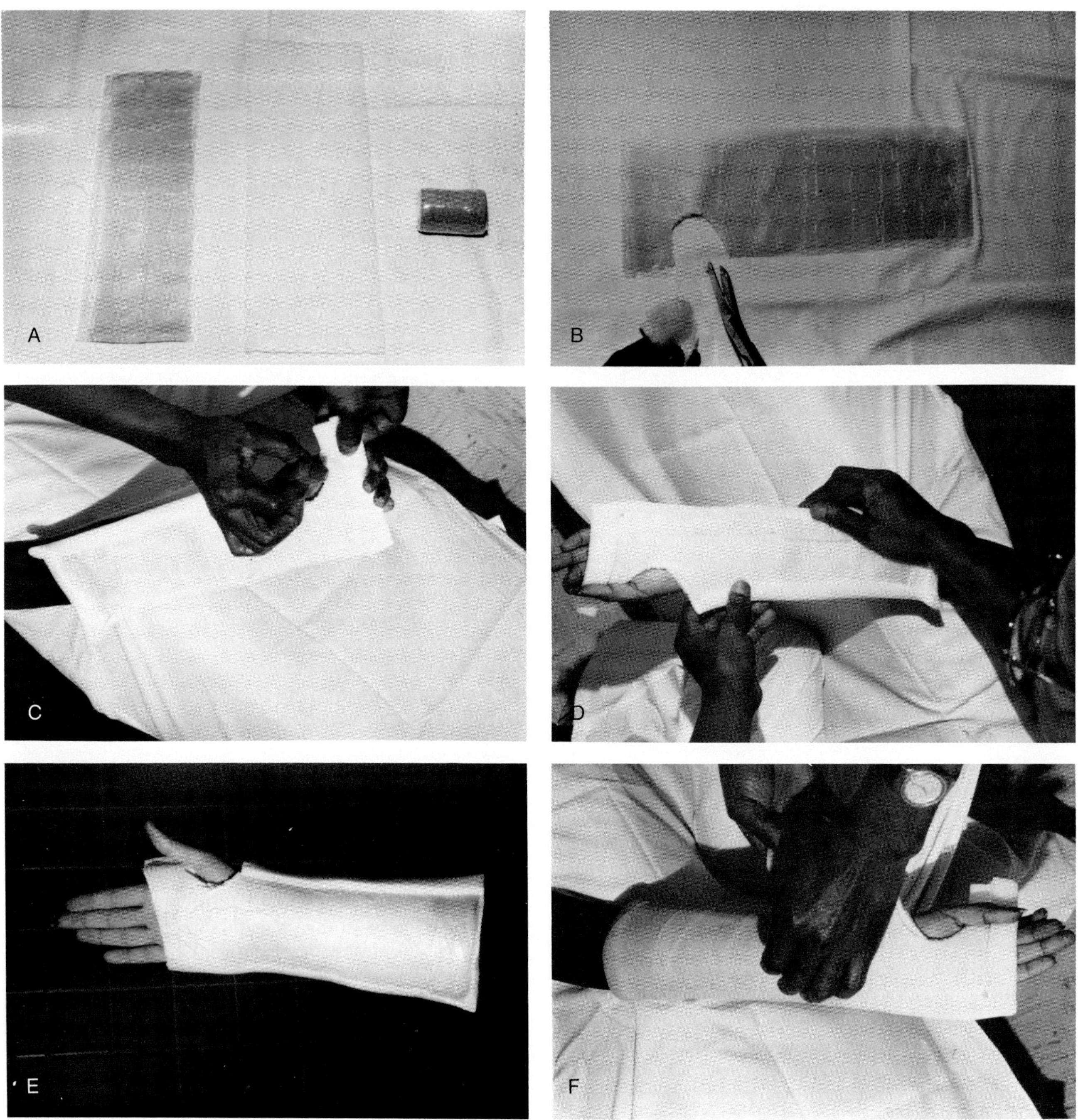

Fig. 5–25. Materials and technique for making a fiberglass volar wrist splint. *A*, Fiberglass splint, adhesive-backed foam rubber sheet, and Ace bandage. *B*, The foam rubber sheet has been applied to the fiberglass splint, and a thumb opening has been cut out of one side of the splint. *C*, *D*, *E*, The splint is applied to the volar aspect of the wrist and forearm. *F*, An Ace bandage is used to hold the wrist splint closely to the volar aspect of the wrist and forearm.

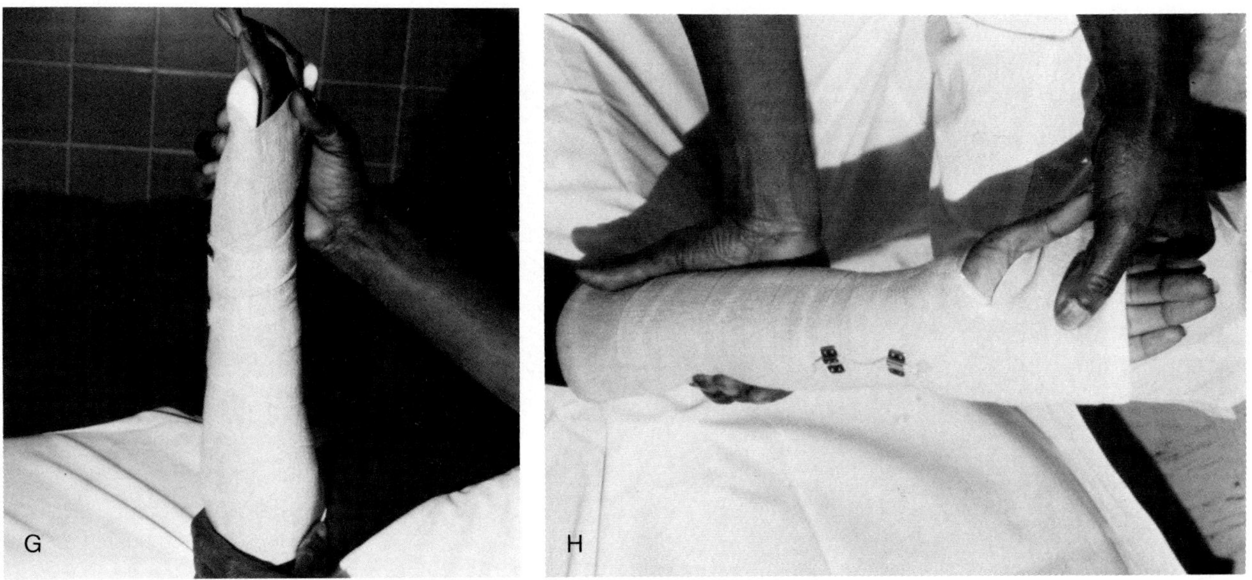

Fig. 5–25 (cont.). *G, H,* The cast technician should carefully mold the splint to fit the contour of the palm and the volar aspect of the wrist and forearm.

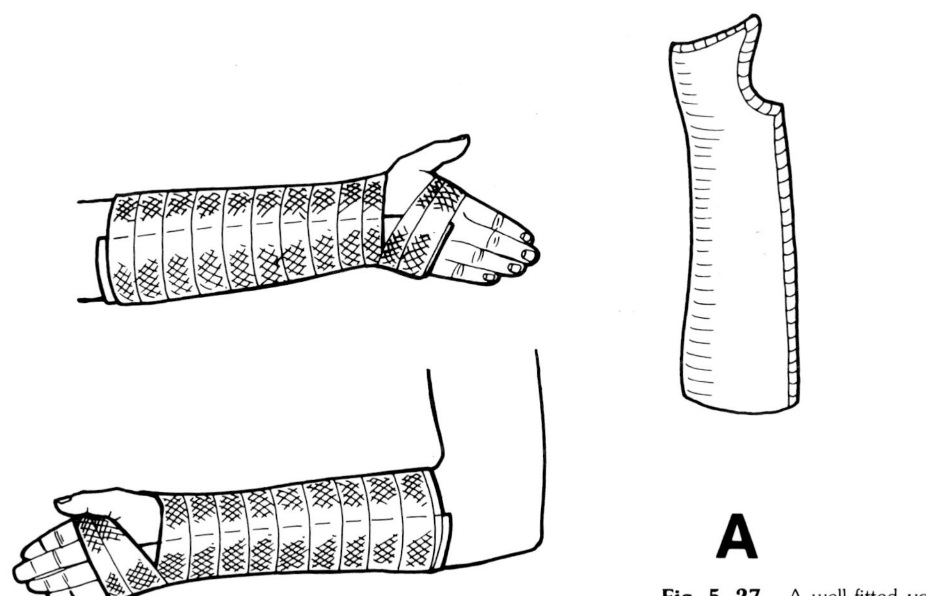

Fig. 5–26. An excellent ulnar gutter wrist splint can be obtained by longitudinally splitting a short-arm cast along the midline of its volar and dorsal surfaces and discarding the top half of the cast.

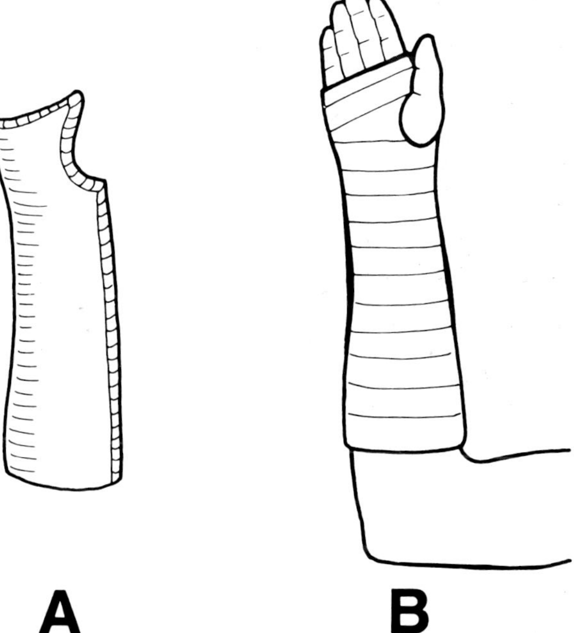

Fig. 5–27. A well-fitted volar wrist splint (*A*) can be made by splitting a short-arm cast along its radial and ulnar borders, lining the volar half of the cast, and returning the lined volar half of the cast to its original position, where it is held with an Ace bandage (*B*).

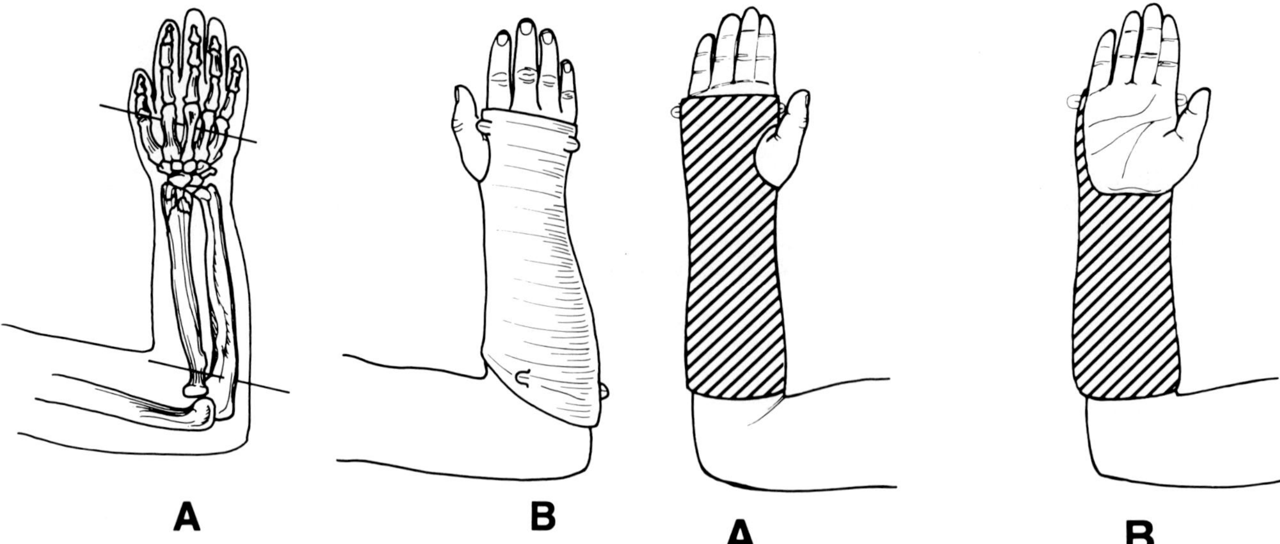

Fig. 5–28. Short-arm cast with bipolar K-wires. *A*, Two K-wires have been driven through the second and third metacarpals and the olecranon. *B*, A short-arm cast incorporating the two K-wires has been applied.

Fig. 5–29. Volar view of two short-arm casts with bipolar K-wires. *A*, The palm is enclosed by the distal end of the cast. *B*, The entire volar aspect of the hand is exposed.

CHAPTER 6. LONG-ARM CAST, LONG-ARM CYLINDER CAST, LONG-ARM CAST-BRACES, AND LONG-ARM SPLINTS

LONG-ARM CAST

Indications

A long-arm cast (Fig. 6-1) is used for dislocations of the wrist and elbow joints and for fractures of the radius, ulna, and humerus.

Cast Materials Needed

Plaster Long-Arm Cast

3″ stockinet

3 rolls of 3″ Webril

4 rolls of 4″ plaster bandage

Fiberglass Long-Arm Cast

3″ stockinet

3 rolls of 3″ Webril

1 roll of 4″ fiberglass bandage

2 rolls of 3″ fiberglass bandage

Patient's Position

A long-arm cast is best applied with the patient in a supine position for maximal control of the arm. The elbow should be flexed to 90°. Two persons should be available to apply the cast, one to maintain proper arm position and reduction and the other to apply the cast.

To maintain the proper reduction of different fractures, the cast is often applied in two stages. For instance, if the fracture is below the elbow, the short-arm portion of the cast should be applied first to stabilize the fracture, and then the above-elbow extension of the cast can be added (Fig. 6-2). If the fracture or dislocation involves the elbow joint or the humerus, a long-arm cylinder cast should be applied first to stabilize the reduced fracture or dislocation before the cast is extended to cover the wrist and hand (Fig. 6-3).

Technique for Applying a Long-Arm Cast

Stockinet

A 3″ stockinet with a thumbhole is used to cover the arm from the bases of the fingers to the armpit. The large transverse wrinkle in front of the elbow should be cut out with a pair of plaster scissors (Fig. 6-4A,B).

Webril

3″ Webril is wrapped from the level of the distal palmar crease to the upper portion of the arm. The Webril should be torn about 75% of its width before it is wrapped around the thumb webspace. The anterior aspect of the elbow region should be wrapped in an overlapping figure-8 fashion, and the posterior aspect of the elbow should be covered with overlapping strips of Webril in order to eliminate all wrinkles (Fig. 6-4C,D).

Plaster Bandage

The first 3 rolls of 4″ plaster bandage are evenly rolled onto the arm from the proximal palmar crease to the upper portion of the arm. To strengthen the distal end of the cast, the first turn of the plaster bandage over the first webspace should be twisted to produce a plaster rope and then wrapped around the palm at the level of the proximal palmar crease. The subsequent layers of plaster across the first webspace should be cut through about 75% of their widths to produce an even distal cast end and to provide room for free motion of the thumb. The proximal and distal ends of the stockinet are then folded down over the cast ends, and a new roll of 4″ plaster is used to go over the entire cast. The finished cast should be rubbed thoroughly to make it smooth and strong (Fig. 6-4E,F,G).

Fiberglass Bandage

The 2 rolls of 3″ fiberglass bandage are rolled onto the arm from the proximal palmar crease to the upper arm region. The bandage should be cut about 75% of its width before it is wrapped over the first webspace to avoid wrinkles in the distal end of the cast. The proximal and distal ends of the stockinet are folded down over the 2 cast ends, and a roll of 4″ fiberglass bandage is wrapped over the entire cast to finish it (Fig. 6-5).

LONG-ARM CYLINDER CAST

Indications

A long-arm cylinder cast is used for fractures and dislocations of the elbow region.

Cast Materials Needed

Materials needed for a long-arm cylinder cast are the same as for a long-arm cast.

Patient's Position

The patient's position is the same as a for a long-arm cast.

Technique for Applying a Long-Arm Cylinder Cast

Stockinet

A 3″ stockinet with a thumb-hole is applied from the level of the metacarpal heads to the upper arm region (Fig. 6-6A). The large transverse wrinkle in front of the elbow is cut out with a pair of plaster scissors.

Webril

Three rolls of 3″ Webril are evenly wrapped around the arm from the level of the radial and ulnar styloid processes to the upper arm region (Fig. 6-6B).

Plaster or Fiberglass Bandage

Three rolls of 4″ plaster bandage or 2 rolls of 3″ fiberglass bandage are evenly wrapped around the arm from the wrist to the upper arm region. The stockinet ends are then folded down over the cast ends, and a roll of 4″ plaster or fiberglass bandage is used to go over the entire cast (Fig. 6-6C,D). The finished cast should be thoroughly rubbed with the palms of both hands to make it smooth and strong.

LONG-ARM CAST-BRACE WITH ELBOW HINGES

Indications

A long-arm cast-brace with elbow hinges is used for fractures of the humerus, radius, ulna, and wrist.

Cast Materials Needed

Plaster Long-Arm Cast-Brace with Elbow Hinges

3″ stockinet

3 rolls of 3″ Webril

4 rolls of 4″ plaster bandage

1 role of 3″ plaster bandage

2 polycentric elbow hinges

Fiberglass Long-Arm Cast-Brace with Elbow Hinges

3″ stockinet

3 rolls of 3″ Webril

2 rolls of 3″ fiberglass bandage

1 roll of 4″ fiberglass bandage

1 roll of 2″ fiberglass bandage

2 polycentric elbow hinges

Patient's Position

The patient's position is the same as for a long-arm cast.

Technique for Applying a Long-Arm Cast-Brace with Elbow Hinges

First, a standard plaster or fiberglass long-arm cast is applied. Next, a cast saw is used to make 2 transverse cuts, perpendicular to the longitudinal axes of the forearm and the arm, about 3″ above and below the elbow flexion crease on both the medial and lateral aspects of the cast, to facilitate subsequent removal of the elbow section of the cast. Two polycentric elbow hinges are placed over the medial and lateral aspects of the elbow joint and are fixed to the cast with 3″ plaster or 2″ fiberglass bandage. The cast material between the 4 transverse cuts is completely removed by completing the transverse cuts in a circumferential manner and longitudinally splitting the freed elbow section of the cast. The underlying Webril is now removed, and the stockinet is cut transversely. Four slits are then made in the medial and lateral aspects of the 2 free ends of the stockinet. These stockinet ends are pulled down over the cut ends of the cast and fixed to the cast-brace with plaster or fiberglass bandages so that they will not be caught by the elbow hinges (Figs. 6-7, 6-8).

LONG-ARM CAST-BRACE WITH ELBOW AND WRIST HINGES

Indications

A long-arm cast-brace with elbow and wrist hinges is used for fractures of the humerus, radius, and ulna.

Cast Materials Needed

Plaster Long-Arm Cast-Brace with Elbow and Wrist Hinges

3″ stockinet

3 rolls of 3″ Webril

4 rolls of 4″ plaster bandage

1 roll of 3″ plaster bandage (for elbow hinges)

1 roll of 2″ plaster bandage (for wrist hinge)

2 polycentric elbow hinges

1 small gate hinge

Fiberglass Long-Arm Cast-Brace with Elbow and Wrist Hinges

3″ stockinet

3 rolls of 3″ Webril

2 rolls of 3″ fiberglass bandage

1 roll of 4″ fiberglass bandage

2 rolls of 2″ fiberglass bandage (for elbow and wrist hinges)

2 polycentric elbow hinges

1 small gate hinge

Patient's Position

The patient's position is the same as for a long-arm cast.

Technique for Applying a Long-Arm Cast-Brace with Elbow and Wrist Hinges

The technique for applying a long-arm cast-brace with elbow hinges has been described in detail in the previous section, and application of a dorsal wrist hinge has been described in Chapter 5. Addition of hinges to a long-arm cast is shown in Figs. 6-9 and 6-10.

HANGING CAST

A hanging cast is a long-arm cast with a small loop attached to its wrist region. An adjustable sling passes through the loop and around the neck.

Indications

A hanging cast is used for a wide variety of humeral fractures. The weight of the cast provides mild extrinsic traction to maintain reasonable alignment of a humeral fracture, however, a very heavy hanging cast can distract the humeral fracture to delay or prevent union. If a hanging cast is to be effective during sleeping hours, the patient should sleep in a sitting position so that gravity can constantly pull on the fracture site to maintain its alignment. In addition, the axillary region of an obese patient should be heavily padded to prevent development of skin ulcer caused by the superomedial aspect of the hanging cast.

Cast Materials Needed

The materials needed for making a hanging cast are the same as for a long-arm cast.

Patient's Position

The patient's position is the same as for a long-arm cast.

Technique for Applying a Hanging Cast

The technique for applying a hanging cast is the same as for applying a long-arm cast except for the wrist loop. The site of the loop is determined by the nature of the displacements of the humeral fractures. For example, a loop at the dorsum of the wrist tends to correct lateral angulation of a humeral fracture, whereas a loop at the volar aspect of the wrist tends to correct medial angulation of a humeral fracture (Fig. 6-11). Lengthening of the sling can correct posterior angulation of a humeral fracture, and shortening of the sling can correct anterior angulation of a humeral fracture (Fig. 6-12).

SUGAR-TONG ARM SPLINT

Indications

A sugar-tong arm splint (Fig. 6-13) is used for fractures of the humerus.

Cast Materials Needed

Plaster Sugar-Tong Arm Splint

Plaster cast materials—2 5″ × 30″ plaster splints or 1 roll of 6″ plaster bandage

Padding—Adhesive-backed foam rubber sheet, felt, or multiple layers of 6″ Webril

Ace bandage—2 rolls of 4″ Ace bandage

Fiberglass Sugar-Tong Arm Splint

Fiberglass cast materials—1 4″ × 30″ fiberglass splint or 1 roll of 4″ fiberglass bandage

Padding—Adhesive-backed foam rubber sheet, felt, or multiple layers of 5″ Webril

Ace bandage—2 rolls of 4″ Ace bandage

Patient's Position

The sugar-tong arm splint can be applied while the patient is either sitting or standing. The elbow joint should be flexed to 90°, and the whole arm should be internally rotated.

Technique for Applying a Sugar-Tong Arm Splint

The exact length of splint material required for a sugar-tong arm splint can be determined by running a tape measure from the armpit down and round the olecranon and then up to the top of the shoulder. The plaster or fiberglass splint is cut to the length measured. If a plaster or fiberglass bandage is used, it should be folded back and forth on itself until the desired thickness is obtained. The splint is then padded with foam rubber sheet, felt, or several layers of Webril, the margins of the padding material extending about $\frac{1}{2}$ inch beyond the plaster or fiberglass splint. The padding material is folded smoothly over the edges of the splint.

The padded splint is soaked in water, and while it is still wet and soft, it should be applied to the arm, starting from the armpit, going down to the olecranon region, and then extending up to the top of the shoulder. It should be molded gently to conform to the general contour of the arm. A 4″ Ace bandage is used to bind the splint to the arm (Fig. 6-14).

BIVALVING OF A LONG-ARM CAST

A long-arm cast can be bivalved either along its radial and ulnar borders (Fig. 6-15) or along the midline of its anterior and posterior surfaces (Fig. 6-16). After the underlying Webril and stockinet have been cut longitudinally, the margins of the two halves of the cast are lined with moleskin. The two halves of the cast are then reapplied to the extremity, where they are held together with several Velcro straps or webbings with attached buckles.

LONG-ARM SPLINTS

Long-arm splints (Fig. 6-17) can either immobilize the wrist or leave the wrist free. Although plaster or fiberglass splints are often used to make long-arm splints, the ideal long-arm splint can only be obtained by bivalving a long-arm cast or a long-arm cylinder cast and keeping the bottom half of the cast (Fig. 6-18).

BIBLIOGRAPHY

Alexander, A.H.: Bilateral traumatic dislocation of the radioulnar joint, ulna dorsal: Case report and review of the literature. Clin. Orthop., *129*:238, 1977.

Bacorn, R.W., and Kurtzke, J.F.: Colles' fracture: A study of two thousand cases from the New York State Workmen's Compensation Board. J. Bone Joint Surg. [Am.], *35*:634, 1953.

Balfour, G.N., Mooney, V., and Ashby, M.: Diaphyseal fractures of the humerus treated with a ready-made fracture brace. J. Bone Joint Surg. [Am.], *64*:11, 1982.

Barquet, A., et al.: Dislocation of the shoulder with fracture of the ipsilateral shaft of the humerus. Injury, *16*:300, 1985.

Berstein, S.M., King, J.D., and Sanderson, R.A.: Fractures of the medial epicondyles of the humerus. Contemp. Orthop., *3*:637, 1981

Blount, W.P.: Fractures in Children. Huntington, NY, Robert E. Krieger, 1977.

Boyd, H.B., and Boals, J.C.: The Monteggia lesion. A review of 159 cases. Clin. Orthop., *66*:94, 1969.

Bradford, C.H., Adams, R.W., and Kilfoyle, R.M.: Fractures of both bones of the forearm in adults. Surg. Gynecol. Obstet., *96*:240, 1953.

Brown, R.F., and Morgan, R.G.: Intercondylar T-shaped fractures of the humerus. J. Bone Joint Surg. [Br.], *53*:425, 1971.

Bryan, R.S.: Fractures about the elbow in adults. American Academy of Orthopaedic Surgeons Instructional Course Lectures, *30*:200, 1981.

Caldwell, J.A.: Treatment of fractures of the shaft of the humerus by hanging cast. Surg. Gynecol. Obstet., *70*:421, 1940.

Charnley, J.: The closed treatment of common fractures. 3rd. Ed. Edinburgh, Churchill Livingstone, 1974.

Collert, S.: Surgical management of fracture of capitellum humeri. Acta. Orthop. Scand., *48*:603, 1977.

Compere, E.L., Bank, S.W., and Compere, C.L.: Pictorial Handbook of Fracture Treatment. 5th Ed. Chicago, Year Book Medical Publishers, 1963.

D'Ambrosia, R.D.: Supracondylar fractures of the humerus—prevention of cubitus varus. J. Bone Joint Surg. [Am.], *54*:60, 1972.

Depalma, A.F., and Cantilli, R.A.: Fractures of the upper end of the humerus. Clin. Orthop., *20*:73, 1961.

Durig, M., Muller, W., Ruedi, T.P., and Gauer, E. F.: The operative treatment of elbow dislocation in the adult. J. Bone Joint Surg. [Am.], *61*:239, 1979.

Ellis, J.: Smith's and Barton's fractures: A method of treatment. J. Bone Joint Surg. [Br.], *47*:724, 1965.

Evans, E.M.: Rotational deformity in the treatment of fractures of both bones of the forearm. J. Bone Joint Surg., *27*:373, 1945.

Galbraith, K.A., and McCullough, C.J.: Acute nerve injury as a complication of closed fractures or dislocations of elbow. Injury, *11*:159, 1979.

Garcia, A., and Maeck, B.H.: Radial nerve injuries in fractures of the shaft of the humerus. Am. J. Surg., *99*:625, 1960.

Gartsman, G.M., Sculo, T.P., and Otis, J.C.: Operative treatment of olecranon fractures: Excision or open reduction with internal fixation. J. Bone Joint Surg. [Am.], *63*:718, 1981.

Grantham, S.A., Norris, T.R., and Bush, D.C.: Isolated fracture of the humeral capitellum. Clin. Orthop., *161*:262, 1981.

Grantham, S.A., and Tietjen, R.: Transcondylar fracture-dislocation of the elbow. J. Bone Joint Surg. [Am.], *58*:1030, 1976.

Grimer, R.J., and Brooks, S.: Brachial artery damage accompanying closed posterior dislocation of the elbow. J. Bone Joint Surg. [Br.], *67*:378, 1985.

Hallet, J.: Entrapment of the median nerve after dislocation of the elbow. A case report. J. Bone Joint Surg. [Br.], *63*:408, 1981.

Heidt, R.S., Jr., and Stern, P.J.: Isolated posterior dislocation of the radial head. A case report. Clin. Orthop., *168*:136, 1982.

Horne, G.: Supracondylar fractures of the humerus in adults. J. Bone Joint Surg. [Br.], *61*:246, 1979.

Horne, J.G., and Tanzer, T.L.: Olecranon fractures: A review of 100 cases. J. Trauma, *21*:469, 1981.

Jupiter, J.B., Neff, U., Holzach, P., and Allgower, M.: Intercondylar fractures of the humerus. An operative approach. J. Bone Joint Surg. [Am.], *67*:226, 1985.

King, T.I., II.: Plaster splinting as a means of reducing elbow flexor spasticity: A case study. Am. J. Occup. Ther., *36*:671, 1982.

Kolb, L.W., and Moore, R.D.: Fractures of the supracondylar process of the humerus: Report of two cases. J. Bone Joint Surg. [Am.], *49*:532, 1967.

Lange, R.H., and Foster, R.J.: Skeletal management of humeral shaft fractures associated with forearm fractures. Clin. Orthop., *195*:173, 1985.

Latta, L., Sarmiento, A., and Tarr, R.R.: The rationale of functional bracing of fractures. Research experiences. Clin. Orthop., *146*:28, 1980.

Louis, D.S., Riciardi, J.E., and Spengler, D.M.: Arterial injury: A complication of posterior elbow dislocation. A clinical and anatomical study. J. Bone Joint Surg. [Am.], *56*:1631, 1974.

McDougall, A., and White, J.: Subluxation of the inferior radio-ulnar joint complicating fracture of the radial head. J. Bone Joint Surg. [Br.], *39*:278, 1957.

McMaster, W.C., Tivnon, M.C., and Waugh, T.R.: Cast brace for the upper extremity. Clin. Orthop., *109*:126, 1975.

Mathenson, M.H., and McCreath, S.W.: Tension band wiring in the treatment of olecranon fractures. J. Bone Joint Surg. [Br.], *57*:399, 1975.

Mathur, N., and Sharma, C.S.: Fracture of the head of the radius treated by elbow cast. Acta Orthop. Scand., *55*:567, 1984.

Mikic, Z.D.: Galeazzi fracture dislocations. J. Bone Joint Surg. [Am.], *57*:1071, 1975.

Niemann, K.M.W.: Condylar fractures of distal humerus in adults. South. Med. J., *70*:915, 1977.

Papavasiliou, V., and Nenopoulos, S.: Ipsilateral injuries of the elbow and forearm in children. J. Pediatr. Orthop., *6*:58, 1986.

Ralston, E.L., Shands, A.R., Jr., Lehr, H.B., and Pitts, F.W.: Hand Book of Fractures. St. Louis, C.V. Mosby, 1967.

Robertson, R.C., and Bogart, F.B.: Fracture of the capitellum and trochlea, combined with fracture of the external humeral condyle. J. Bone Joint Surg., *15*:206, 1933.

Rooney, P.J., and Cockshott, W.P.: Pseudarthrosis following proximal humeral fractures: A possible mechanism. Skeletal Radiol., *15*:21, 1986.

Rosacker, J.A., and Kopta, J.A.: Both bone fractures of the forearm: A review of surgical variables associated with union. Orthopedics, *4*:1353, 1981.

Sarmiento, A. Cooper, J.S., and Sinclair, W.F.: Forearm fractures. Early functional bracing—a preliminary report. J. Bone Joint Surg. [Am.], *57*:297, 1975.

Sarmiento, A., et al.: Functional bracing of fractures of the shaft of the humerus. J. Bone Joint Surg. [Am.], *59*:596, 1977.

Shmueli, G., and Herold, H.Z.: Compression screwing of displaced fractures of head of the radius. J. Bone Joint Surg. [Br.], *63*:535, 1981.

Smaill, G.B.: Long term follow-up of Colles' fractures. J. Bone Joint Surg. [Br.], *47*:80, 1965.

Soltampur, A.: Anterior supracondylar fracture of the humerus (flexion type). J. Bone Joint Surg. [Br.], *60*:383, 1978.

Sovio, O.M., and Tredwell, S.J.: Divergent dislocation of the elbow in a child. J. Pediatr. Orthop., *6*:96, 1986.

Stewart, M.J., and Hundley, J.M.: Fractures of the humerus. A comparative study in methods and treatment. J. Bone Joint Surg. [Am.], *37*:681, 1955.

Swanson, A.B., Jaeger, S.H., and Rochelle, D.L.: Comminuted fractures of the radial head. The role of silicone-implant replacement arthroplasty. J. Bone Joint Surg. [Am.], *63*:1039, 1981.

Thompson, H.C., III, and Garcia, A.: Myositis ossificans (aftermath of elbow injuries). Clin. Orthop., *50*:129, 1967.

Wilson, J.N.: The treatment of fractures of the medial epicondyle of the humerus. J. Bone Joint Surg. [Br.], *42*:778, 1960.

Young, T.B., and Wallace, W.A.: Conservative treatment of fractures and fracture-dislocation of the upper end of humerus. J. Bone Joint Surg. [Br.], *67*:373, 1985.

Zuckerman, J.D., Flugstad, D.L., Teitz, C.C., and King, H.A.: Axillary artery injury as a complication of proximal humeral fractures. Two case reports and a review of the literature. Clin. Orthop., *189*:234, 1984.

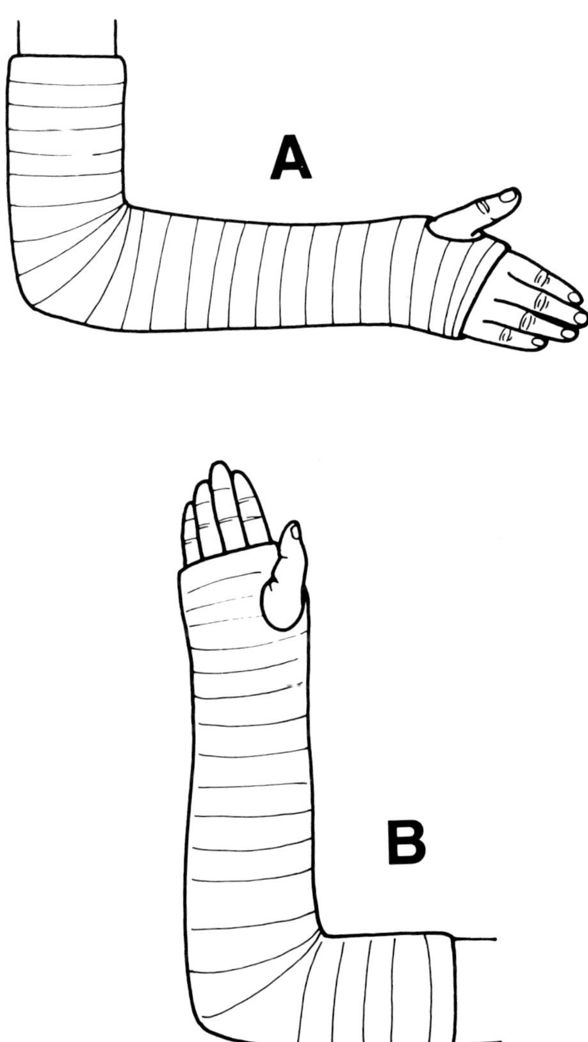

Fig. 6–1. Lateral (*A*) and medial (*B*) views of a long-arm cast.

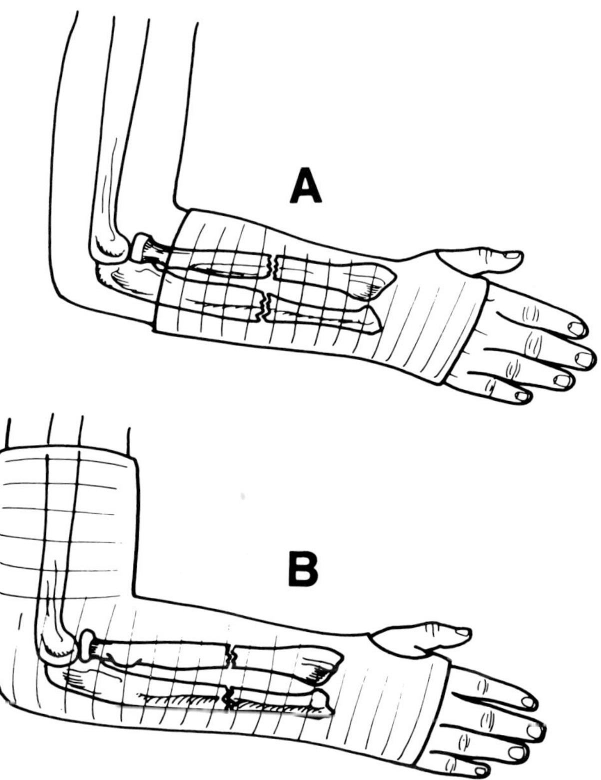

Fig. 6–2. In treatment of fractures of both bones of the forearm, a short-arm cast is applied first to stabilize the fractures (*A*), and then an above-elbow extension is added (*B*).

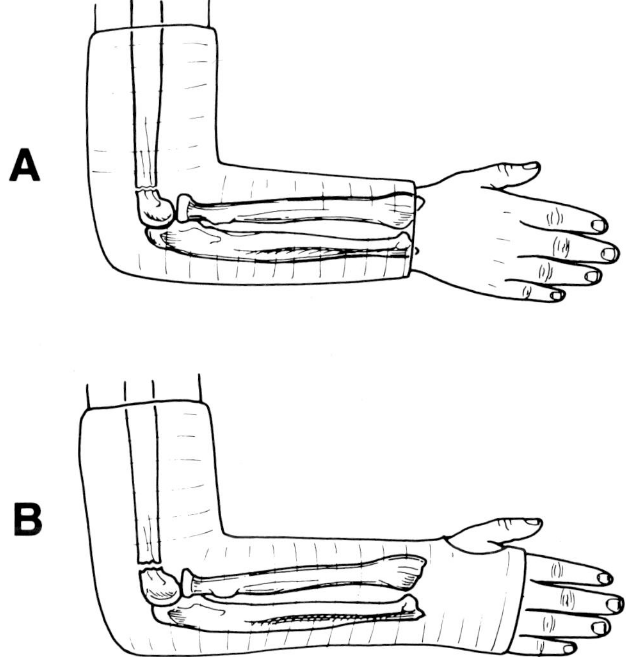

Fig. 6–3. In treatment of a supracondylar fracture of the humerus with a long-arm cast, a long-arm cylinder cast should be applied first to stabilize the supracondylar fracture (*A*). Then the cast can be extended to cover the wrist and hand (*B*).

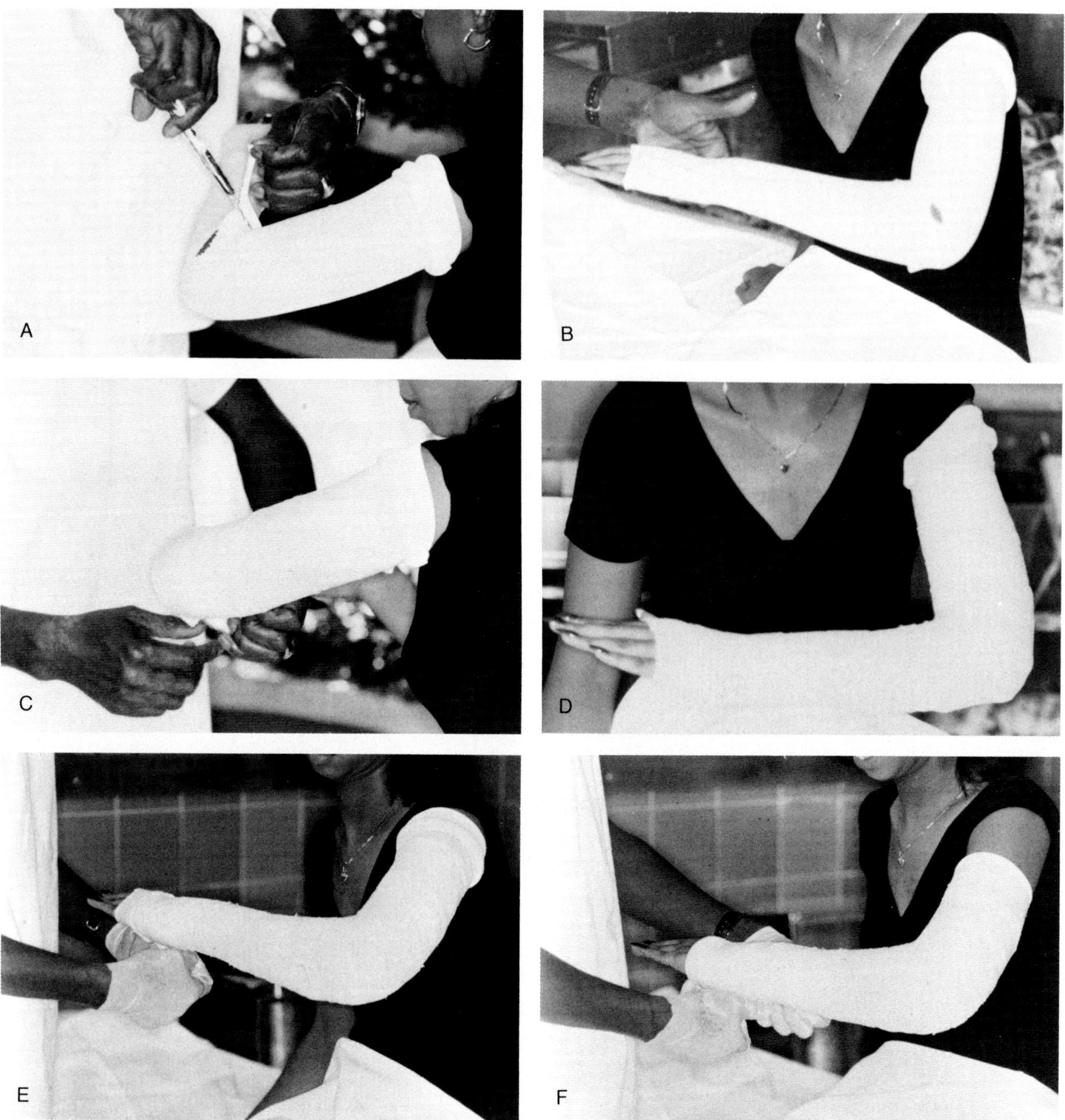

Fig. 6–4. The making of a plaster long-arm cast. *A, B,* The large transverse wrinkle of the stockinet in front of the elbow is cut out with a pair of plaster scissors. *C, D,* Three rolls of 3″ Webril are wrapped around the arm from the distal palmar crease to the upper arm region. *E,* Three rolls of 4″ plaster bandage have been applied to the whole arm. *F,* The stockinet ends have been pulled down over the cast ends, and a new roll of 4″ plaster bandage has been wrapped around the cast.

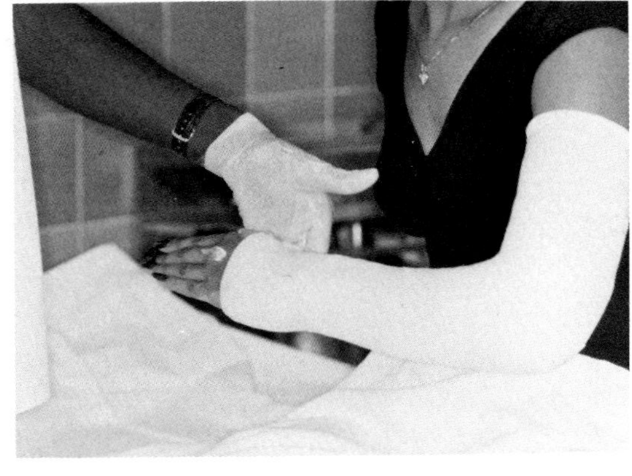

G

Fig. 6–4 (cont.). *G*, The palms of both hands are used to rub the cast to make it smooth and strong.

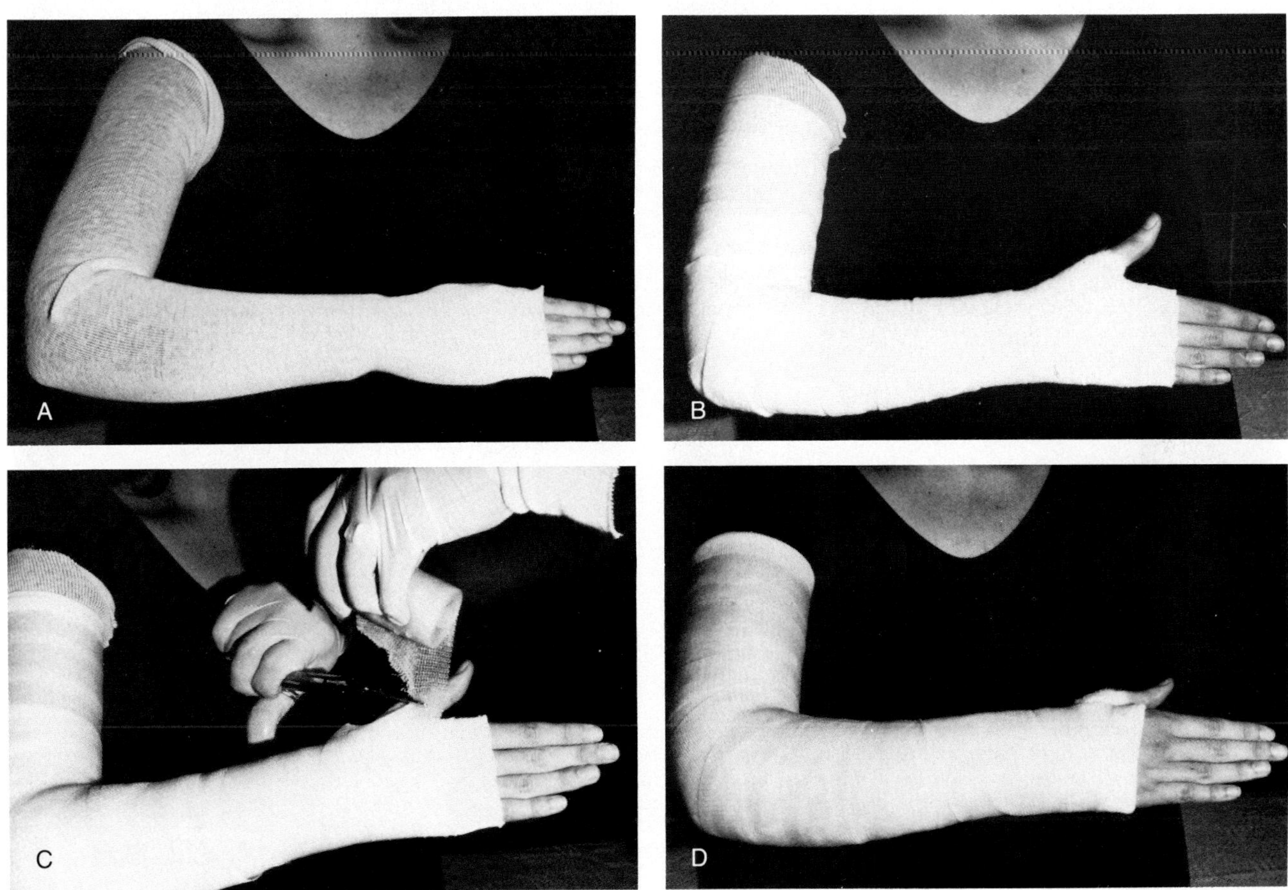

Fig. 6–5. The making of a fiberglass long-arm cast. *A*, A 3″ stockinet with a thumbhole has been applied to the arm. The transverse wrinkle in front of the elbow should be cut out. *B*, Three rolls of 3″ Webril have been applied, from the distal palmar crease to the upper arm region. *C*, Two rolls of 3″ fiberglass bandage are being applied to the arm. Note the 75% cut through the width of the bandage before it is wrapped across the first webspace. *D*, After the ends of the stockinet have been turned down over the proximal and distal cast ends, a roll of 4″ fiberglass bandage is applied over the cast to complete it.

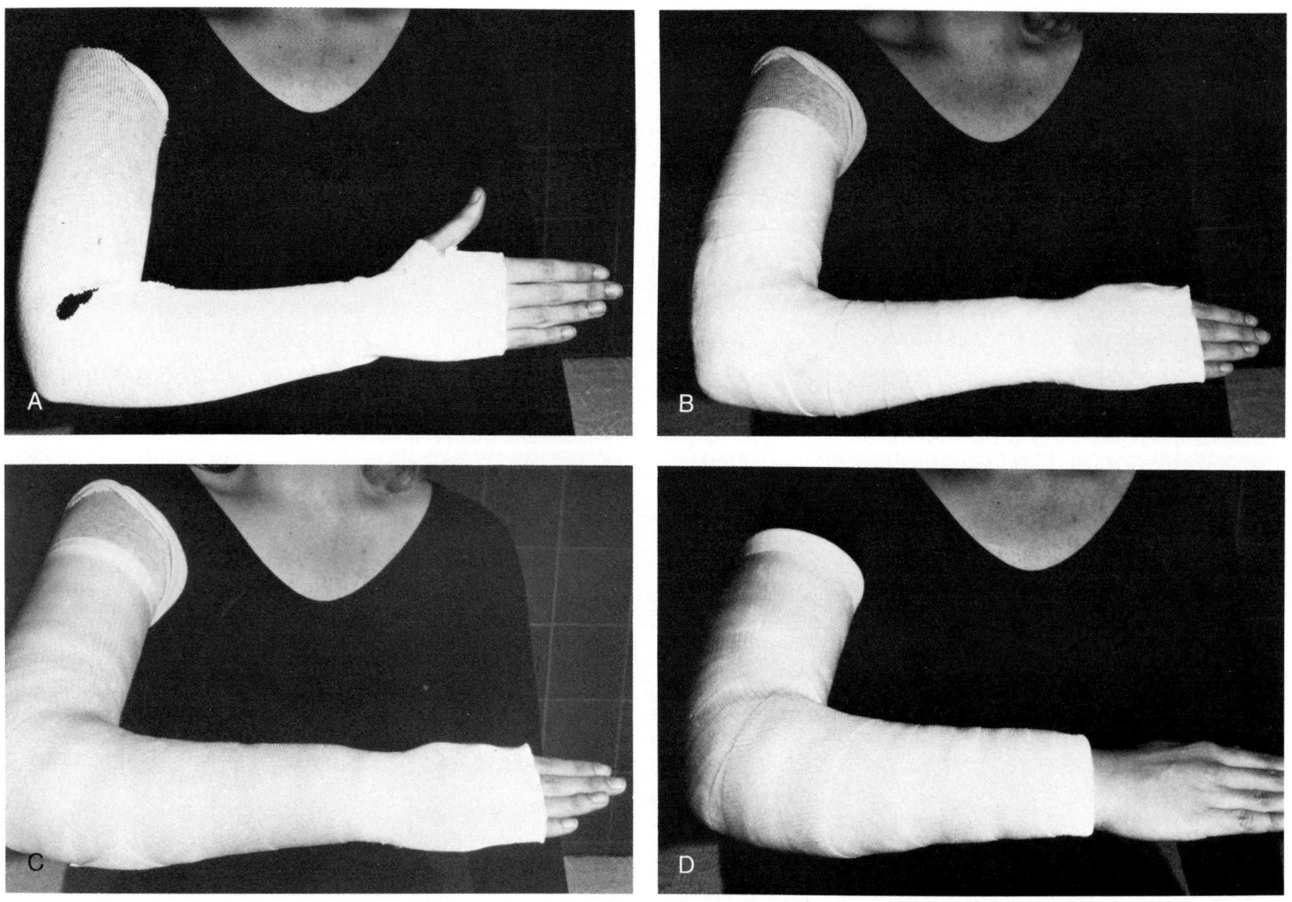

Fig. 6–6. The making of a long-arm cylinder cast. *A*, A 3″ stockinet with a thumbhole has been applied to the arm, and the transverse wrinkle in front of the elbow has been removed. *B*, Three rolls of 3″ Webril have been applied to the arm from the wrist to the upper arm region. *C*, Two rolls of 3″ fiberglass bandage have been wrapped around the arm from the wrist to the upper arm region. *D*, After the stockinet ends have been pulled down tightly over the proximal and distal cast ends, a roll of 4″ fiberglass bandage is used to cover the entire cast to complete it.

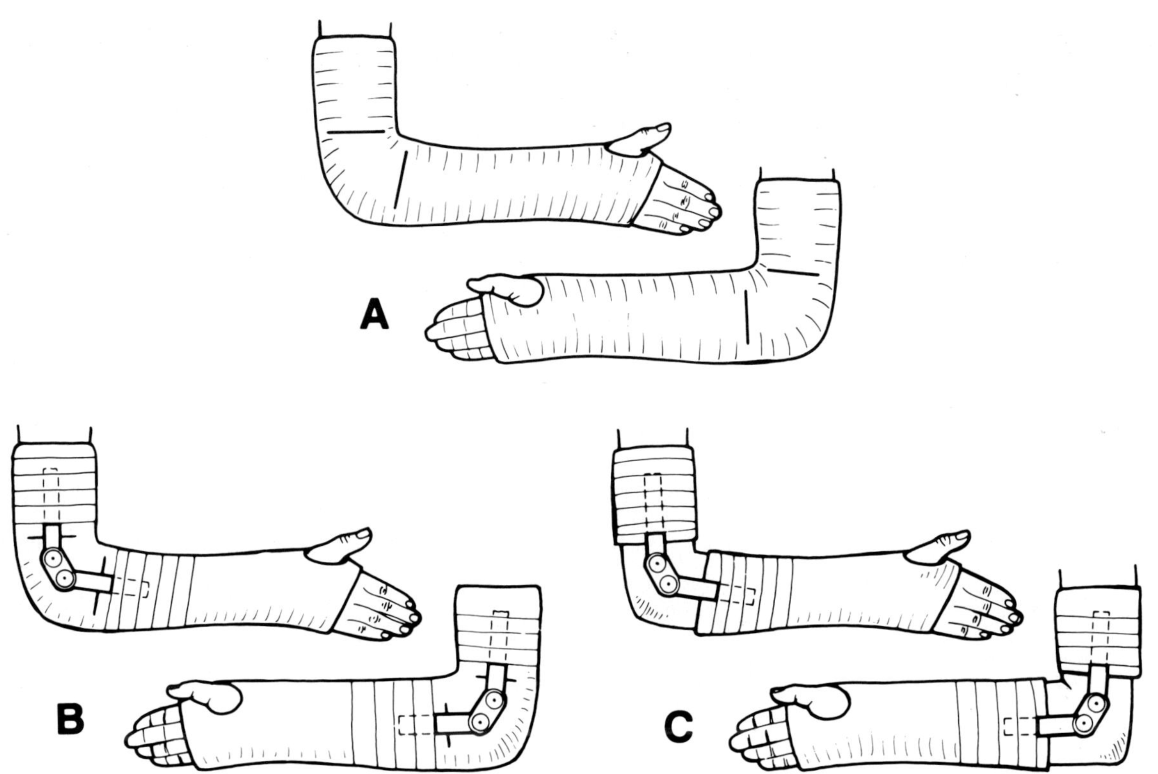

Fig. 6–7. Fitting a long-arm cast with elbow hinges. *A*, Four transverse cuts are made perpendicular to the longitudinal axes of forearm and arm about 3″ from the elbow flexion crease on the medial and lateral aspects of the elbow region of the cast. *B*, The 2 polycentric elbow hinges have been attached to the medial and lateral aspects of the elbow. *C*, The elbow section of the cast between the 4 transverse cuts has been removed, the underlying Webril removed, and the stockinet transversely divided and pulled down over the 2 cast ends of the elbow region, to be fixed to the cast-brace with new plaster or fiberglass bandage.

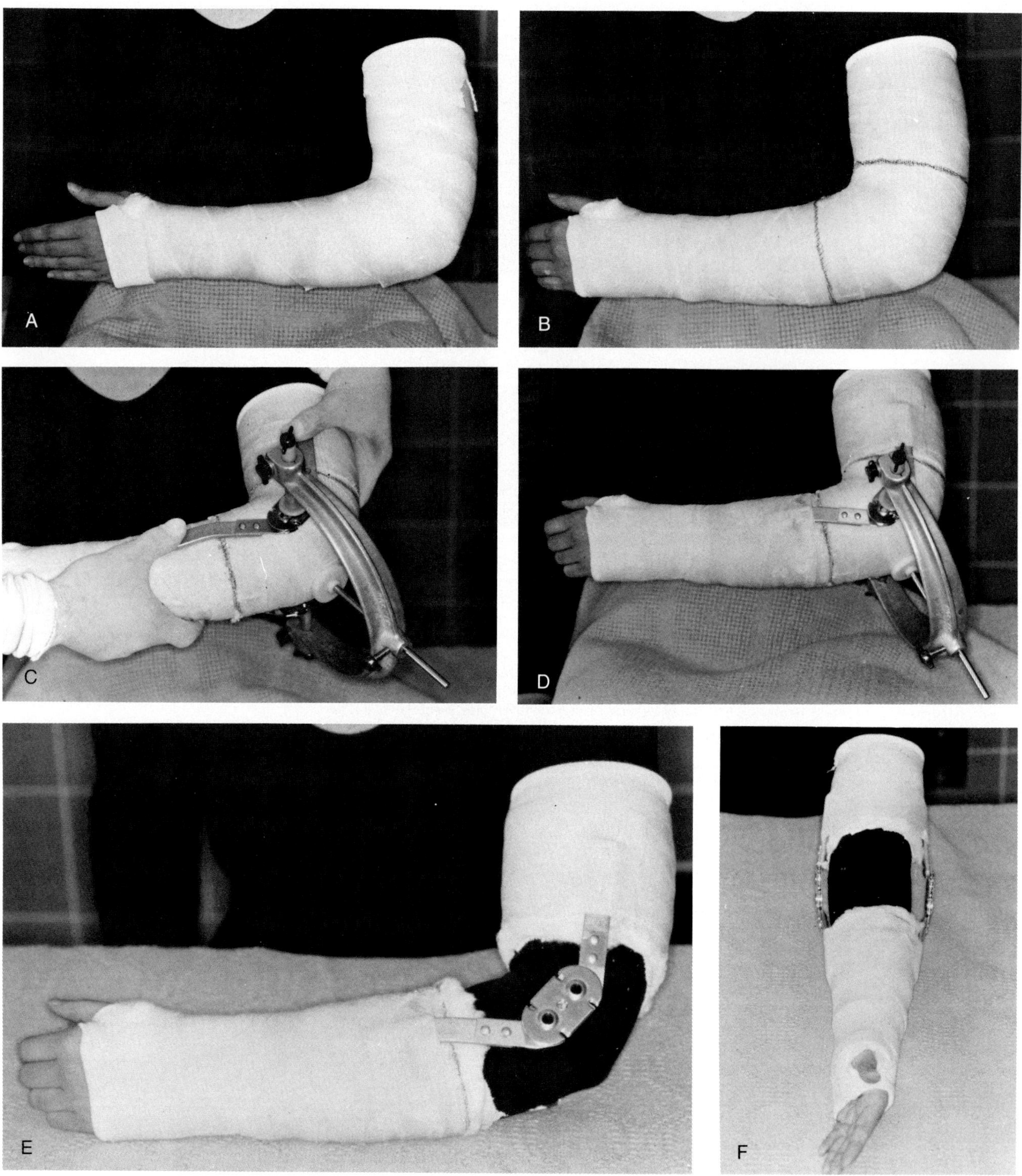

Fig. 6–8. The making of long-arm cast braces with elbow hinges. *A*, A long-arm cast has been applied. *B*, Four transverse cuts, above and below the elbow joint, will be made on the lines marked with wax pencil. *C*, The two polycentric elbow hinges are being held with a fracture-brace alignment fixture. *D*, The polycentric elbow hinges have been fixed to the cast. *E*, *F*, Good elbow motion following removal of the cast materials between the transverse cuts.

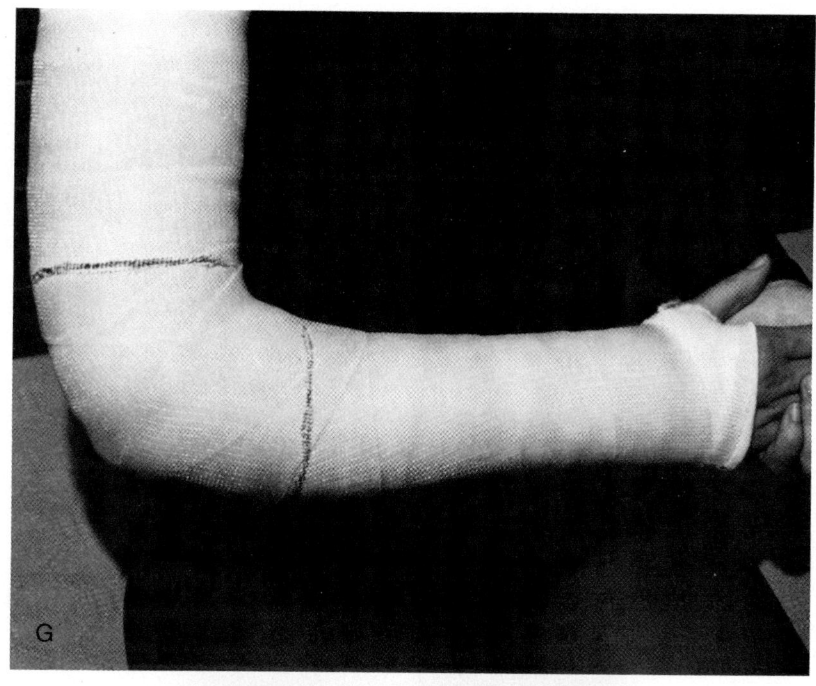

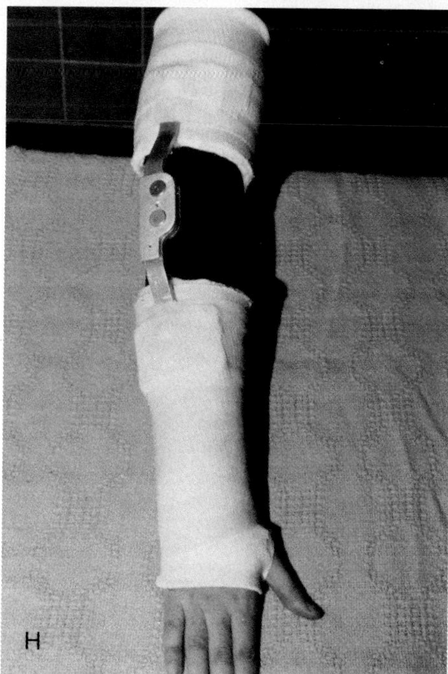

Fig. 6–8 (cont.). *G*, Another long-arm cast has been applied and marked with wax pencil. *H*, Two different polycentric elbow hinges have been fixed to the cast, and the cast material between the transverse cuts has been removed.

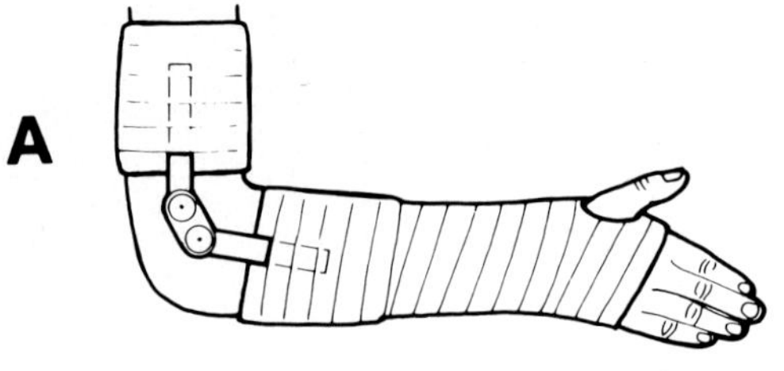

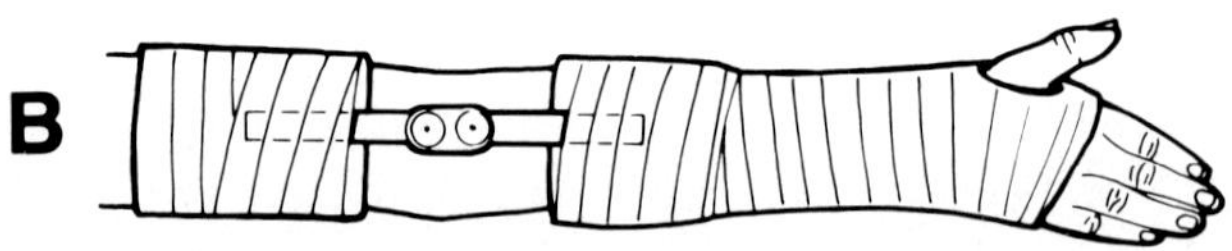

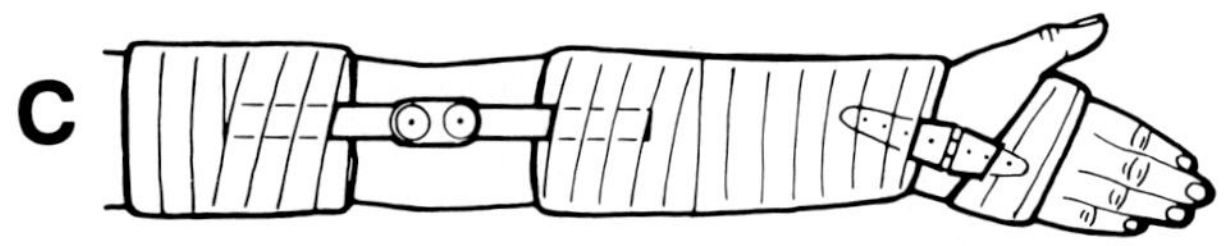

Fig. 6–9. The major steps in converting a long-arm cast to a long-arm cast-brace with elbow hinges and dorsal wrist hinge. *A*, *B*, Installation of the two polycentric elbow hinges. *C*, Installation of a dorsal wrist hinge.

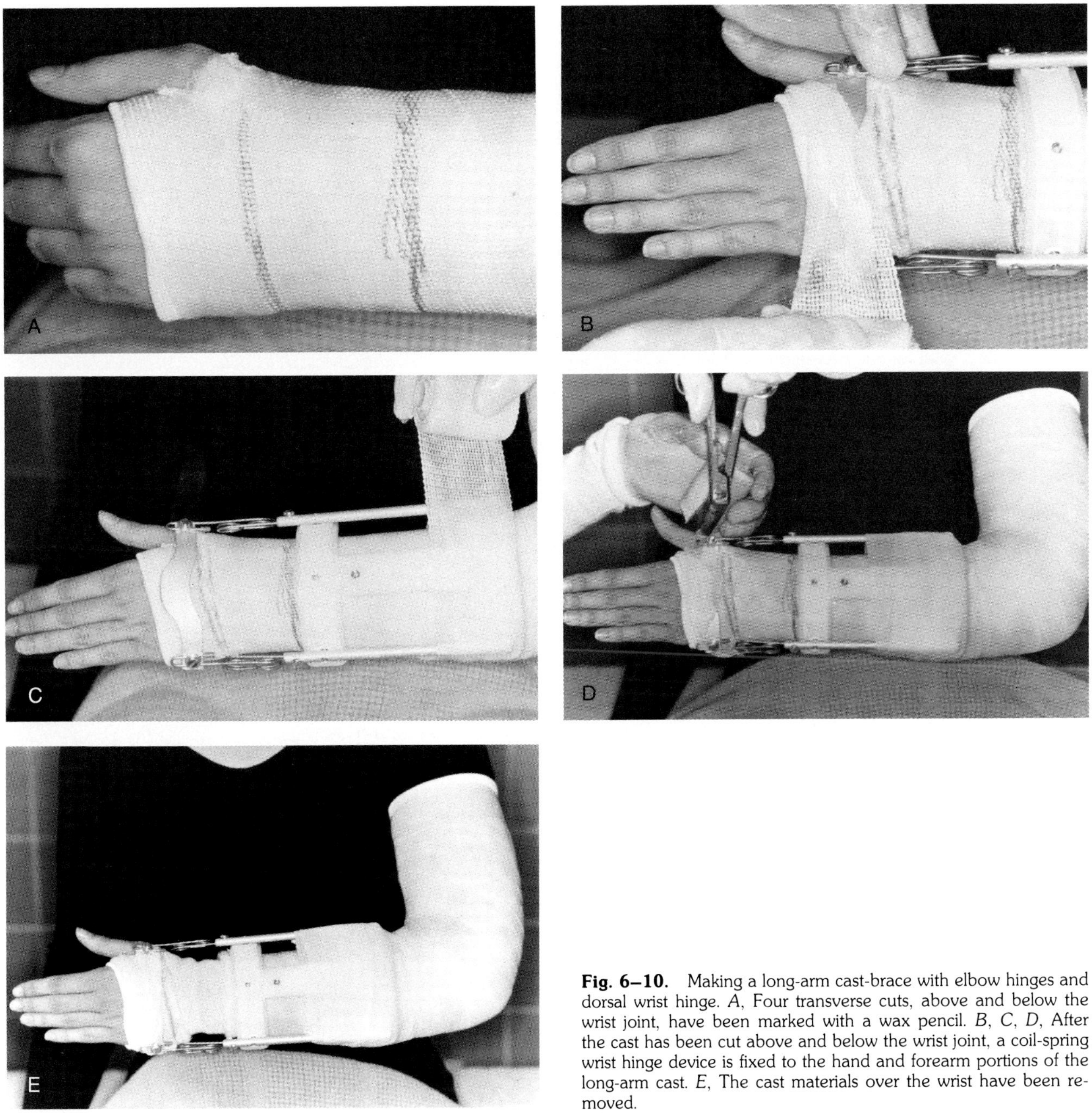

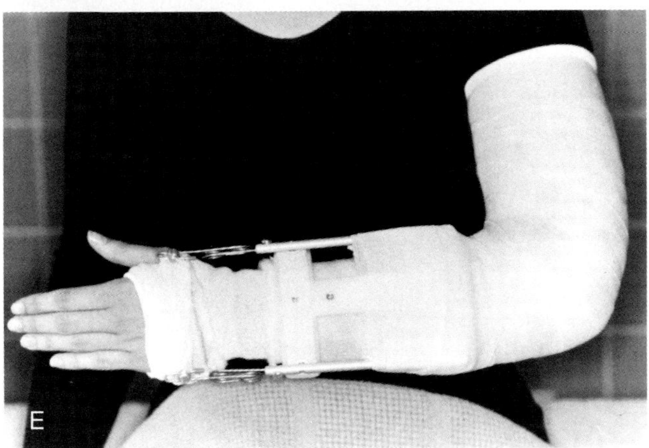

Fig. 6–10. Making a long-arm cast-brace with elbow hinges and dorsal wrist hinge. *A*, Four transverse cuts, above and below the wrist joint, have been marked with a wax pencil. *B*, *C*, *D*, After the cast has been cut above and below the wrist joint, a coil-spring wrist hinge device is fixed to the hand and forearm portions of the long-arm cast. *E*, The cast materials over the wrist have been removed.

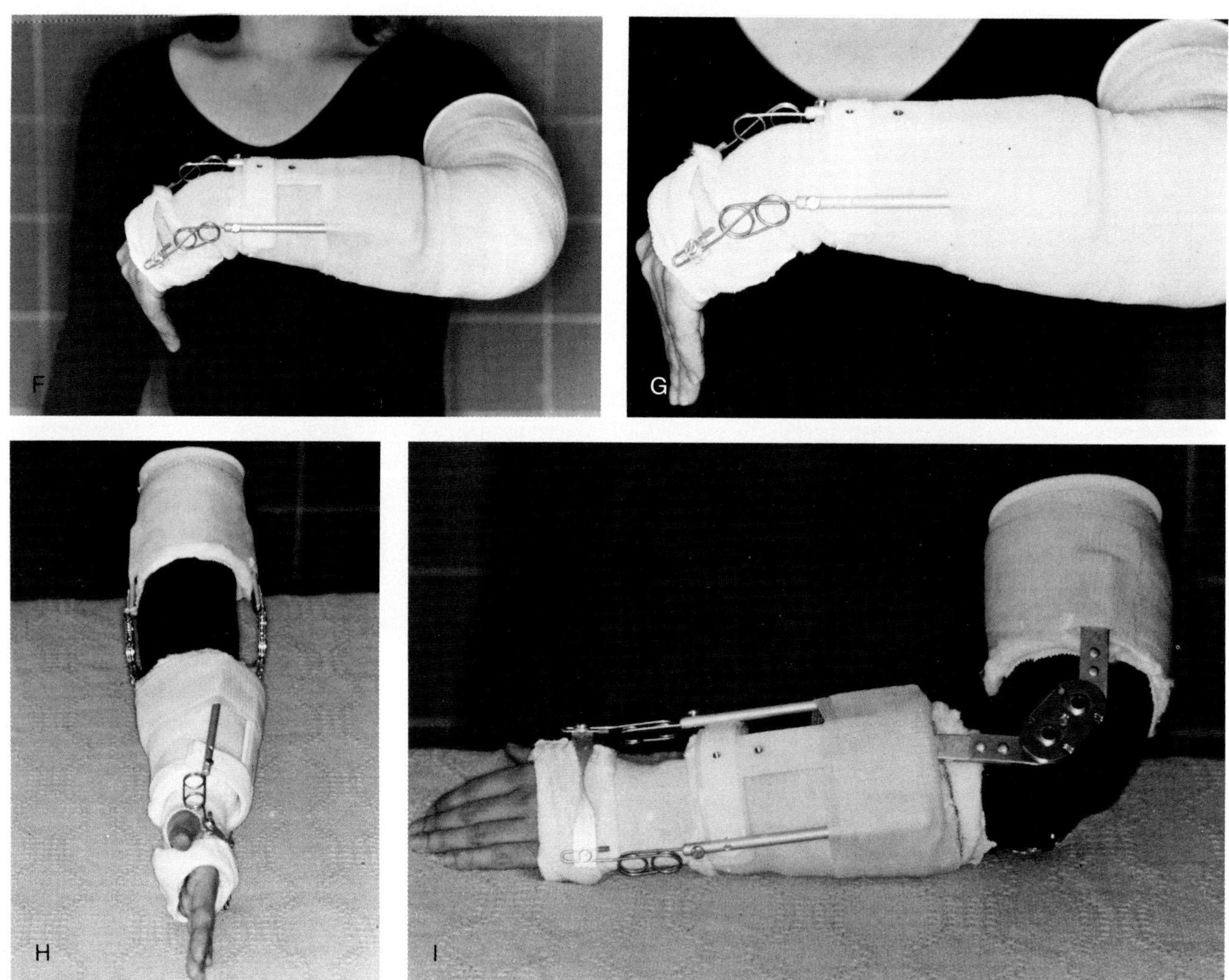

Fig. 6–10 (cont.). *F*, *G*, Standard and close-up views of the same cast showing the amount of wrist flexion. A gate hinge could have been used instead of the coil-spring hinge device. *H*, *I*, A completed long-arm cast-brace, showing good range of motion of the elbow joint.

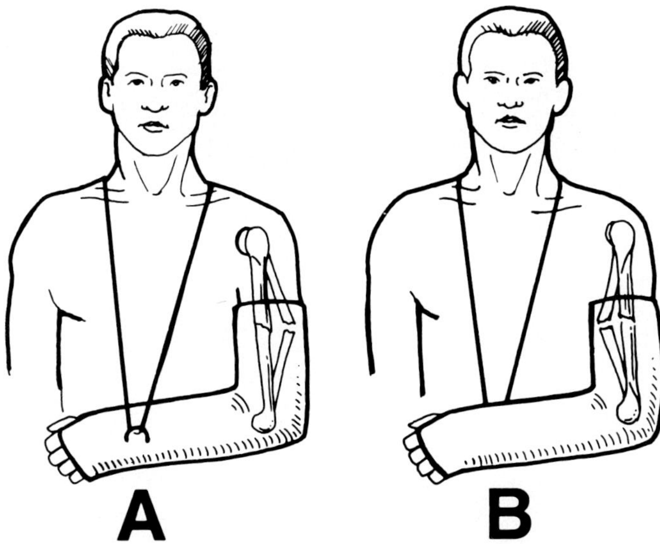

Fig. 6–11. Correction of medial and lateral angulation of a humeral fracture by means of a hanging cast. *A*, A loop at the dorsum of the wrist tends to correct lateral angulation of a humeral fracture. *B*, A loop at the volar aspect of the wrist tends to correct medial angulation of a humeral fracture.

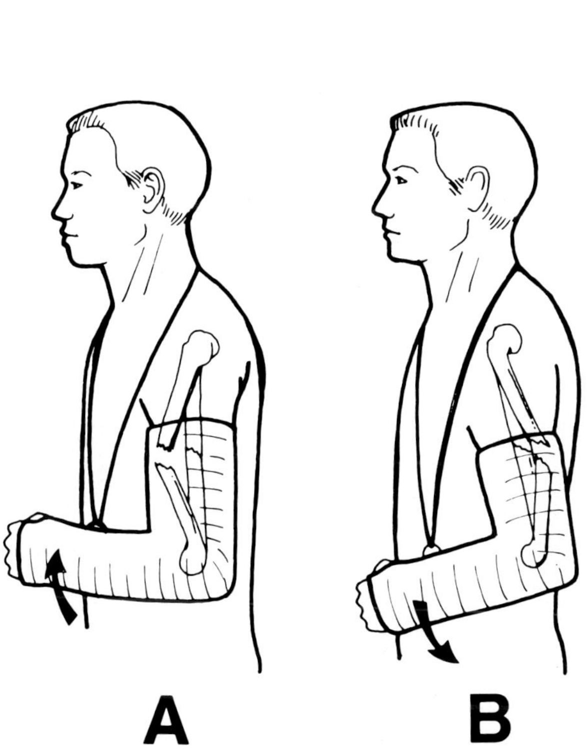

Fig. 6–12. Correction of anterior and posterior angulations of humeral fractures by changing the length of a sling. *A*, Shortening of the sling tends to correct anterior angulation of a humeral fracture. *B*, Lengthening of the sling tends to correct posterior angulation of a humeral fracture.

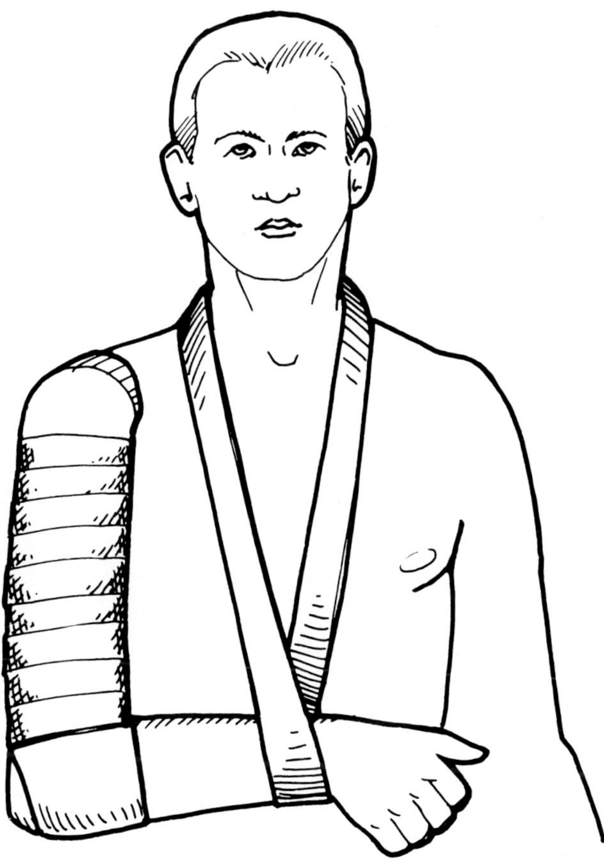

Fig. 6–13. A sugar-tong arm splint has been used to immobilize a humeral fracture, and a sling is used to support the arm.

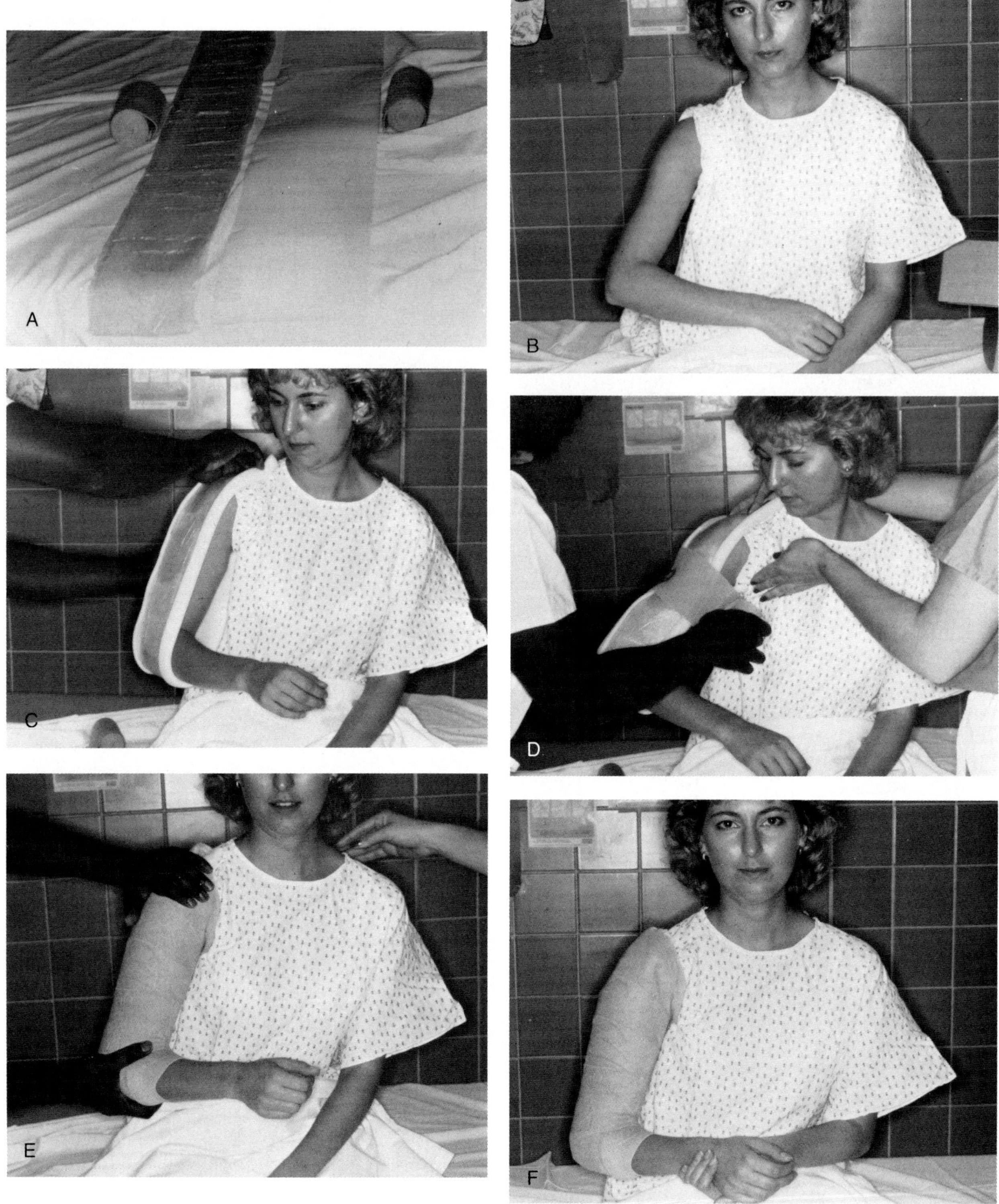

Fig. 6–14. Application of a sugar-tong arm splint. *A*, A 4″ × 30″ fiberglass splint, a foam rubber padding sheet, and 2 rolls of 4″ Ace bandage. *B*, The patient is sitting with her elbow flexed 90° and her arm internally rotated. *C*, A well-padded fiberglass splint has been applied from the armpit down to the elbow and then up to the top of the shoulder. *D*, *E*, *F*, Two rolls of 4″ Ace bandage are used to hold the splint to the arm and elbow, including the top of the shoulder. While the splint is hardening, gentle and even hand pressure is systematically applied to the whole splint to make it conform to the contours of the underlying shoulder, arm, and elbow.

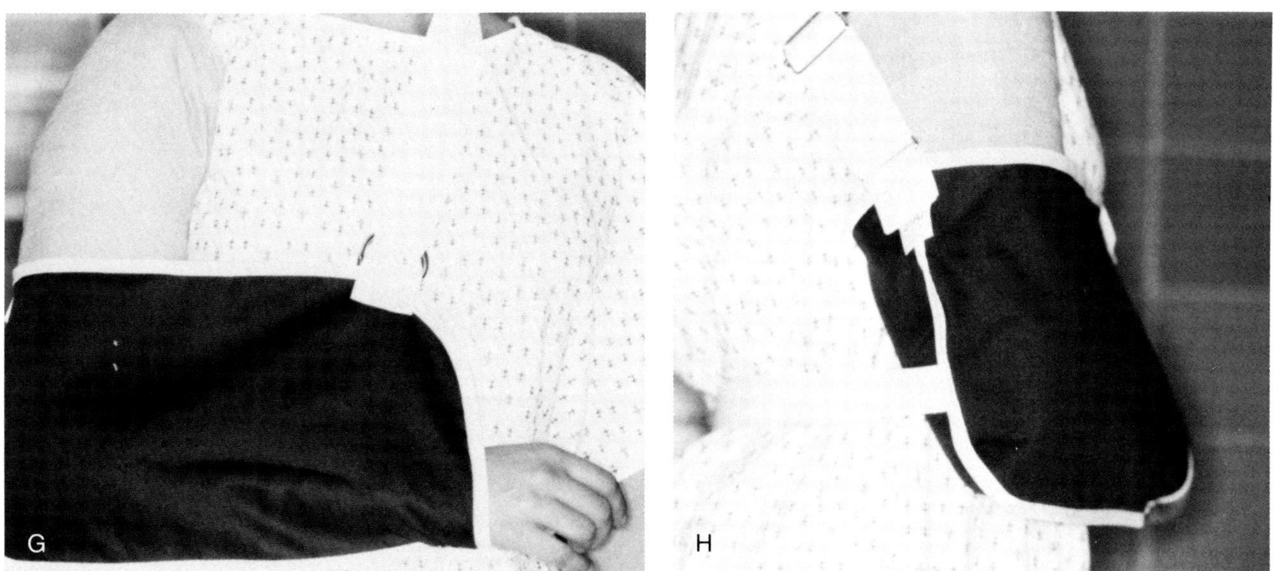

Fig. 6–14. *G*, *H*, A shoulder immobilizer is used to support the arm.

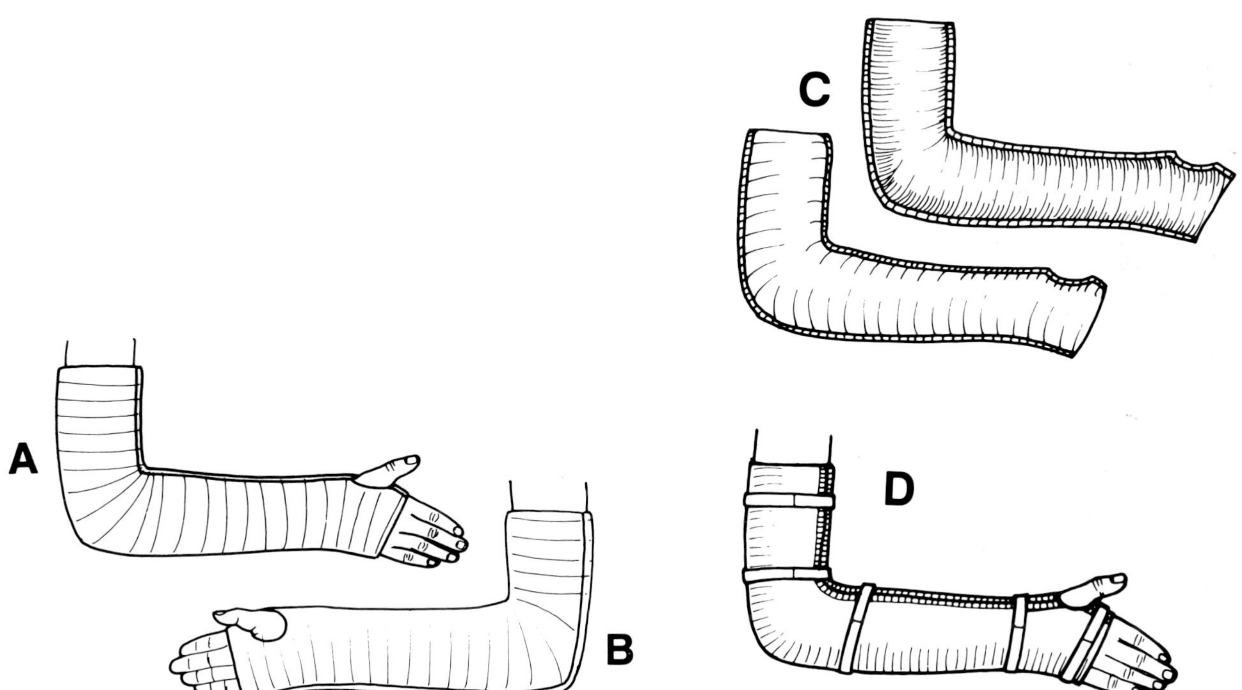

Fig. 6–15. Bivalving of a long-arm cast. *A*, A cut is made through the radial border of the cast. *B*, A cut is made through the ulnar border of the cast. *C*, The margins of the two halves of the cast are lined with moleskin. *D*, The bivalved cast is reapplied to the arm. The two halves of the cast are held together with Velcro straps or webbings and buckles.

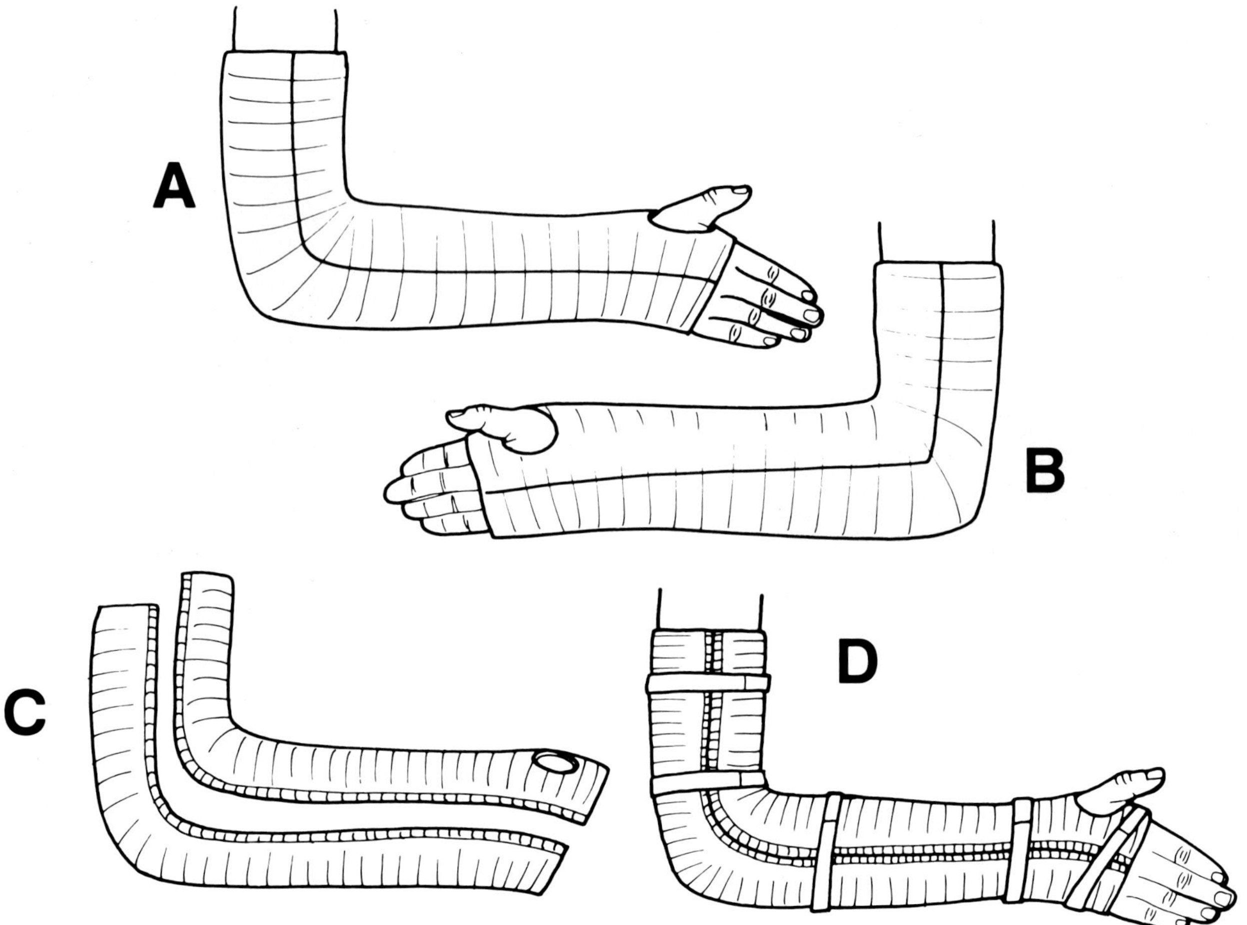

Fig. 6–16. An alternative method for bivalving a long-arm cast. *A*, A longitudinal cut is made along the midline of the posterior surface of the cast. *B*, A longitudinal cut is made along the midline of the anterior surface of the cast. *C*, The margins of the two halves of the cast are lined with moleskin. *D*, The bivalved cast is reapplied to the arm, and the two halves are held together with Velcro straps or webbings and buckles.

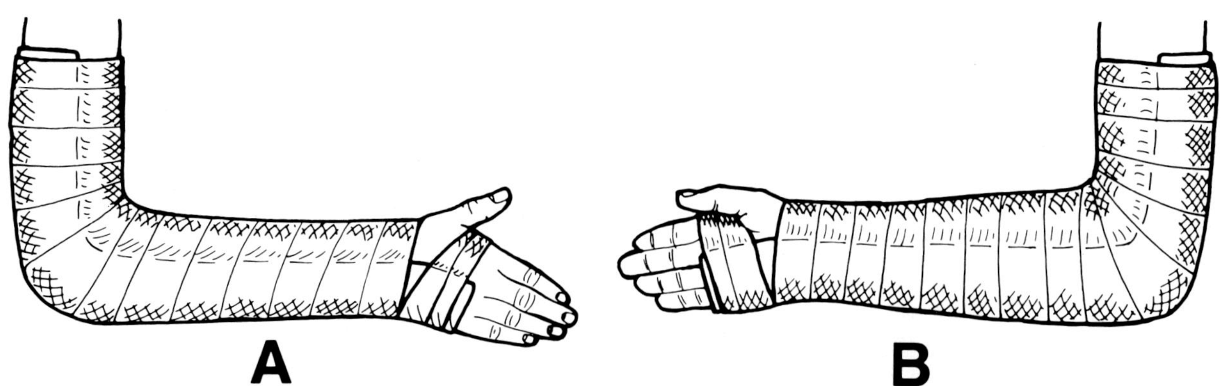

Fig. 6–17. A long-arm splint that extends from the proximal palmar crease along the ulnar border of the forearm to the posterior aspect of the upper arm region.

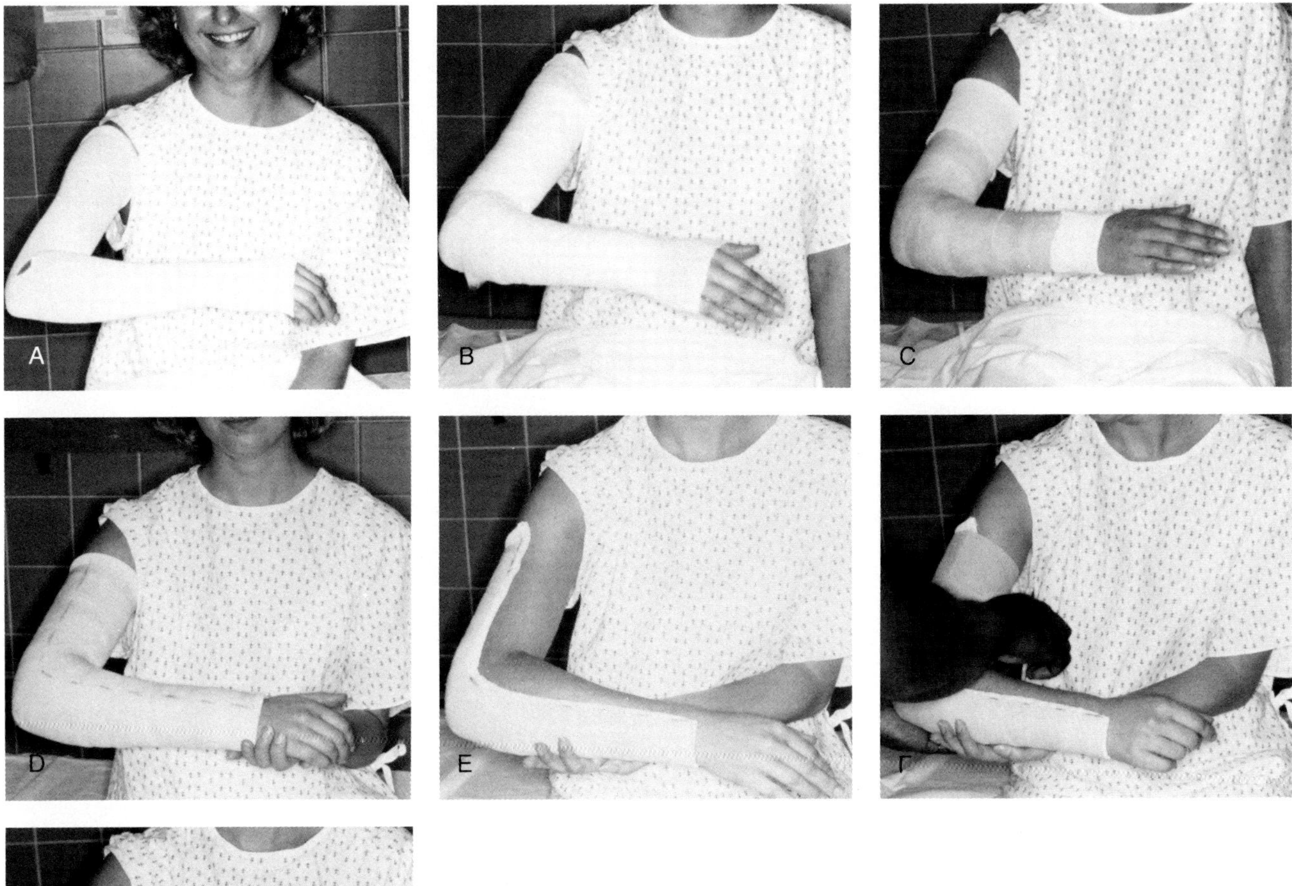

Fig. 6–18. The making of a well-fitted long-arm splint. *A*, A 3″ stockinet has been applied to the arm, and the transverse wrinkle in front of the elbow has been removed. *B*, Three rolls of 3″ Webril have been wrapped around the arm from the wrist to the upper arm region. *C*, Two rolls of 3″ fiberglass bandage have been wrapped around the whole arm, and the stockinet ends have been turned down over the cast ends. *D*, A roll of 4″ fiberglass bandage has been added to finish the cast, and the cast has been marked with a wax pencil along the midline of the dorsal and volar surfaces of the forearm portion of the cast and the mid-lateral and mid-medial aspects of the upper arm portion of the cast. *E*, The cast has been bivalved, and the upper half has been discarded. *F*, *G*, The bottom half of the cast is reapplied to the arm and held in place with Ace bandages.

CHAPTER 7. SHOULDER SPICA CASTS

CONVENTIONAL SHOULDER SPICA CAST

Indications

A conventional shoulder spica cast (Fig. 7-1) is used for unstable fractures and dislocations of the shoulder, shoulder fusion, and post-operative immobilization of a repaired rotator cuff.

Cast Materials Needed

Plaster Shoulder Spica Cast

10″ or 12″ stockinet for the body

3″ or 4″ stockinet for the arm

1 roll of 3″ Webril

3 rolls of 4″ Webril

6 rolls of 6″ Webril

1 box of 5″ × 30″ plaster splints (10 splints)

4 rolls of 6″ plaster bandage

7 rolls of 4″ plaster bandage

1 wooden bar about 12″ in length

Felt pads—1 shoulder pad, 2 anterior iliac crest pads, and 1 coccygeal pad

Fiberglass Shoulder Spica Cast

10″ or 12″ stockinet for the body

3″ or 4″ stockinet for the arm

1 roll of 3″ Webril

3 rolls of 4″ Webril

6 rolls of 6″ Webril

4 rolls of 5″ fiberglass bandage

6 rolls of 4″ fiberglass bandage

1 wooden bar about 12″ in length

Felt pads—1 shoulder pad, 2 iliac crest pads, and 1 coccygeal pad

Patient's Position

The patient can either sit or stand, with the elbow flexed to 90° and the arm in 50° abduction, 25° flexion, and 25° internal rotation.

Technique for Applying a Plaster Shoulder Spica Cast

Circular armholes about 6″ in diameter should be cut from both sides of the body stockinet approximately 9″ from 1 end. The body stockinet is worn like a T-shirt, with the patient's arms sticking out through the armholes. A 6″ longitudinal cut should be made above and below the armhole for the injured arm. Next, the 3″ or 4″ stockinet is applied to the whole arm, and a longitudinal cut of about 6″ is made along the medial and lateral aspects of the proximal end of the stockinet. The 4 cut ends of the arm stockinet are lapped over the adjacent cut ends of the body stockinet, and a roll of 3″ Webril is used to secure the cut ends. The whole arm, from the distal palmar crease to the axillary region, is then covered with 3 rolls of 4″ Webril, and the body is covered with 6 rolls of 6″ Webril. Five or 6 overlapping strips of 6″ Webril are used to cover the junction between the arm and the body to provide even coverage throughout the cast.

The body portion is covered evenly with 2 rolls of 6″ plaster bandage, and the arm with 2 rolls of 4″ plaster bandage. One whole box of 5″ × 30″ plaster splints is applied to the body portion of the cast in a vertical (or so-called barrel-stave) manner, and a 5″ × 30″ plaster splint is applied to the arm from the base of the neck, across the top of the shoulder, and along the posterior aspect of the arm and forearm to the wrist. One roll of 4″ plaster bandage is wrapped around the entire arm to cover the turned-down distal stockinet end and to incorporate the long-arm splint. In a similar manner, 2 rolls of 6″ plaster bandage are wrapped around the body portion of the cast to incorporate the vertical plaster splints.

The 12″ wooden bar is fixed to the medial aspect of the mid-forearm and the anterior iliac crest region by means of 2 rolls of 4″ plaster bandage, which should also be wrapped around the entire wooden bar. Excess plaster should be trimmed from the upper end of the cast to allow free movement of the neck and opposite shoulder joint, and the stockinet should be pulled down over the upper end of the cast and fixed to the cast with a roll of 4″ plaster bandage.

An ideal trimming of the lower end of the cast should include making a pubic projection to provide better fixation, trimming the cast to the level of the padded anterior iliac crests to allow good hip flexion, allowing the lower margins of the cast to go down to the level of the greater trochanters for better stabilization, and then crossing the buttock to the padded coccygeal region, where pressure relief can be provided by removing the plaster cast substance directly over the coccyx (Fig. 7-2).

Technique for Applying a Fiberglass Shoulder Spica Cast

Application of stockinet and Webril bandages is the same as for a plaster shoulder spica cast. Because of the superior strength of fiberglass, however, no splints are needed, and only 3 rolls of 5″ bandage are required for the body portion of the cast and 3 rolls of 4″ bandage for the arm. One roll of 5″ fiberglass bandage is used to fix the stockinet to the lower end of the cast, and 3 rolls of 4″ bandage are used to fix the stockinet to the upper end of the cast and to attach the wooden bar.

OPEN-SHOULDER SHOULDER SPICA CAST

Indications

An open-shoulder shoulder spica cast is used for unstable shoulder fractures and dislocations in association with open shoulder wounds.

Cast Materials Needed

Plaster Open-Shoulder Shoulder Spica Cast

10″ or 12″ stockinet for the body

3″ or 4″ stockinet for the arm

3 rolls of 4″ Webril

2 rolls of 6″ Webril

3 rolls of 6″ plaster bandage

6 rolls of 4″ plaster bandage

2 wooden bars

2 felt pads for anterior iliac crests

Fiberglass Open-Shoulder Shoulder Spica Cast

10″ or 12″ stockinet for the body

3″ or 4″ stockinet for the arm

3 rolls of 4″ Webril

2 rolls of 6″ Webril

2 rolls of 5″ fiberglass bandage

4 rolls of 4″ fiberglass bandage

2 rolls of 3″ fiberglass bandage

2 wooden bars

2 felt pads for anterior iliac crests

Patient's Position

The position of the patient is the same as for a conventional shoulder spica cast.

Technique for Applying a Plaster Open-Shoulder Shoulder Spica Cast

The 3″ or 4″ stockinet, 3 rolls of 4″ Webril, and 3 rolls of 4″ plaster bandage are applied to the arm to produce a long-arm cast in the regular manner. The 10″ or 12″ stockinet is then applied to the body like a corset, and 2 rolls of 6″ Webril are used to wrap the lower part of the body from the mid-buttock level to the lower thoracic region. After the 2 felt pads have been placed over the anterior iliac crests, 3 rolls of 6″ plaster bandage are wrapped around the lower part of the body and carefully molded over the iliac crests. The upper and lower ends of the body part of the cast are trimmed, and the ends of the stockinet are folded down over the ends of the cast, to be secured with 1 roll of 4″ plaster bandage. The arm is then held in a position of 50° of abduction, 25° of flexion, and 25° of internal rotation, and 2 wooden bars are bound in place with 2 rolls of 4″ plaster bandage, one from the medial aspect of the elbow region to the ipsilateral anterior iliac crest and the other from the medial aspect of the mid-forearm region to the contralateral anterior iliac crest of the body part of the cast. The plaster bandages should also individually and completely cover the 2 wooden bars.

Technique for Applying a Fiberglass Open-Shoulder Shoulder Spica Cast

The technique for applying a fiberglass open-shoulder shoulder spica cast is identical to that for applying a plaster open-shoulder shoulder spica cast except that 3 rolls of fiberglass bandage are used to make the long-arm cast, 2 rolls of 5″ fiberglass bandage and 1 roll of 4″ fiberglass bandage are used to produce the body part of the cast, and 2 rolls of 3″ fiberglass bandage are used to bind the long-arm cast and the body part of the cast together by means of the two wooden bars (Fig. 7-3).

BIBLIOGRAPHY

Anderson, D., Zvirbulis, R., and Ceullo, J.: Scapular manipulation for reduction of anterior shoulder dislocations. Clin. Orthop., *164:*181, 1982.

Aston, J.W., and Gregory, C.F.: Dislocation of the shoulder with significant fracture of the glenoid. J. Bone Joint Surg. [Am.], *55:*1531, 1973.

Baker, D.M.: Fractures of the humeral shaft associated with ipsilateral fracture dislocation of the shoulder: Report of a case. J. Trauma, *11:*532, 1971.

Barth, E. and Hagen, R.: Surgical treatment of recurrent dislocation of the sternoclavicular joint. Acta Orthop. Scand., *53:*709, 1982.

Bernard, T.N., Jr., Brunet, M.E., and Haddad, R.J.: Fractured coracoid process in acromioclavicular dislocations. Clin. Orthop., *175:*227, 1983.

Brett, A.L.: A new method of arthrodesis of the shoulder joint, incorporating the control of the scapula. J. Bone Joint Surg., *15:*969, 1933.

Brown, F.W., and Navigato, W.J.: Rupture of the axillary artery and brachial plexus palsy associated with anterior dislocation of the shoulder—report of a case with successful vascular repair. Clin. Orthop., *60:*195, 1968.

Brown, J.T.: Nerve injuries complicating dislocation of the shoulder. J. Bone Joint Surg. [Br.], *34*:526, 1952.

Darrow, J.C., Smith, J.A., and Lockwood, R.C.: A new conservative method for treatment of Type III acromioclavicular separations. Orthop. Clin. North Am., *11*:727, 1980.

Dingley, A., and Denham, R.: Fracture-dislocation of the humeral head: A method of reduction. J. Bone Joint Surg. [Am.], *55*:1299, 1973.

Drury, J.K., and Scullion, J.E.: Vascular complications of anterior dislocation of the shoulder. Br. J. Surg., *67*:579, 1980.

Elting, J.J.: Retrosternal dislocation of the clavicle. Arch Surg., *104*:35, 1972.

Gardham, J.R.C., and Scott, J.E.: Axillary artery occlusion with erect dislocation of the shoulder. Injury, *11*:155, 1980.

Gill, A.B.: A new operation for arthrodesis of the shoulder. J. Bone Joint Surg., *13*:287, 1931.

Hawkins, R.J., and Koppert, G.: The natural history following anterior dislocation of the shoulder in the older patient. J. Bone Joint Surg. [Br.], *64*:255, 1982.

Henry, J.H., and Genung, J.A.: Natural history of glenohumeral dislocation—revisited. Am. J. Sports Med., *10*:135, 1982.

Howard, F.M., and Shafer, S.J.: Injuries to the clavicle with neurovascular complications. J. Bone Joint Surg. [Am.], *47*:1335, 1965.

Kummel, B.M.: Fractures of the glenoid causing chronic dislocation of the shoulder. Clin. Orthop., *69*:189, 1970.

Lev-El, A., and Rubinstein, Z.: Axillary artery injury in erect dislocation of the shoulder. J. Trauma, *21*:323, 1981.

Leyshon, R.L.: Closed treatment of fractures of the proximal humerus. Acta Orthop. Scand., *55*:48, 1984.

McLaughin, H.: Dislocations of the shoulder with tuberosity fracture. Surg. Clin. N. Am., *43*:1615, 1963.

Neviaser, J.S.: Injuries of the clavicle and its articulations. Orthop. Clin. North Am., *11*:233, 1980.

Putti, V.: Arthrodesis for tuberculosis of the knee and of the shoulder. Chir. Org. Movimento, *18*:217, 1933.

Rowe, C.R.: An atlas of anatomy and treatment of mid-clavicular fractures. Clin. Orthop., *58*:29, 1968.

Simonet, W.T., and Cofield, R.H.: Prognosis in anterior shoulder dislocation. Am. J. Sports Med., *12*:19, 1984.

Sondergard-Petersen, P., and Mikkelsen, P.: Posterior acromioclavicular dislocation. J. Bone Joint Surg. [Br.], *64*:52, 1982.

Watson-Jones, R.: Extra-articular arthrodesis of the shoulder. J. Bone Joint Surg., *15*:862, 1933.

Zenni, E.J., Kreig, J.K., and Rosen, M.J.: Open reduction and internal fixation of clavicular fractures. J. Bone Joint Surg. [Am.], *63*:147, 1981.

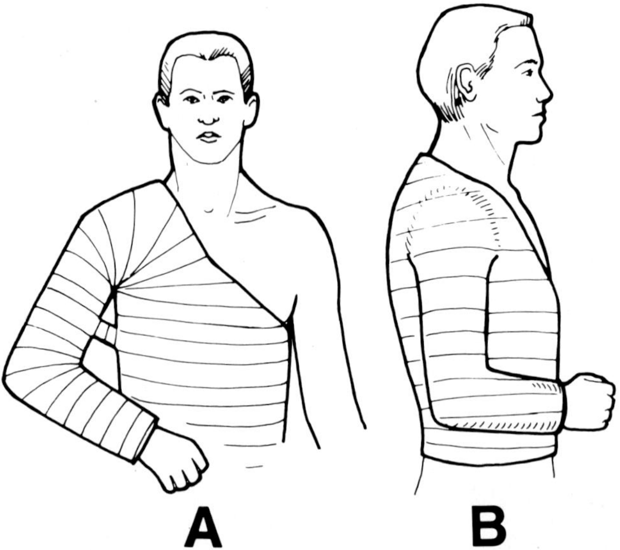

Fig. 7–1. Anterior (*A*) and lateral (*B*) views of a conventional shoulder spica cast.

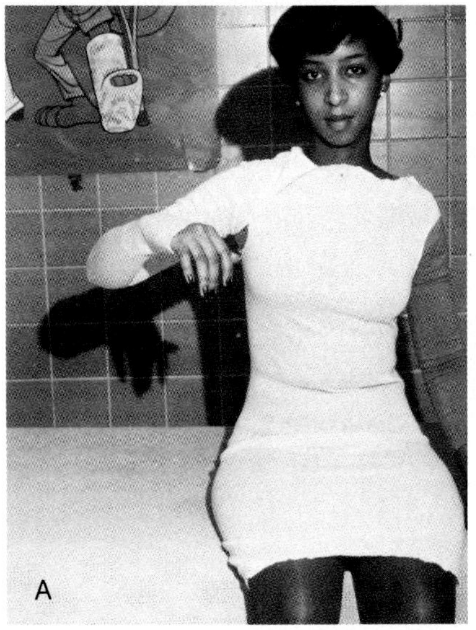
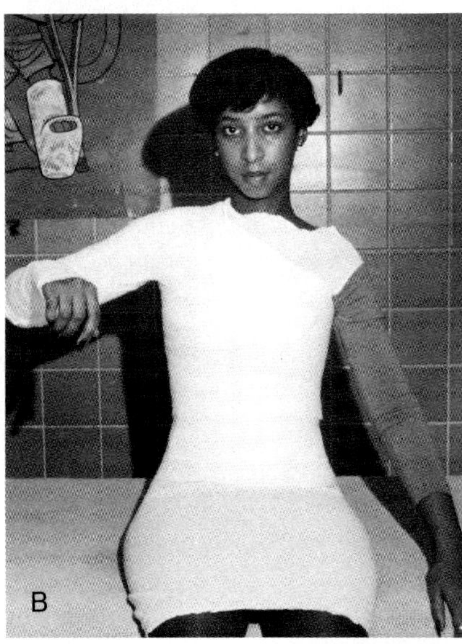
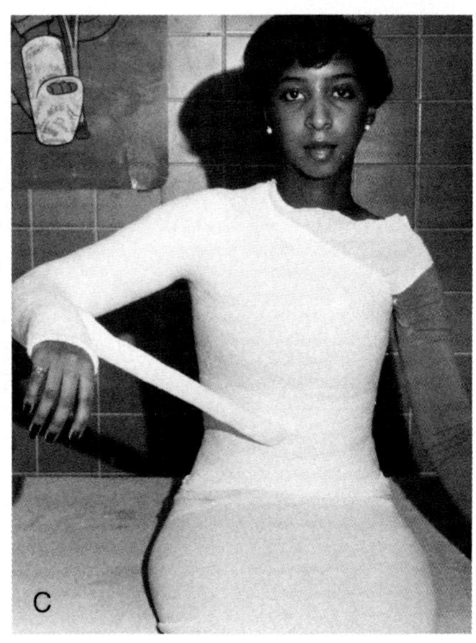
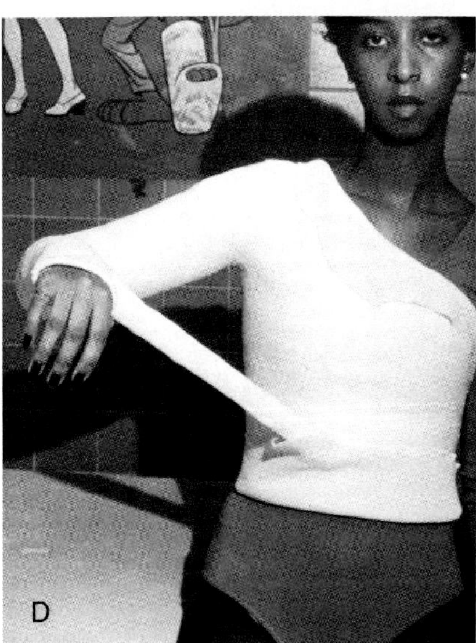
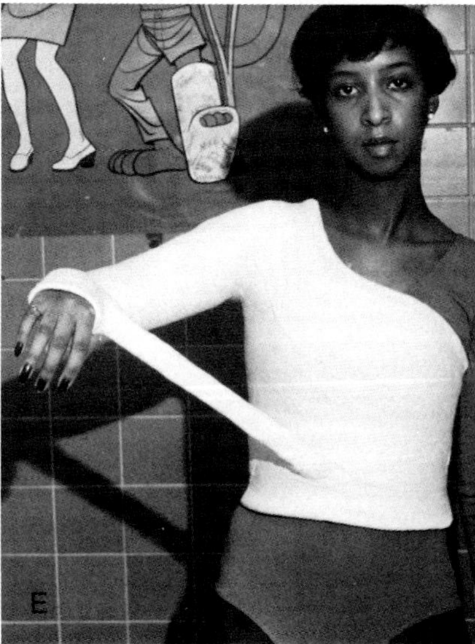

Fig. 7–2. Making a shoulder spica cast. *A*, 10″ and 3″ stockinets have been applied to the body and arm, respectively. *B*, 6″ and 4″ Webril bandages have been wrapped around the body and arm, respectively. *C*, All the necessary plaster bandages and splints have been applied to the arm, shoulder, and body, and a 12″ wooden bar has been fixed between the medial aspect of the mid-forearm and the anterior iliac crest region. *D*, The upper and lower ends of the shoulder spica cast have been trimmed, and the stockinet ends have been folded over the upper and lower cast ends. *E*, The upper and lower stockinet ends have been fixed to the cast with 4″ plaster bandages.

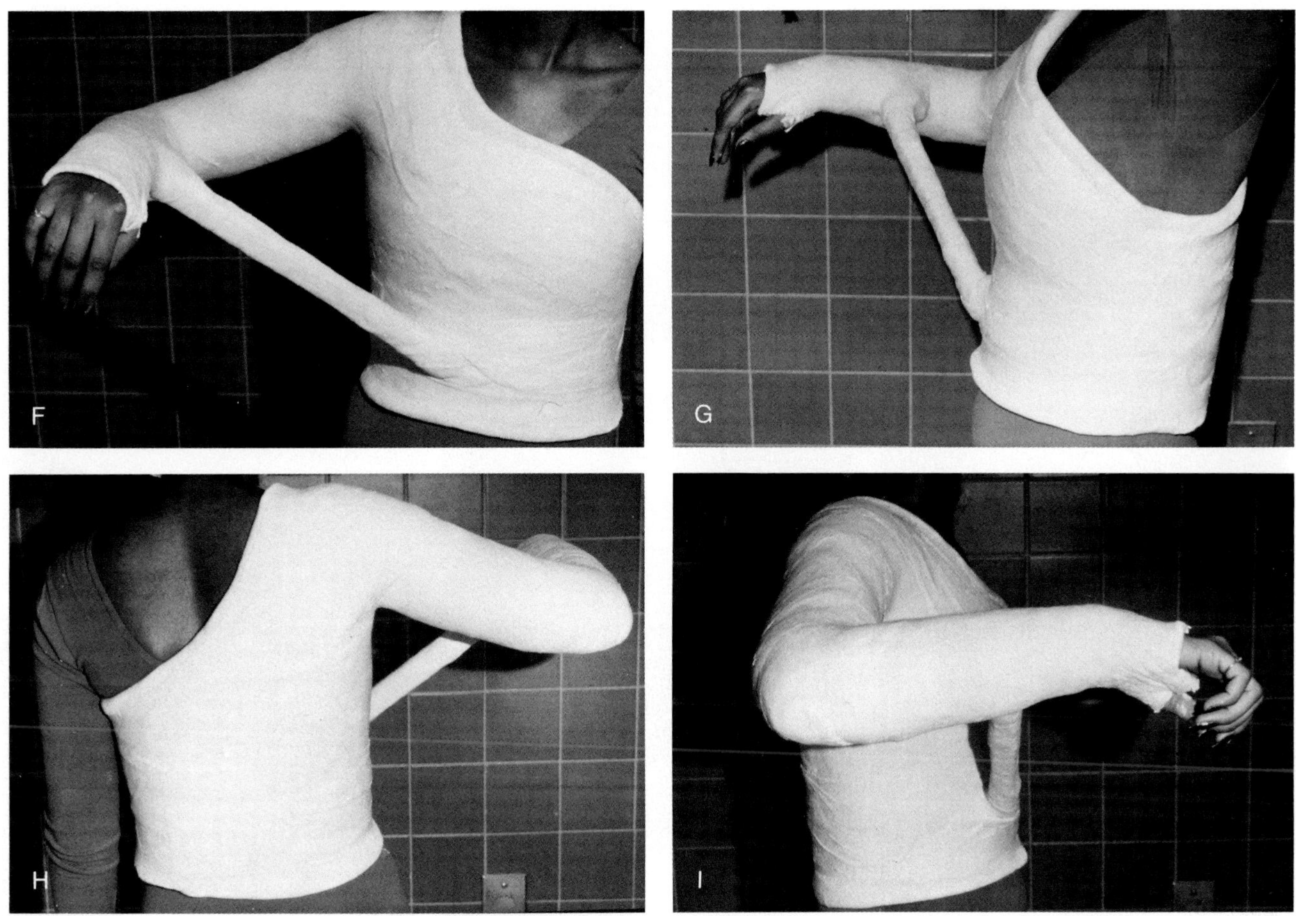

Fig. 7–2 (cont.). *F–I*, Anterior, medial, posterior, and lateral views of the finished plaster shoulder spica cast.

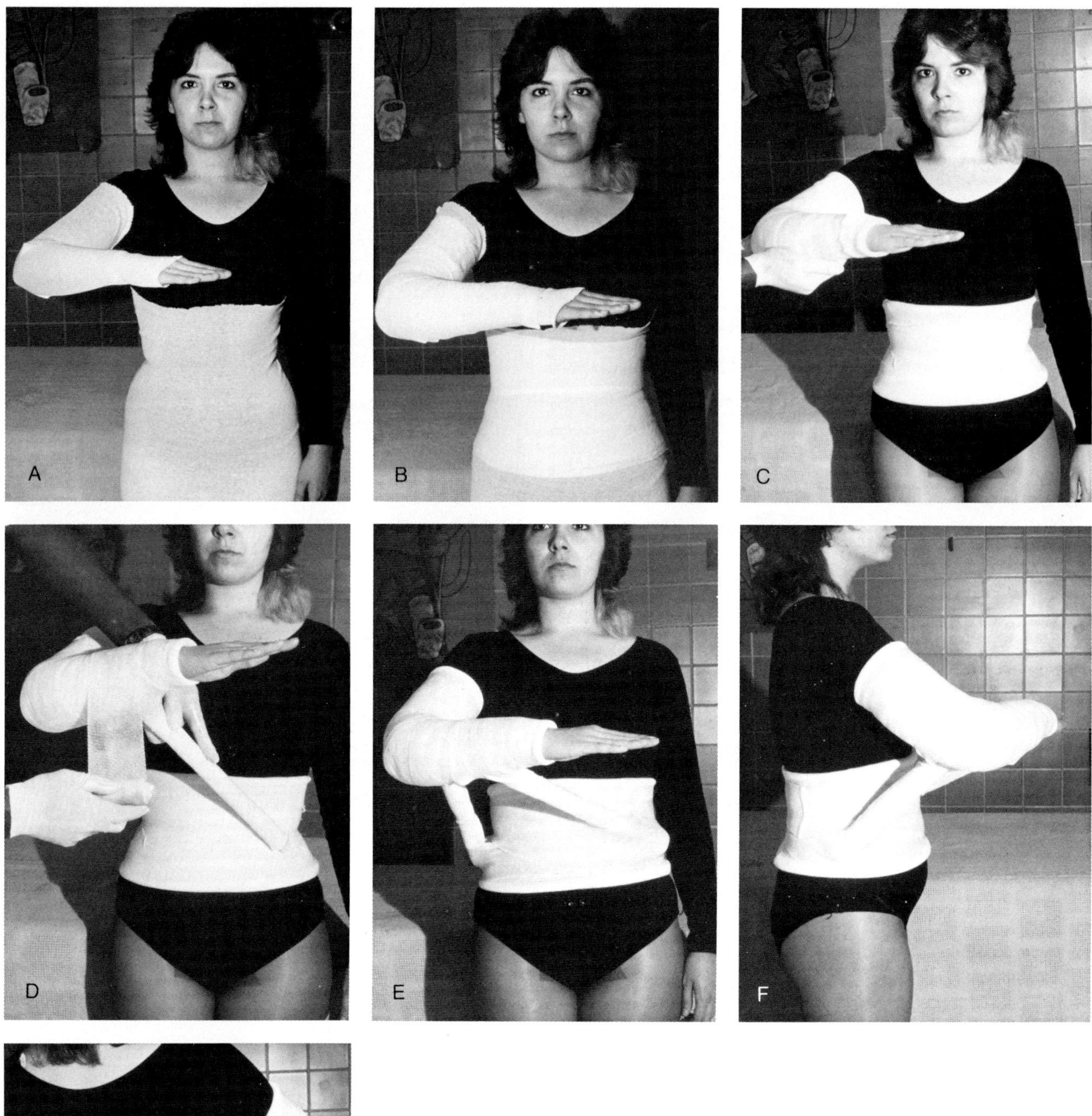

Fig. 7–3. Making an open-shoulder shoulder spica cast. *A*, The 3″ stockinet and 10″ stockinet have been applied to the arm and the lower part of the body, respectively. *B*, Three rolls of 4″ Webril have been applied to the arm, and 2 rolls of 6″ Webril have been applied to the lower part of the body. *C*, Three rolls of 4″ fiberglass bandage have been used to complete the long-arm cast, and 2 rolls of 5″ fiberglass bandage and 1 roll of 4″ fiberglass bandage have been employed to finish the body part of the cast. *D*, *E*, Two wooden bars are used to bind the long-arm cast and the body part of the cast together by means of 2 rolls of 3″ fiberglass bandage. *F*, *G*, Lateral and posterior views of the finished cast.

CHAPTER 8. SHORT-LEG CASTS, CAST-BRACE AND SPLINTS, AND PATELLAR-TENDON-BEARING (PTB) CASTS

SHORT-LEG CAST

Indications

A short-leg cast (Fig. 8-1) is used for stable ankle fractures and fractures and dislocations of the tarsal and metatarsal bones.

Cast Materials Needed

Plaster Short-Leg Cast

4″ stockinet

3 rolls of 4″ Webril

2 rolls of 6″ plaster bandage

2 5″ × 30″ plaster splints

Fiberglass Short-Leg Cast

4″ stockinet

3 rolls of 4″ Webril

3 rolls of 4″ fiberglass bandage

Patient's Position

A short-leg cast is best applied with the patient in a sitting position with the knee flexed to 90° to relax the powerful gastrocnemius muscle and to use gravity to help maintain the fracture reduction. If the patient is unable to sit up, the leg should be hung over the side of the casting table. To avoid casting a foot in an equinus position, one can use a metal foot stand to support the foot and to keep the ankle in a neutral position.

Technique for Applying a Plaster Short-Leg Cast

Stockinet

The 4″ stockinet should cover the lower leg from the toes to the knee, and the large transverse wrinkle in front of the ankle should be cut off (Fig. 8-2A).

Webril

Three rolls of Webril are wrapped evenly around the whole lower leg. In the ankle region, the Webril is applied in an overlapping figure-8 fashion, and the bare heel area is covered uniformly with overlapping strips of 4″ Webril.

Plaster Bandage

One roll of 6″ plaster bandage is applied to the lower leg from the proximal ends of the toe webspaces to a level either above or below the fibular neck, where the common peroneal nerve is particularly vulnerable to cast pressure. The 2 5″ × 30″ plaster splints are applied to the posterior aspect of the lower leg and the bottom portion of the foot, and the terminal 2″ or so of the distal end of the plaster splint should be folded back on itself at the level of the metacarpophalangeal joint to strengthen the distal end of the cast. The stockinet ends are pulled tightly over the cast ends, and a roll of 6″ plaster bandage is used to finish the cast. The cast should be rubbed thoroughly with the palms of both hands to make it smooth and strong (Fig. 8-2B–F).

Technique for Applying a Fiberglass Short-Leg Cast

Application of a fiberglass short-leg cast is similar to application of a plaster short-leg cast except that no splint is needed and only 3 rolls of 4″ fiberglass bandage are used. Two or 3 extra layers of fiberglass bandage should be applied to the ankle and foot region of the cast, which has to withstand the most stress from weight-bearing (Fig. 8-3).

Technique for Making a Toe Guard for a Short-Leg Cast

After the plaster or fiberglass cast has hardened, a 1-inch-wide padded aluminum splint is bent in such a way that it is only $^1/_3$ inch distal to the ends of the toes. The ends of the aluminum splint are held tightly against the medial and lateral sides of the foot portion of the cast, and a 3″ plaster or fiberglass bandage is used to fix the toe guard to the foot portion of the cast (Fig. 8-4). We routinely use a toe guard to protect protruding K-wires used to treat fractures and dislocations of the phalanges and metatarsals.

Technique for Making a Short-Leg Cast with a Toe Plate

A toe plate provides support for the toes and metatarsals and consists of an extension of the bottom part of the foot portion of a cast to a level slightly distal to the ends of all 5 toes. The cast is applied like a short-leg cast except that both the Webril and plaster or fiberglass bandages are allowed to extend beyond the tips of the toes. The soft plaster or fiberglass cast substance over the dorsal aspect of the toes should be trimmed back to the level of the proximal ends of the toe webspaces. The distal end of the stockinet is pulled tightly over the distal cast end and is fixed to the cast with 3″ plaster or fiberglass bandage (Fig. 8-5).

Univalving a Short-Leg Cast

A short-leg cast is occasionally univalved to give additional room for postoperative or posttraumatic swelling to take place. The cast is split longitudinally along the midline of its anterior surface, and the underlying Webril and stockinet should be split in a similar manner (Fig. 8-6).

Bivalving a Short-Leg Cast

The best way to bivalve a short-leg cast is to split the cast along its medial and lateral aspects (Fig. 8-7). The margins of the bivalved cast should be lined with moleskin. The fully lined bivalved cast is reapplied to the injured leg and is held in place with Velcro or webbings and buckles (Fig. 8-8).

SHORT-LEG WALKING CAST

The indications for a short-leg walking cast (Fig. 8-9) are similar to those for a short-leg cast. Many fractures and dislocations of the ankle and foot are initially treated in a short-leg cast, and subsequently in a short-leg walking cast. A short-leg cast can be converted easily into a short-leg walking cast by applying a cast cushion to the bottom of it or by using a cast sandal.

Technique for Making a Plaster Short-Leg Walking Cast

A folded 5″ × 30″ plaster splint about 7½ inches in length is applied to the bottom of the heel, and the cast cushion is firmly seated in the wet plaster parallel to the bottom of the foot. A roll of 4″ plaster bandage is used to fix the cast cushion to the bottom of the cast: first it is wound through the transverse groove, then the 2 diagonal grooves, and finally the anterior and posterior lips of the cast cushion. The remaining plaster bandage can be wrapped around the sides of the cast cushion as well as the bottom part of the cast, to fix it firmly to the bottom of the cast (Fig. 8-10).

Technique for Making a Fiberglass Short-Leg Walking Cast

The technique for making a fiberglass short-leg walking cast is identical to that for making a plaster short-leg walking cast except that 1 roll of folded 3″ fiberglass bandage is used under the cast cushion, and another roll of 3″ fiberglass bandage is used to bind the cast cushion to the bottom of the cast.

SHORT-LEG CYLINDER CAST WITH ANKLE HINGES AND HEEL CUP (SHORT-LEG CAST-BRACE)

Indications

A short-leg cylinder cast with ankle hinges and heel cup is used for incompletely healed tibial and fibular fractures that require more time to achieve further consolidation. The principal benefit of this cast is that it permits early knee and ankle motion.

Cast Materials Needed

Plaster Short-Leg Cylinder Cast with Ankle Hinges and Heel Cup

4″ stockinet

2 rolls of 4″ Webril

2 rolls of 6″ plaster bandage

1 roll of 3″ plaster bandage

1 heel cup with attached ankle hinges

Fiberglass Short-Leg Cylinder Cast with Ankle Hinges and Heel Cup

4″ stockinet

2 rolls of 4″ Webril

2 rolls of 4″ fiberglass bandage

1 roll of 3″ fiberglass bandage

Patient's Position

The patient's position is the same as for a short-leg cast.

Technique for Applying a Fiberglass Short-Leg Cylinder Cast with Ankle Hinges and Heel Cup

Stockinet

The 4″ stockinet is applied to the leg from the foot to the knee (Fig. 8-11A).

Webril

Two rolls of 4″ Webril are wrapped around the leg from the supramalleolar region to the knee (Fig. 8-11B).

Fiberglass Bandage

The first roll of 4″ fiberglass bandage is applied to the leg from the supramalleolar region to the level of the proximal end of the fibula, and the stockinet ends are folded down over the proximal and distal cast ends (Fig. 8-11C). The heel cup is applied to the foot, and its 2 attached ankle hinges are secured to the distal portion of the cast by means of a roll of 3″ fiberglass bandage (Fig. 8-11D,E,F).

Technique for Applying a Plaster Short-Leg Cylinder Cast with Ankle Hinges and Heel Cup

The technique for applying a plaster short-leg cylinder cast with ankle hinges and heel cup is similar to that for its fiberglass counterpart except that 2 rolls of 6″ plaster bandage are wrapped around the lower leg and a roll of 3″ plaster bandage is used to attach the ankle hinges to the lower part of the cast.

SHORT-LEG CYLINDER CAST WITH BIMALLEOLAR FLANGES

Indications

A short-leg cylinder cast with bimalleolar flanges is used for incompletely healed tibial and fibular fractures requiring more time and protection to heal properly. The main advantage of this cast is that it allows early knee and ankle motion.

Cast Materials and Patient's Position

Cast materials and patient's position are the same as for a short-leg cast.

Technique for Applying a Fiberglass Short-Leg Cylinder Cast with Bimalleolar Flanges

Stockinet

A 4″ stockinet is applied to the leg from the mid-foot region to the knee (Fig. 8-12A).

Webril

Three rolls of 4″ Webril are wrapped around the lower leg from the mid-foot level to the knee (Fig. 8-12B).

Fiberglass Bandage

Two rolls of 4″ fiberglass bandage are applied to the leg from the mid-foot to the knee. At least 3 layers of bandage should be wrapped around the malleolar region, and the cast should be molded carefully around the medial and lateral malleoli. The medial and lateral malleolar flanges and the 2 circular anterior and posterior supramalleolar notches are then marked on the ankle region of the cast with a wax pencil. The distal portion of the cast is removed by following the wax pencil mark with a cast saw. After the redundant Webril has been removed, the stockinet is split longitudinally along its anterior and posterior aspects. The 2 malleolar flanges and the adjacent portion of the cast are painted liberally with plastic adhesive, and the cut stockinet ends are pulled tightly over the distal cast end and allowed stick to the malleolar flanges and the distal portion of the cast. The opposite stockinet end is similar folded down over the proximal cast end, and a third roll of 4″ fiberglass bandage is used to go over the whole cast to finish it (Fig. 8-12C–G).

Technique for Applying a Plaster Short-Leg Cylinder Cast with Bimalleolar Flanges

Application of a plaster short-leg cylinder cast with bimalleolar flanges is similar to application of a fiberglass cast with bimalleolar flanges except that 2 rolls of 6″ plaster bandage are first applied to the lower leg from the mid-foot region to the knee. After the 2 malleolar flanges have been carved out and the 2 stockinet ends have been turned down, a roll of 4″ plaster bandage is used to finish the cast.

DR. WU'S BUNION BOOT

Dr. Wu's bunion boot (Fig. 8-13) is designed for use often a Mitchell's bunionectomy has been performed. The boot is worn for approximately 10 days, until the standard postoperative Mitchell's bunionectomy cast can be applied. The boot is very bulky because it is applied over a bulky postoperative dressing consisting of 4 conform bandages, 3 tongue blades, 1 Kerlix bandage, and 1 3″ Ace bandage (Fig. 8-14). The bunion boot is usually applied the third day after a Mitchell's bunionectomy.

Cast Materials Needed

Plaster Bunion Boot

4″ stockinet

4 rolls of 4″ Webril

1 roll of 6″ plaster bandage

Fiberglass Bunion Boot

4″ stockinet

4 rolls of 4″ Webril

1 roll of 4″ fiberglass bandage

1 roll of 5″ fiberglass bandage

Patient's Position

The patient usually sits on a cast table with the leg hung over the side of the cast table and the ankle in a neutral position.

Technique for Applying a Bunion Boot

Stockinet

A 4″ stockinet is applied from the upper calf region to a level beyond the tips of toes.

Webril

Four rolls of 4″ Webril are wrapped evenly around the lower leg from the mid-calf level to a point about 1 inch distal to the tips of the toes.

Bandages for Plaster Boot. One roll of 6″ plaster bandage is rolled onto the lower leg from the mid-calf level to a point about 1 inch distal to the toes. The 2 stockinet ends are folded down over the 2 cast ends, and a second roll of 6″ plaster bandage is applied over the whole cast to finish it. Either a cast sandal or an attached cast cushion can be used to permit full weight-bearing.

Bandages for Fiberglass Boot. One roll of 4″ fiberglass bandage is applied from the mid-calf region to a level slightly distal to the tips of the toes. The 2 stockinet ends are turned down over the 2 cast ends, and a roll of 5″ fiberglass bandage is applied over the whole cast to finish it. Sometimes a half-moon-shaped cut has to be made in the anterosuperior aspect of the cast to eliminate skin irritation by the upper cast end (Fig. 8-13). A cast sandal is worn routinely with a fiberglass bunion boot.

SHORT-LEG GREAT TOE SPICA CAST

Indications

A short-leg great toe spica cast (Fig. 8-15) is used for fractures and dislocations of the first metatarsal and its corresponding phalanges. I use this cast mainly to protect the distal osteotomy of the first metatarsal after performing a Mitchell's bunionectomy.

Cast Materials Needed

Plaster Short-Leg Great Toe Spica Cast

4″ stockinet

3 rolls of 4″ Webril

1 roll of 1″ Webril (by splitting a roll of 2″ Webril into 2 halves with a scalpel)

2 rolls of 6″ plaster bandage

1 roll of 2″ plaster bandage

2 5″ × 30″ plaster splints

For application of a cast cushion:

1 5″ × 30″ plaster splint

1 cast cushion

1 roll of 4″ plaster bandage

Fiberglass Short-Leg Great Toe Spica Cast

4″ stockinet

3 rolls of 4″ Webril

1 roll of 1″ Webril

3 rolls of 4″ fiberglass bandage

1 roll of 2″ fiberglass bandage

Patient's Position

The cast is best applied with the patient in a recumbent position. A leg rest should be used to elevate the leg and to bend the knee so that the ankle can be held easily in a neutral position.

Technique for Applying a Short-Leg Great Toe Spica Cast

The technique for applying a short-leg great toe spica cast is illustrated in Figs. 8-16 and 8-17.

Stockinet

After the 4″ stockinet has been applied from the toes to the knee, the double layers of stockinet between the great and second toes should be cut longitudinally. The 2 cut ends of the stockinet immediately lateral to the great toe are lapped over the lateral side of the great toe, and 1″ Webril is used to wrap the great toe and the distal portion of the foot.

Webril

Three rolls of 4″ Webril are applied evenly to the lower leg from the metatarsal head region to the upper calf.

Bandages

Bandages for Plaster Cast. One roll of 6″ plaster bandage is applied to the lower leg from the bases of the toes to the upper calf. The 2 5″ × 30″ plaster splints are applied to the posterior aspect of the lower leg and the bottom portion of the foot. A 2″ plaster bandage is wrapped once around the distal portion of the cast, and as it approaches the first toe webspace, a 1-inch transverse cut is made in the bandage so that it can be wrapped smoothly around the great toe. After the bandage has been wrapped twice around the great toe, it is brought to the medial aspect of the great toe, where it is folded back and forth on itself 3 times to reinforce the junction of the toe spica and the short-leg cast. The bandage is then wrapped around the great toe 2 more times before applying the remaining portion of the cast. The stockinet ends are pulled over the cast ends, and a second roll of 6″ plaster bandage is applied over the whole cast to complete it. The cast cushion is applied as in the short-leg walking cast.

Bandages for Fiberglass Cast. The method for applying fiberglass bandages is similar to the method for applying plaster bandages for a great toe spica cast except that the splints are omitted and 3 rolls of 4″ fiberglass bandage are substituted for the 2 rolls of 6″ plaster bandage. A cast sandal is routinely applied, but a cast cushion can also be used if the need should arise (the technique for applying a cast cushion to a fiberglass cast has been described in the section dealing with the short-leg walking cast).

SHORT-LEG GREAT TOE SPICA CAST WITH TOE GUARD

A short-leg great toe spica cast with toe guard (Fig. 8-18) is used primarily in the postoperative management of Mitchell's bunionectomy and concurrent hammertoe correction, which often requires insertion of 1 or more K-wires. This cast can also be used for fractures and dislocations of the first metatarsal and its associated phalanges, and concurrent fractures and dislocations of the metatarsals and phalanges of the lesser toes. A 1-inch padded aluminum splint is bent to shape, and then its 2 ends are fixed to the distal portion of the cast with a roll of 3″ fiberglass or plaster bandage (Fig. 8-19).

SHORT-LEG INVERSION-EVERSION SPLINTS

Short-leg inversion-eversion splints are usually used in treating ankle sprains or in protecting incompletely healed ankle fractures and dislocations.

Technique for Applying a Fiberglass Short-Leg Inversion-Eversion Splint

The technique for applying a fiberglass short-leg inversion-eversion splint is illustrated in Fig. 8-20. A 4″ stockinet is applied to the lower leg. The adhesive-backed foam rubber sheet is applied to a 4″ × 30″ fiberglass splint, and the splint is applied to the lower leg along its medial and lateral aspects and to the bottom of the foot. A roll of 4″ Ace bandage is used to hold the splint snugly to the lower leg. The patient is asked to put full body weight on the splint, and the splint is molded to fit the contour of the lower leg. To produce a removable short-leg inversion-eversion splint, 2 webbings with attached buckles are riveted to the splint so that it can be worn or removed with ease (Fig. 8-21).

Technique for Applying a Plaster Short-Leg Inversion-Eversion Splint

The technique for applying a plaster short-leg inversion-eversion splint is similar to that for applying a fiberglass splint except that the single 4″ × 30″ fiberglass splint is replaced with 2 or 3 5″ × 30″ plaster splints, which should be padded with felt, foam rubber sheet, or several layers of Webril before they are applied to the lower leg and held in place with a roll of 4″ Ace bandage.

POSTERIOR SHORT-LEG SPLINT

A posterior short-leg splint can best be made by applying a plaster or fiberglass short-leg cast and then bivalving it along its medial and lateral aspects. The margins of the lower half of the cast should be lined with moleskin. The fully lined bottom half of the cast is reapplied to the leg and held in place with a roll of Ace bandage (Fig. 8-22).

PTB CAST

Indications

A PTB cast (Fig. 8-23) is used for fractures and dislocations of the ankle and fractures of the tibia and fibula. A PTB cast allows motion of the knee joint but severely restricts motion of the tibia, fibula, and the ankle joint and can thus replace a long-leg cast in many instances.

Cast Materials Needed

Plaster PTB Cast

4″ stockinet

3 rolls of 4″ Webril

3 5″ × 30″ plaster splints

2 rolls of 6″ plaster bandage

1 roll of 4″ plaster bandage

Fiberglass PTB Cast

4″ stockinet

3 rolls of 4″ Webril

3 rolls of 5″ fiberglass bandage

1 roll of 3″ fiberglass bandage

Patient's Position

A PTB cast should be applied with the patient in a sitting position with the knee joint at 90° of flexion.

Technique for Applying a Fiberglass PTB Cast

Stockinet

A 4″ stockinet is applied from the mid-thigh to the toes (Fig. 8-24A).

Webril

Three rolls of 4″ Webril are applied to the leg from the bases of the toes to the mid-thigh region (Fig. 8-24B).

Fiberglass Bandages

Three rolls of 5″ fiberglass bandage are applied evenly to the leg from the metatarsal head level to the mid-thigh region. While the cast is still soft, both thumbs should be used to make a transverse indentation directly over the patellar tendon, and both index fingers should be used to make another transverse indentation about 2″ below the popliteal crease. The cast should also be molded closely to the medial and lateral femoral condyles (Fig. 8-24C,D).

A wax pencil is used to mark the upper margins of the cast by starting at the center of the transverse cast indentation over the patellar tendon, going proximally along the medial and lateral borders of the patella to its superior pole, where the 2 lines follow the upper ends of the medial and lateral condyles to the posterior aspect of the distal femur, where the lines are extended in a posterior and distal direction to join the transverse cast indentation below the popliteal crease (Fig. 8-24E,F). A cast saw is used to cut the cast along the wax pencil line to remove redundant cast material (Fig. 8-24G,H,I). After the redundant Webril has been removed and split longitudinally and the 2 supracondylar flanges and adjacent upper ends of the cast have been painted with plastic adhesive, the upper and lower stockinet ends are pulled over the 2 cast ends and a roll of 3″ fiberglass bandage is used to wrap the cast from its distal end to the bases of the 2 supracondylar flanges (Fig. 8-24J,K,L). A cast sandal is added to allow immediate weight bearing (Fig. 8-24M,N,O).

Technique for Applying a Plaster PTB Cast

After the 4″ stockinet and 3 rolls of 4″ Webril have been applied to the leg, a roll of 6″ plaster bandage is applied from the metatarsal head region to the mid-thigh region. Two 5″ × 30″ plaster splints are applied to the posterior aspect of the leg and the bottom portion of the foot, and the third 5″ × 30″ plaster bandage is cut transversely into 2 halves, which are applied to the medial and lateral sides of the supracondylar and knee region. The second roll of 6″ plaster bandage is used to wrap the leg from the bases of the toes to the mid-thigh region. Two transverse indentations are then made in the cast below the patella and popliteal crease, and the 2 supracondylar flanges are carved out of the cast with a cast saw. After the 2 stockinet ends have been folded down over the proximal and distal cast ends, a roll of 4″ plaster bandage is used to cover the cast from its distal end to the bases of the 2 supracondylar flanges to finish the cast.

PTB CAST WITH ANKLE HINGES AND HEEL CUP (PTB CAST-BRACE)

A PTB cast with ankle hinges and heel cup is used primarily in treating tibial and fibular fractures. It allows both knee and ankle motion and can often replace a long-leg cast or even a PTB cast. To produce this cast, a plaster or fiberglass PTB cast should be applied first. The distal portion of the cast below the ankle is then removed. The heel cup is applied to the foot, and the 2 ankle hinges are fixed to the supramalleolar portion of the cast with a 3″ plaster or fiberglass bandage (Fig. 8-25).

BIBLIOGRAPHY

Adams, J.C.: Outline of Fractures. 8th Ed. Edinburgh, Churchill Livingstone, 1983.

Anderson, L.D., and Kutchins, W.C.: Fractures of the tibia and fibula treated with casts and transfixation pins. South. Med. J., *59:*1026, 1966.

Austin, R.T.: The Sarmiento tibial plaster: A prospective study of 145 fractures. Injury, *13:*10, 1981.

Black, H.M., Brand, R.L., and Eichelberger, M.R.: An improved technique for the evaluation of ligamentous injury in severe ankle sprains. Am. J. Sports Med., *6:*276, 1978.

Bleck, E.E.: Metatarsus adductus: Classification and relationship to outcomes of treatment. J. Pediatr. Orthop., *3:*2, 1983.

Brown, D.C., and McFarland, G.B., Jr.: Dislocation of the medial cuneiform bone in tarsometatarsal fracture-dislocation. A case report. J. Bone Joint Surg., [Am.], *57:*858, 1975.

Brown, T.I.S.: Avulsion fracture of the fibular sesamoid in association with dorsal dislocation of the metatarso-phalangeal joint of the hallux. Report of a case and review of the literature. Clin. Orthop., *149:*229, 1980.

Canale, S.T., and Kelly, F.B., Jr.: Fractures of the neck of the talus. Long-term evaluation of seventy-one cases. J. Bone Joint Surg., [Am.], *60:*143, 1978.

Cave, E.F., Burke, J.F., and Boyd, R.J.: Trauma management. Chicago, Year Book Medical Publishers, 1974.

DeBenedetti, M.J., Evanski, P.M., and Waugh, T.R.: The unreducible Lisfranc fracture. Case report and literature review. Clin. Orthop., *136:*238, 1978.

DeLee, J.C., and Curtis, R.: Subtalar dislocation of the foot. J. Bone Joint Surg., [Am.], *64:*433, 1982.

Dockery, G.L., Tozzi, M.A., and Spencer, A.M.: A fiberglass casting material for use in podiatry. J. Am. Podiatry Assoc., *67:*436, 1977.

Drez, D., Jr., Young, J.C., Johnston, R.D., and Parker, W.D.: Metatarsal stress fractures. Am. J. Sports Med., *8:*123, 1980.

Eraltug, U.: Corrective plaster application in the treatment of vertical talus. An analysis of eleven cases. Int. Surg., *46:*246, 1966.

Fleetcroft, J.: Plastering: A combination of old and new. Injury, *13:*131, 1981.

Gans, B.M., Erickson, G., and Simons, D.: Below-knee orthosis: A wrap-around design for ankle-foot control. Arch. Phys. Med. Rehabil., *60:*78, 1979.

Gilbert, B.S.: Metatarsal stress fracture: The use of a posterior plaster of paris splint. A case report. J. Am. Podiatry Assoc., *58:*438, 1968.

Glasgow, M., Jackson, A., and Jamieson, A.M.: Instability of the ankle after injury to the lateral ligament. J. Bone Joint Surg., [Br.], *62:*196, 1980.

Hardcastle, P.H., Reschauer, R., Kutscha-Lissberg, E., and Schoffmann, W.: Injuries to the tarsometatarsal joint. J. Bone Joint Surg., [Br.], *64:*349, 1982.

Hartman, J.T.: Fracture management: A practical approach. Philadelphia, Lea & Febiger, 1978.

Hawkins, L.G.: Fracture of the lateral process of the talus. J. Bone Joint Surg., [Am.], *47:*1170, 1965.

Hedges, J.R., and Anwar, R.A.: Management of ankle sprains. Ann. Emerg. Med., *9:*298, 1980.

Henning, C.E., and Egge, L.N.: Cast brace treatment of acute unstable lateral ankle sprain. A preliminary report. Am. J. Sports Med., *5:*252, 1977.

Heppenstall, R.B., Farahvar, H., Balderston, R., and Lotke, P.: Evaluation and management of subtalar dislocations. J. Trauma, *20:*494, 1980.

Hice, G.A., Solomon, W., and Faschada, P.: The plaster-synthetic cast. J. Am. Podiatry Assoc., *73:*427, 1983.

Hilsinger, E.A.: Partial plaster splint for the sprained ankle. JAMA, *214:*1326, 1970.

Jahss, M.H.: Traumatic dislocations of the first metatarsophalangeal joint. Foot-Ankle, *1:*15, 1980.

Jahss, M.H.: Stubbing injuries to the hallus. Foot-Ankle, *1:*327, 1981.

Jebsen, R.H., Corcoran, P.J., and Simons, B.C.: Clinical experience with a plastic short leg brace. Arch. Phys. Med. Rehabil., *51:*114, 1970.

Jennings, J.J., Miller, W.E., and Dupree, D.N.: A modified solid ankle brace for the treatment of arthritides. South. Med. J., *69:*767, 1976.

Kavanaugh, J.H., Brower, T.D., and Mann, R.V.: The Jones fracture revisited. J. Bone Joint Surg., [Am.], *60:*776, 1978.

Keller, J., and Rasmussen, T.B.: Closed treatment of Achilles tendon rupture. Acta Orthop. Scand., *55*:548, 1984.
Kenwright, J., and Taylor, R.G.: Major injuries of the talus. J. Bone Joint Surg., [Br.], *52*:36, 1970.
Lang-Stevenson, A.I., Sharrard, W.J., Betts, R.P., and Duckworth, T.: Neuropathic ulcers of the foot. J. Bone Joint Surg., [Br.], *67*:438, 1985.
Lildholdt, T., and Munch-Jorgensen, T.: Conservative treatment to Achilles tendon rupture. A follow-up study of 14 cases. Acta Orthop. Scand., *47*:454, 1976.
Mac, S.S., and Kleiger, B.: The early complications of subtalar dislocations. Foot-ankle, *1*:270, 1981.
McCollough, N.C., III., Vinsant, J.E., and Sarmiento, A.: Functional fracture bracing of long bone fractures of the lower extremity in children. J. Bone Joint Surg., [Am.], *60*:314, 1978.
Main, B.J., and Jowett, R.L.: Injuries of the midtarsal joint. J. Bone Joint Surg., [Br.], *57*:89, 1975.
Nadeau, P., and Templeton, J.: Vertical fracture-dislocation of the tarsal navicular. J. Trauma, *16*:669, 1976.
Niedermann, B., et al.: Rupture of the lateral ligaments of the ankle: Operation or plaster cast? A prospective study. Acta Orthop. Scand., *52*:579, 1981.
Persson, A., and Wredmark, T.: The treatment of total ruptures of the Achilles tendon by plaster immobilization. Int. Orthop., *3*:149, 1979.
Pollard, J.P., and Lequesne, L.P.: Method of healing diabetic forefoot ulcers. Br. Med. J., *286*:436, 1983.
Pratt, D.J.: Energy of gait in below-knee casts with different soles. J. Biomed. Eng., *7*:63, 1985.
Rao, J.P., and Banzon, M.T.: Irreducible dislocation of the metatarsophalangeal joints of the foot. Clin. Orthop., *145*:224, 1979.
Rees, D.: Fracture-separation of the lower femoral epiphysis as a complication of the Sarmiento below-knee functional cast: A case report. Injury, *16*:117, 1984.
Salama, R., Benamara, A., and Weissman, S.L.: Functional treatment of intra-articular fractures of the calcaneus. Clin. Orthop., *115*:236, 1976.
Sarmiento, A.: A functional below-the-knee cast for tibial fracture. J. Bone Joint Surg., [Am.], *49*:855, 1967.
Sarmiento, A.: A functional below-knee brace for tibial fractures. J. Bone Joint Surg., [Am.], *52*:295, 1970.
Sarmiento, A.: Functional bracing of tibial and femoral shaft fractures. Clin. Orthop., *82*:2, 1972.
Sarmiento, A.: Functional bracing of tibial fractures. Clin. Orthop., *105*:202, 1974.
Sarmiento, A., Kinman, P.B., and Latta, L.: Fractures of the proximal tibia and tibial condyles. Clin. Orthop., *145*:136, 1979.
Scheck, M.: Treatment of comminuted distal tibial fractures by combined dual pin fixation and limited open reduction. J. Bone Joint Surg., [Am.], *47*:1537, 1965.
Schober, W.R., and Grant, D.L.: Plastic bivalved walking splint for immobilization of an arthritic ankle. Phys. Ther., *51*:785, 1971.
Segal, D., and Wasilewski, S.: Total dislocation of the talus. Case report. J. Bone Joint Surg., [Am.], *62*:1370, 1980.
Sneppen, O., Christensen, S.B., Krogsoe, O., and Lorentzen, J.: Fracture of the body of the talus. Acta Orthop. Scand., *48*:317, 1977.
Svend-Hansen, H., Bremerskov, V., and Ostri, P.: Fracture-suspending effect of the patellar-tendon-bearing cast. Acta Orthop. Scand., *50*:237, 1979.
Trickey, E.L.: Treatment of fractures of the calcaneus. J. Bone Joint Surg., [Br.], *57*:411, 1975.
Viswanath, S.S., and Shephard, E.: Dislocation of the calcaneum. Injury, *9*:50, 1977.
Warrick, C.K., Bremner, A.E.: Fractures of the calcaneum—with an atlas illustrating the various types of fracture. J. Bone Joint Surg., [Br.], *35*:33, 1953.
Weatherwax, R.J.: The plaster slipper cast. Clin. Orthop., *154*:327, 1981.
Yale, J.: A statistical analysis of 3657 consecutive fatigue fractures of the distal lower extremities. J. Am. Podiatry Assoc., *66*:739, 1976.

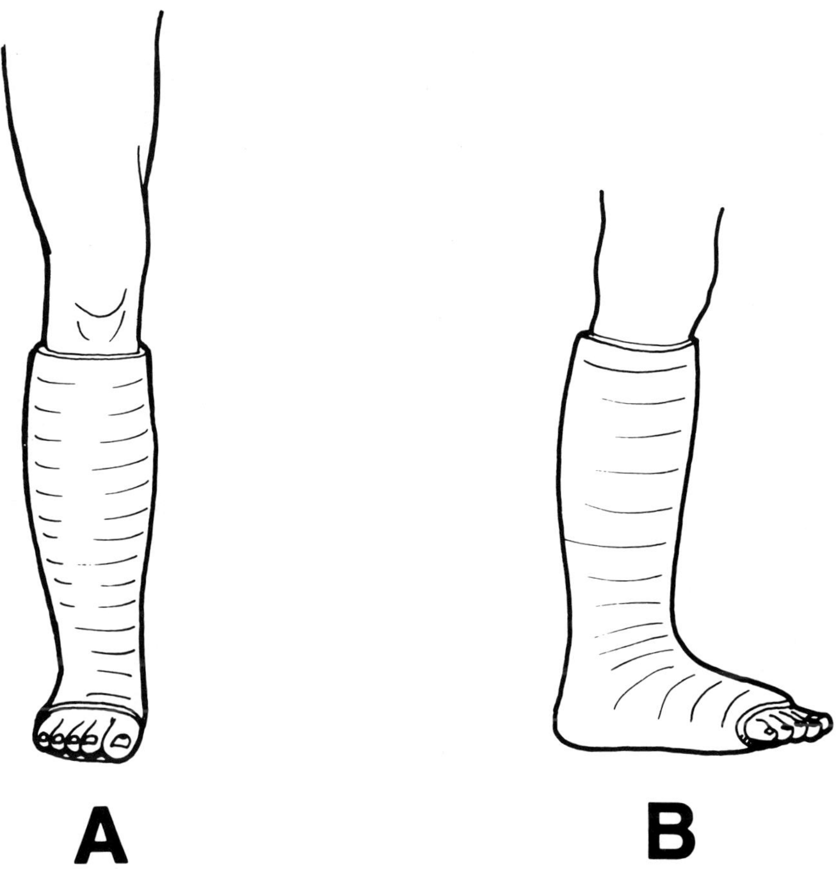

Fig. 8–1. Anterior (*A*) and lateral (*B*) views of a short-leg cast.

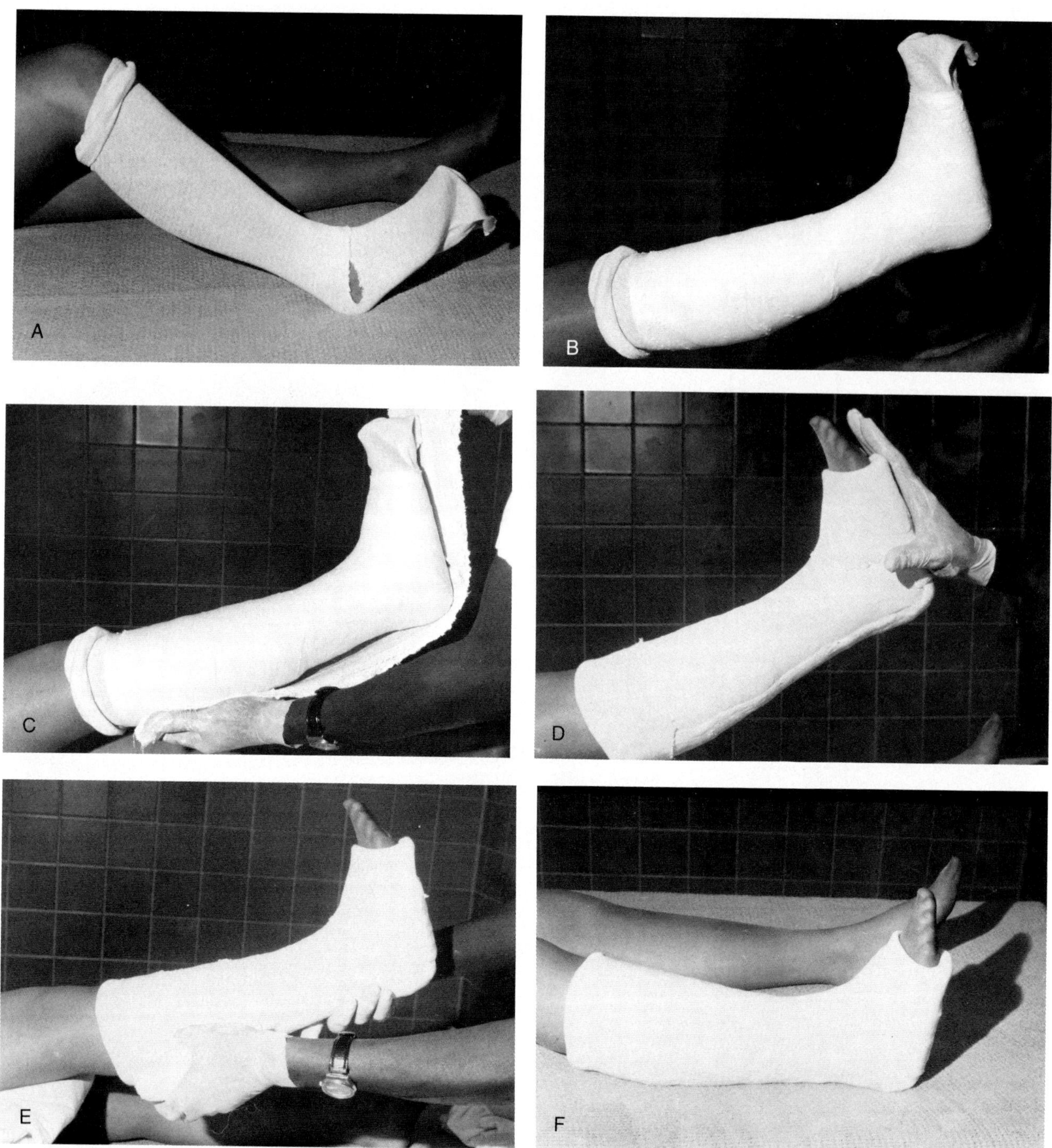

Fig. 8–2. The making of a plaster short-leg cast. *A*, A 4″ stockinet has been applied to the lower leg from the toes to the knee. The large transverse wrinkle in front of the ankle has been cut off. *B*, After 3 rolls of 4″ Webril have been wrapped around the lower leg, a roll of 6″ plaster bandage is used to cover the Webril. *C*, Two 5″ × 30″ plaster splints are applied to the posterior and plantar aspects of the cast. *D*, The 2 plaster splints are molded into the posterior and plantar aspects of the cast, and the 2 stockinet ends are folded over the proximal and distal ends of the cast. *E*, A roll of 6″ plaster bandage is used to cover the cast. *F*, The palms of both hands have been used to rub the whole cast to make it smooth and strong.

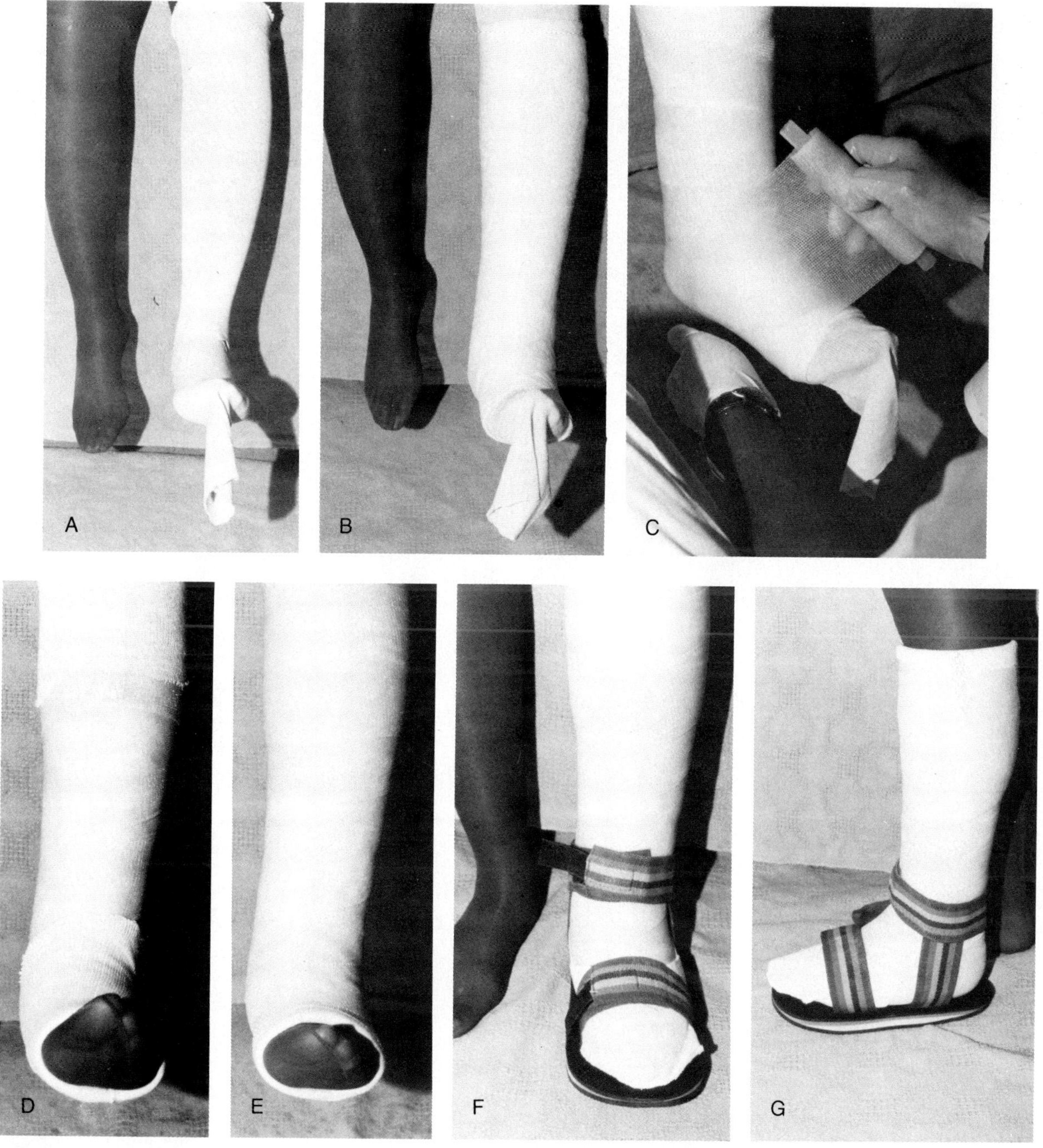

Fig. 8–3. The making of a fiberglass short-leg cast. *A*, A 4″ stockinet has been applied to the lower leg, and the wrinkle in front of the ankle has been removed. *B*, Three rolls of 4″ Webril have been applied to the lower leg. *C*, Two rolls of 4″ fiberglass bandage are being applied to the lower leg. *D*, The 2 stockinet ends are folded down over the proximal and distal ends of the cast. *E*, A new roll of 4″ fiberglass bandage has been used to go over the entire cast to finish it. *F*, *G*, Anterior and lateral views of the fiberglass short-leg cast. A cast sandal and a stockinet toe cap have been applied.

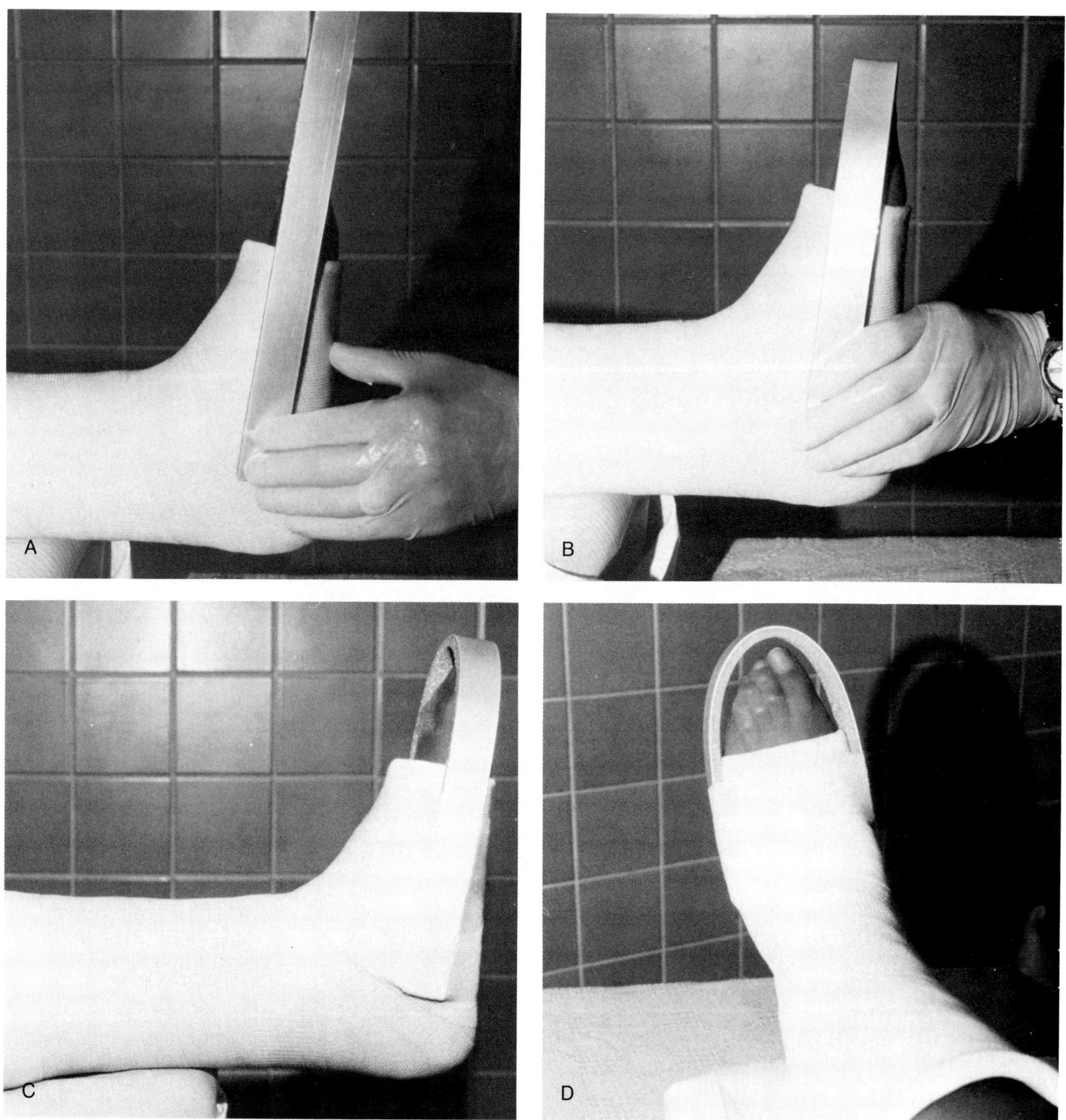

Fig. 8–4. Short-leg cast with toe guard. *A*, A 1-inch-wide padded aluminum splint is held tightly against the medial side of the foot portion of a fiberglass short-leg cast. *B*, The aluminum splint is bent in such a way that it is about $^1/_3$ inch distal to the tips of the toes. *C*, *D*, A roll of 3″ fiberglass bandage is used to fix the 2 ends of the aluminum splint to the medial and lateral aspects of the foot portion of the cast.

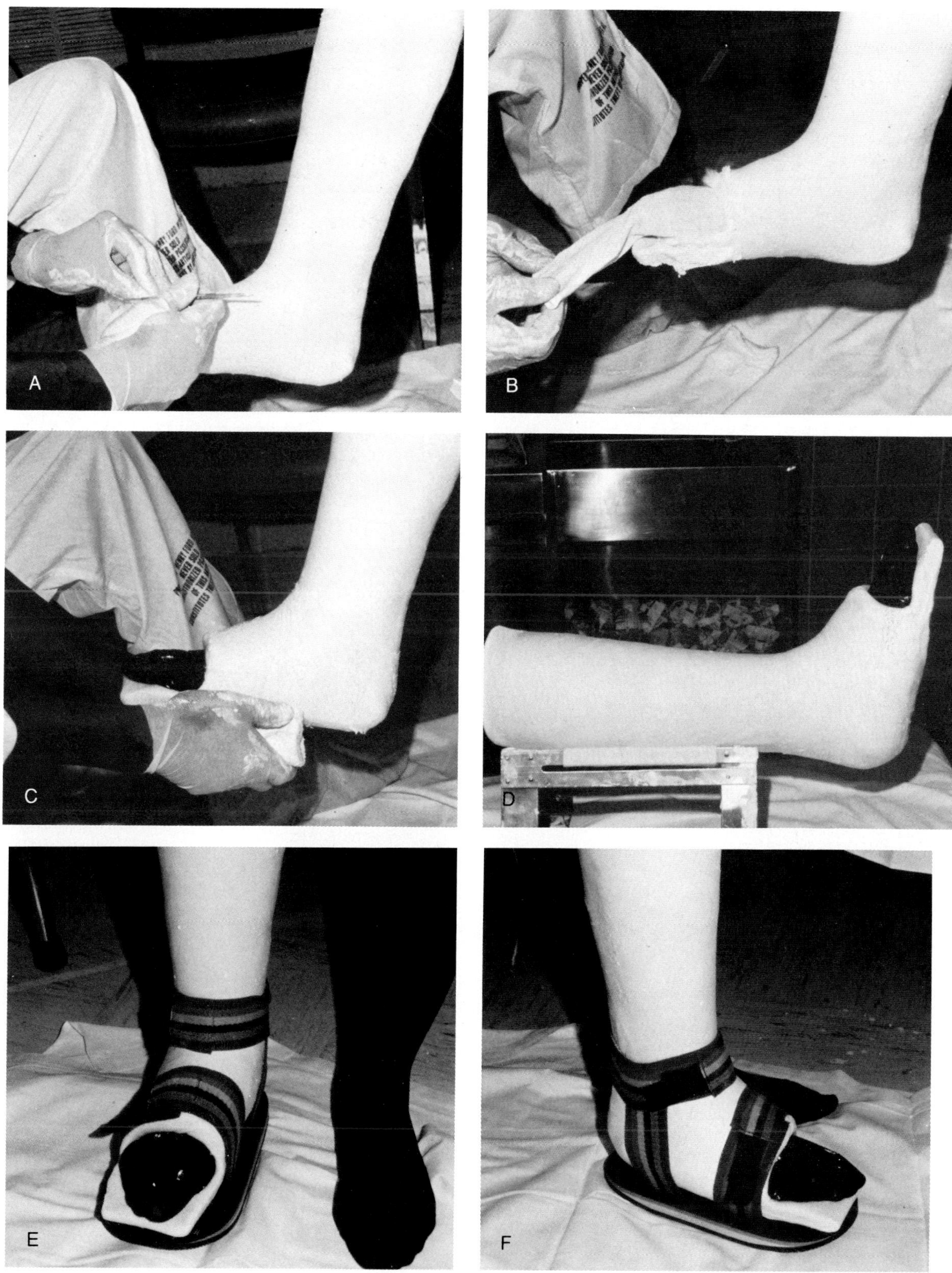

Fig. 8–5. The making of a short-leg cast with a toe plate. *A*, *B*, After a plaster short-leg cast has been made with plaster extending beyond the tips of the toes, a scalpel is used to remove the plaster and Webril over the dorsal aspect of the toes to the level of the proximal ends of the toe webspaces. *C*, *D*, The end of the stockinet is tightly pulled over the distal end of the cast and is fixed to the cast with 3″ plaster bandage. *E*, *F*, Anterior and lateral views of a plaster short-leg cast with a toe plate. A cast sandal is being worn.

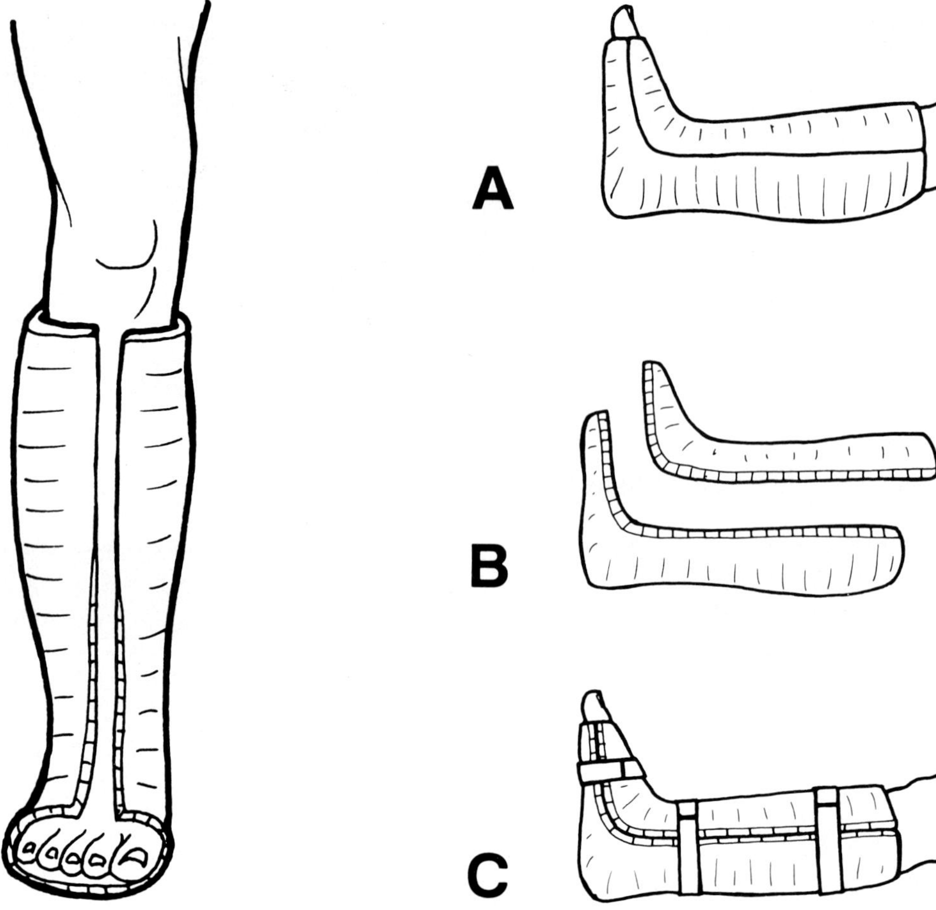

Fig. 8–6. A short-leg cast has been univalved along the midline of its anterior surface.

Fig. 8–7. Bivalving of a short-leg cast. *A*, The short-leg cast is cut along its medial and lateral aspects. *B*, The edges of the bivalved cast are lined with moleskin. *C*, The bivalved cast is reapplied to the leg and is held in place with either Velcro straps or webbings and buckles.

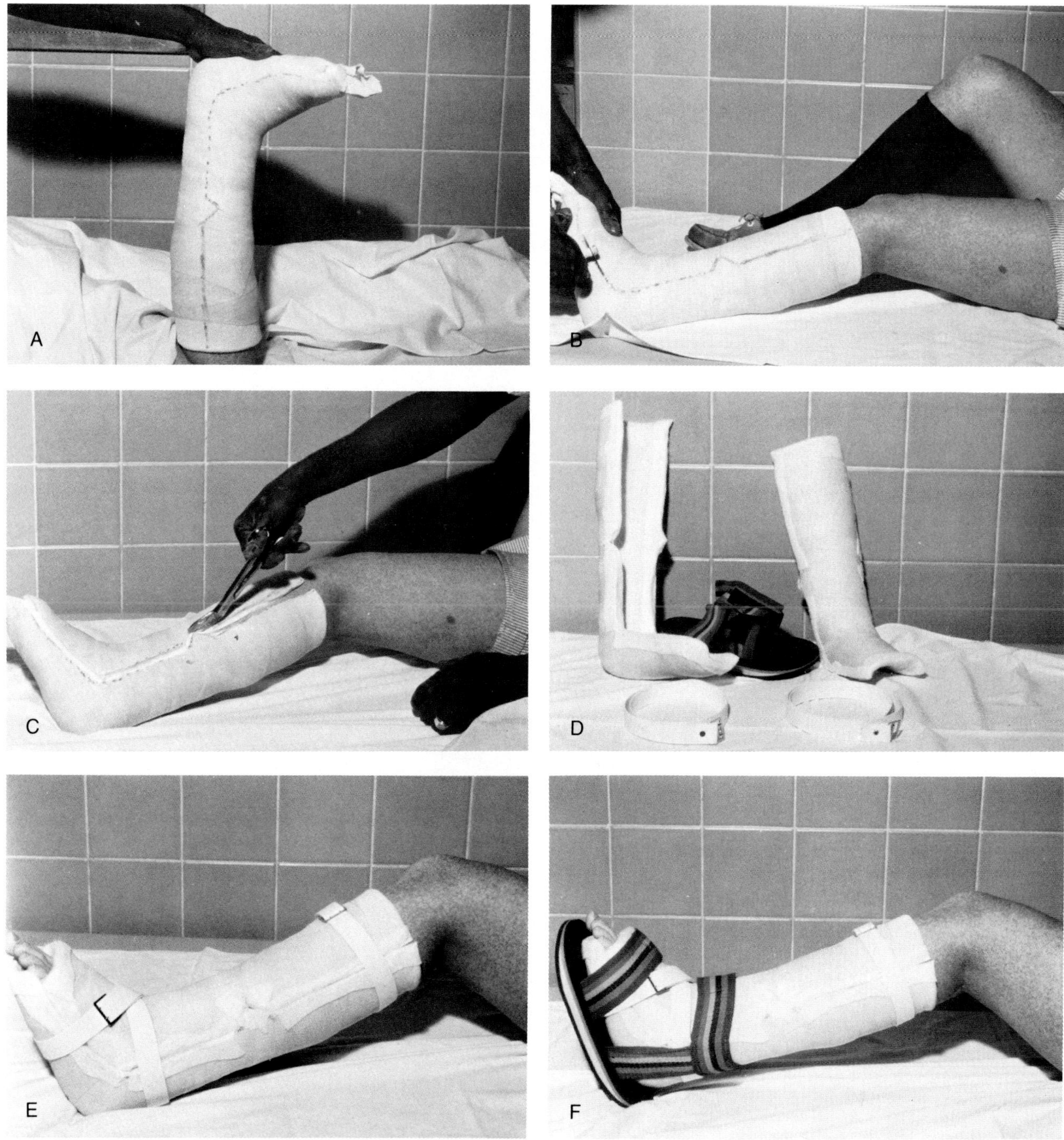

Fig. 8–8. Bivalving a short-leg cast. *A*, The lines for bivalving a fiberglass short-leg cast have been marked on the medial and lateral aspects of the cast. Two triangular notches and matching triangular projections are built into the bivalved area to prevent slippage of the two sections of the cast. *B*, A cast saw is being used to cut the cast. *C*, The Webril and stockinet under the saw cut are cut with a pair of plaster scissors. *D*, The margins of the bivalved cast have been lined with moleskin. A cast sandal and two buckled webbings have been obtained for subsequent application. *E*, The bivalved cast has been reapplied to the injured leg, and buckled webbings hold the bivalved cast in place. *F*, A cast sandal has been applied to the cast.

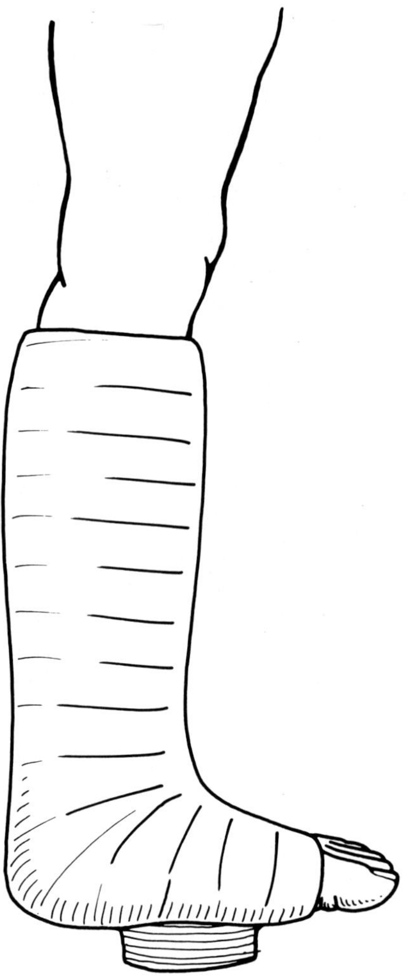

Fig. 8–9. Side view of a short-leg walking cast.

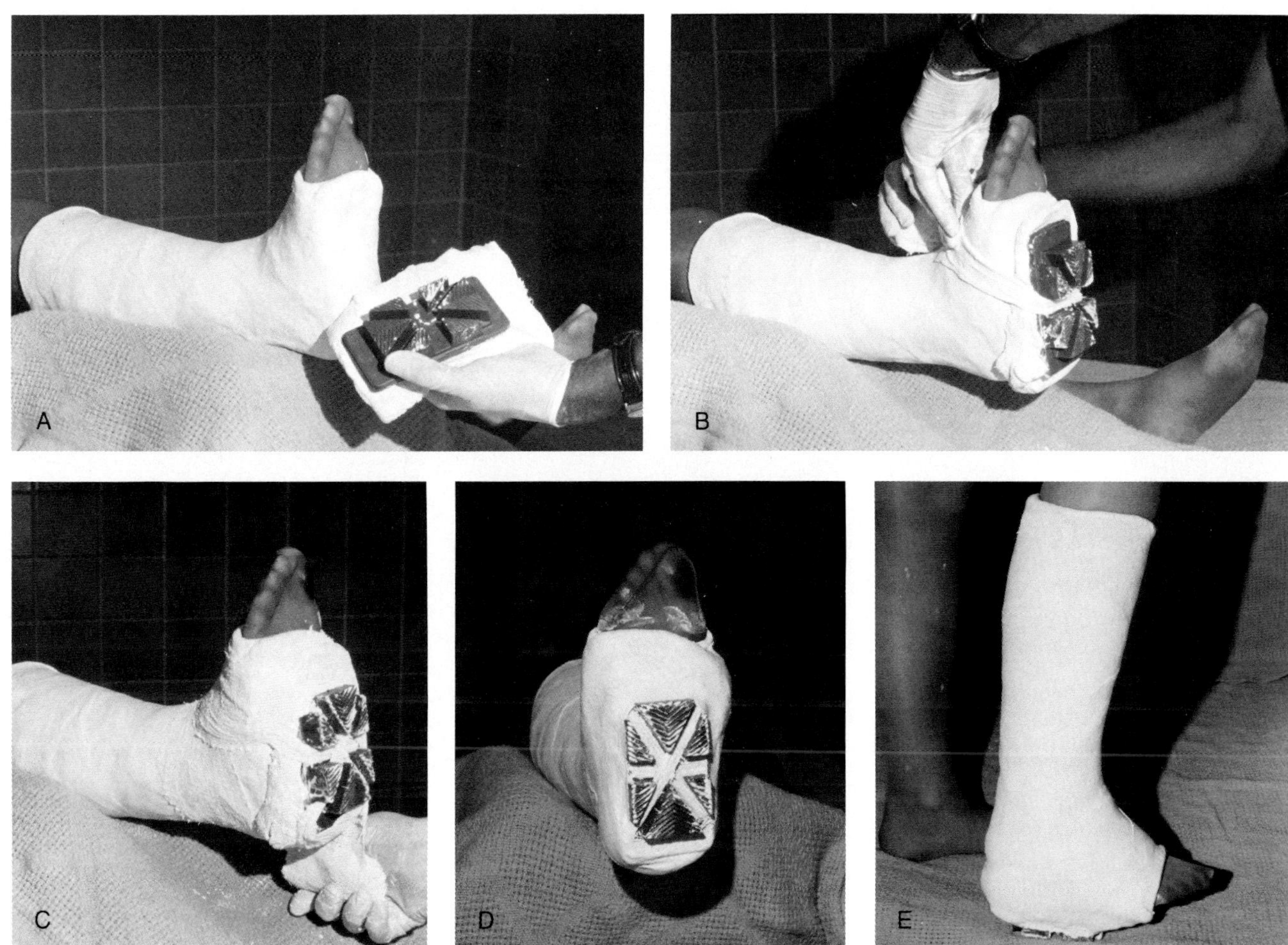

Fig. 8–10. The making of a short-leg walking cast. *A*, A folded 5″ × 30″ plaster splint with a cast cushion on it is ready to be applied to the bottom of a short-leg cast. *B*, The first turn of the 4″ plaster bandage has gone into the transverse groove on the bottom of the cast cushion to anchor the cast cushion to the bottom of the cast. *C*, The plaster bandage is then wound through the 2 diagonal grooves and finally over the anterior and posterior lips of the cast cushion to fix the cast cushion securely to the bottom of the cast. *D*, *E*, Bottom and lateral views of the plaster short-leg walking cast.

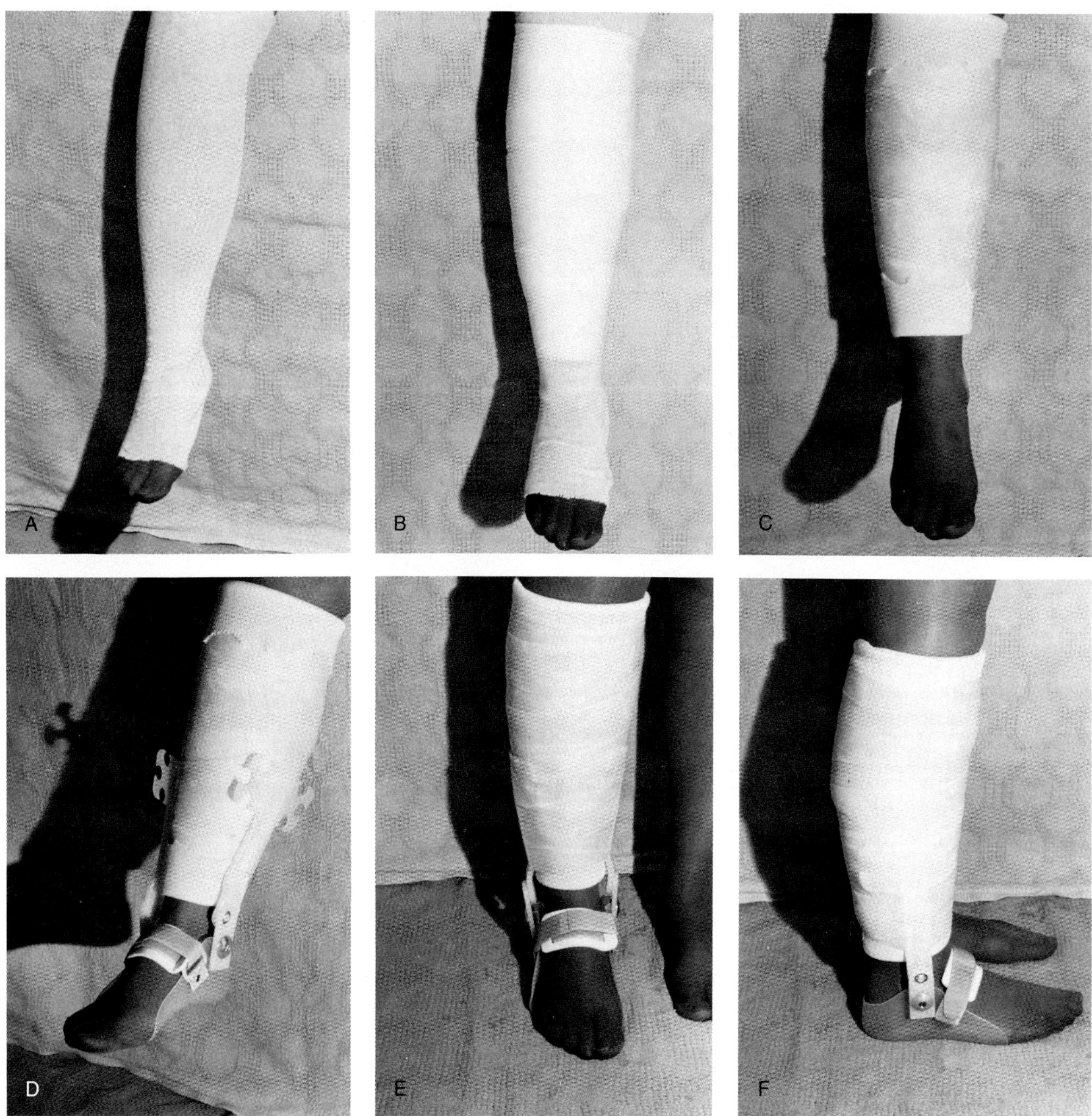

Fig. 8–11. The making of a short-leg cylinder cast with ankle hinges and heel cup. *A*, A 4″ stockinet has been applied to the lower leg. *B*, Two rolls of 4″ Webril have been wrapped around the leg from the supramalleolar region to the knee. *C*, One roll of 4″ fiberglass bandage has been applied to the leg from the supramalleolar level to the proximal end of the fibula, and the ends of the stockinet have been folded down over the proximal and distal ends of the cast. *D*, The heel cup with 2 attached ankle hinges is applied to the foot. *E*, *F*, Anterior and lateral views of the finished cast after the ankle hinges have been fixed to the distal portion of the cast with 1 roll of 3″ fiberglass bandage.

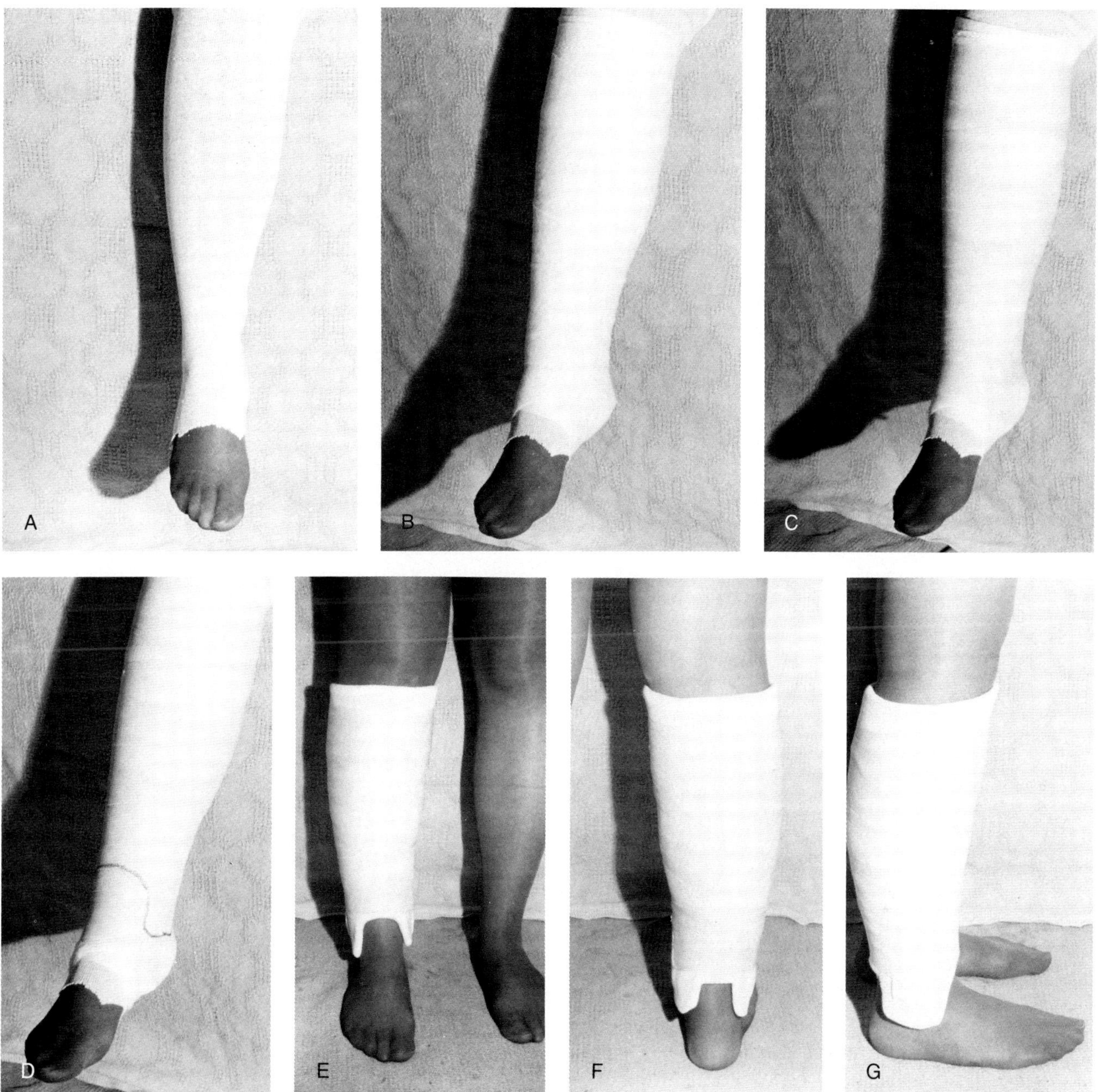

Fig. 8–12. The making of a short-leg cylinder cast with bimalleolar flanges. *A*, A 4″ stockinet has been applied to the leg from the foot to the knee. *B*, Three rolls of 4″ Webril have been applied to the leg from the mid-foot level to the knee. *C*, Two rolls of 4″ fiberglass bandage have been applied to the leg from the mid-tarsal region to the knee. *D*, The medial and lateral malleolar flanges and the anterior and posterior supramalleolar notches have been marked on the cast with a wax pencil. *E*, *F*, *G*, Anterior, posterior, and lateral views of the finished cast after the 2 stockinet ends have been turned down over the proximal and distal ends of the cast and a third roll of 4″ fiberglass bandage has been applied over the whole cast.

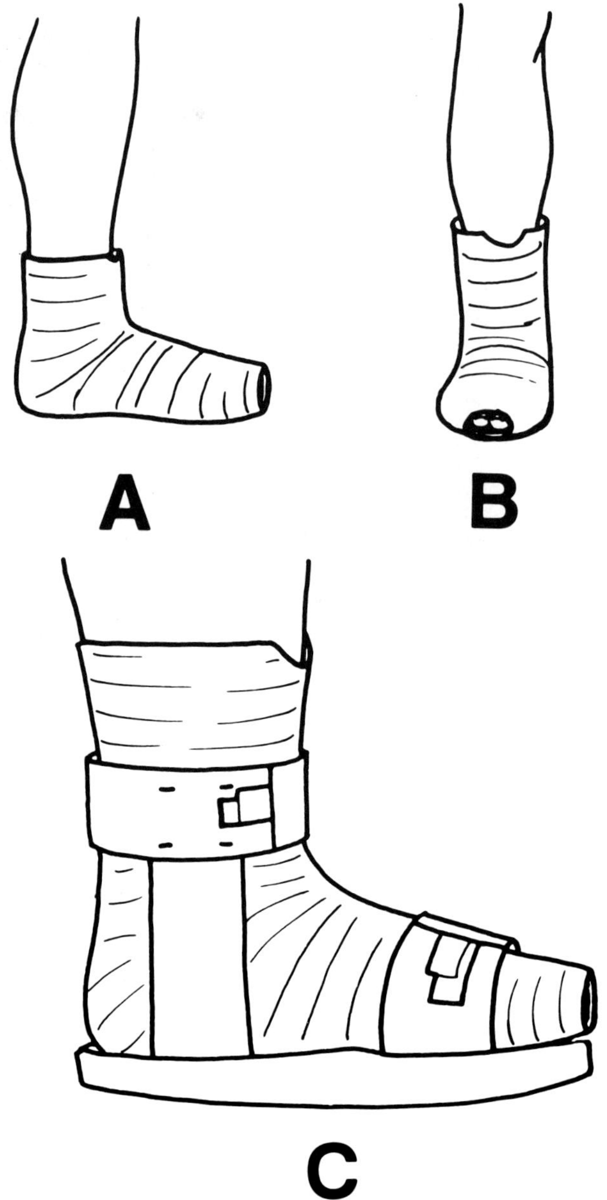

Fig. 8–13. Dr. Wu's bunion boot. *A*, *B*, Lateral and anterior views of the bunion boot. *C*, A bunion boot in a cast sandal.

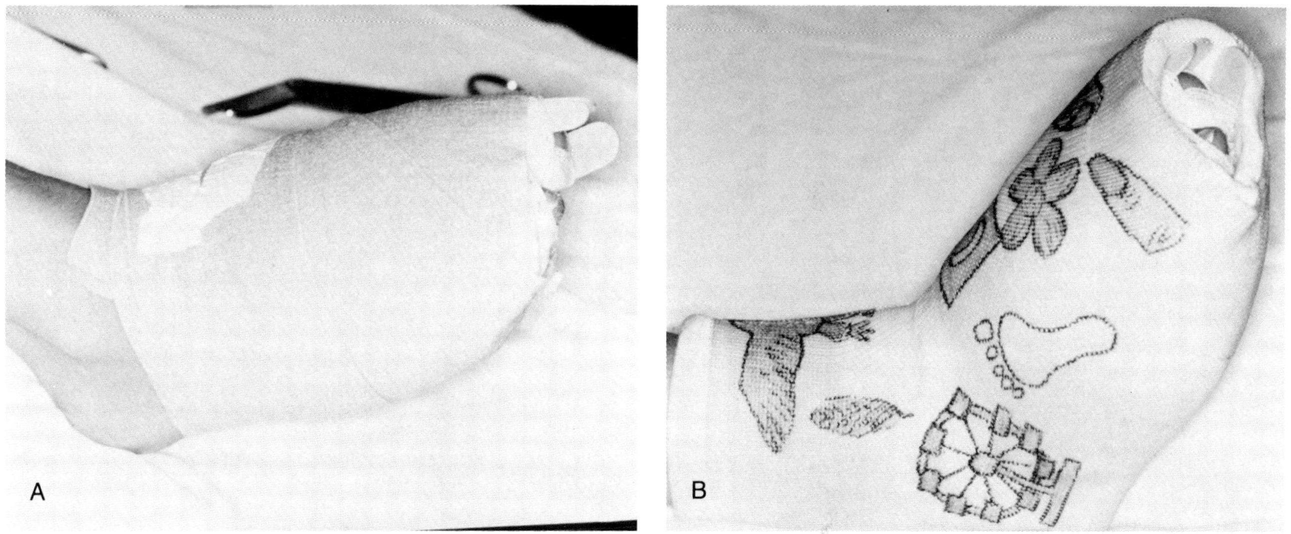

Fig. 8–14. *A*, A foot that has undergone a Mitchell's bunionectomy is protected with three tongue blades around the dorsal, medial, and plantar aspects of the first metatarsal, to prevent accidental displacement of the metatarsal osteotomy site, and a bulky compression dressing to minimize postoperative swelling. We now routinely perform Mitchell's bunionectomies on an outpatient basis. *B*, The same foot after a bunion boot has been applied.

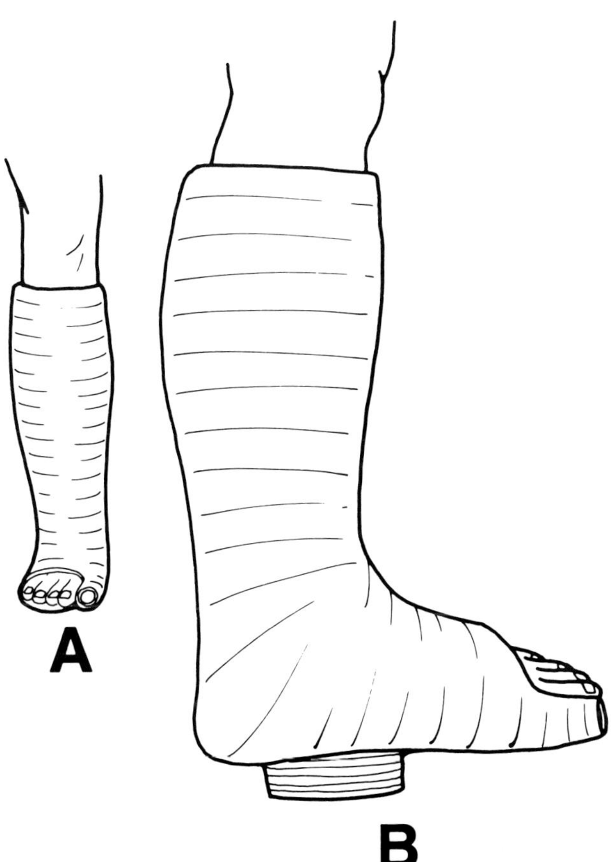

Fig. 8–15. Anterior (*A*) and lateral (*B*) views of a short-leg great toe spica cast with an attached cast cushion.

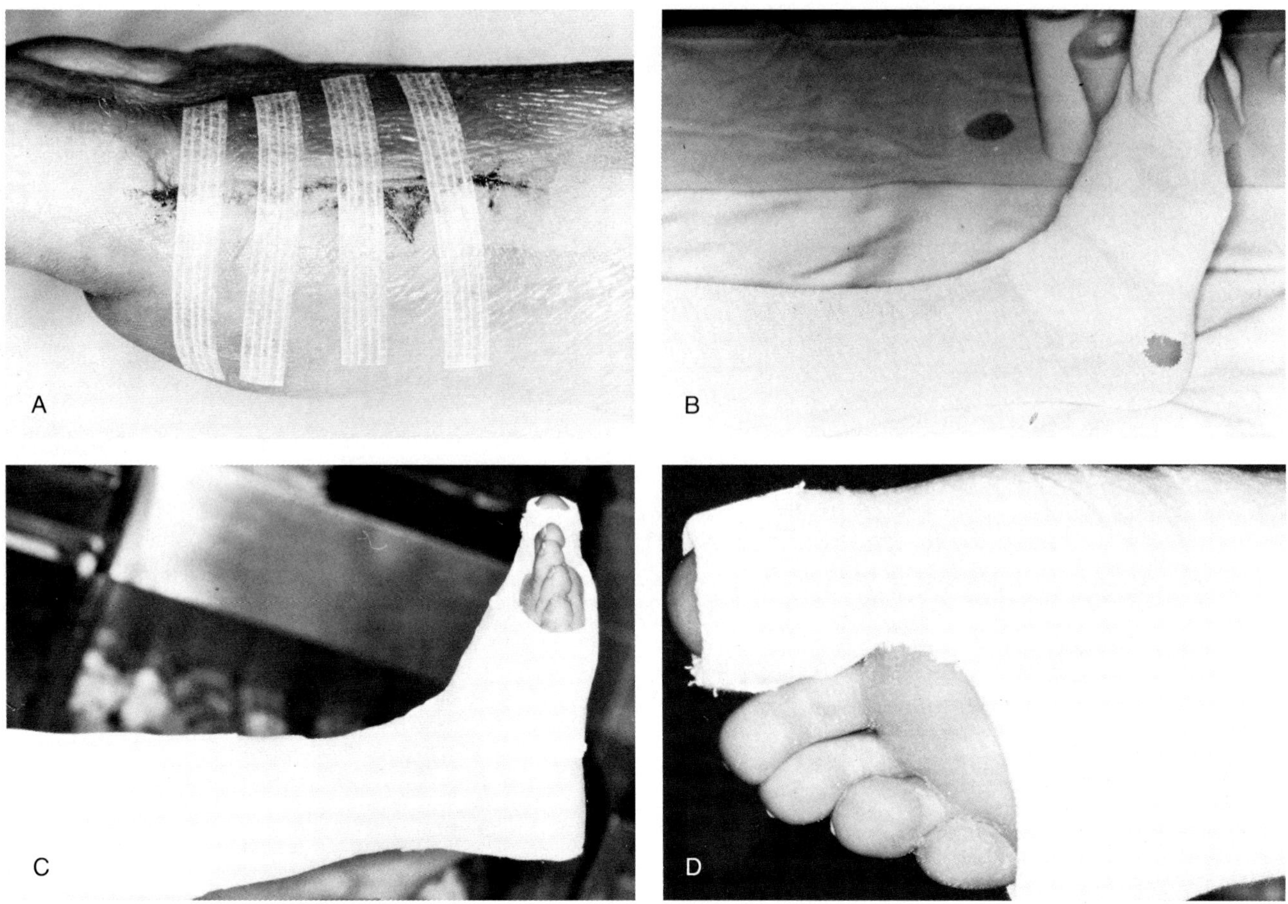

Fig. 8–16. The making of a short-leg great toe spica cast. *A*. Two weeks after a Mitchell's bunionectomy, stitches have been removed and several Steri-Strips have been applied to the incision site. *B*, A 4″ stockinet has been applied to the leg, and the 4″ and 1″ Webril bandages are ready to be applied to the lower leg and great toe. *C*, The 6″ and 1″ plaster bandages and the 2 5″ × 30″ plaster splints have been applied to the whole lower leg. *D*, Bottom view of the finished cast. The great toe is held in a neutral position in order to avoid development of hallux extensus or hallux varus.

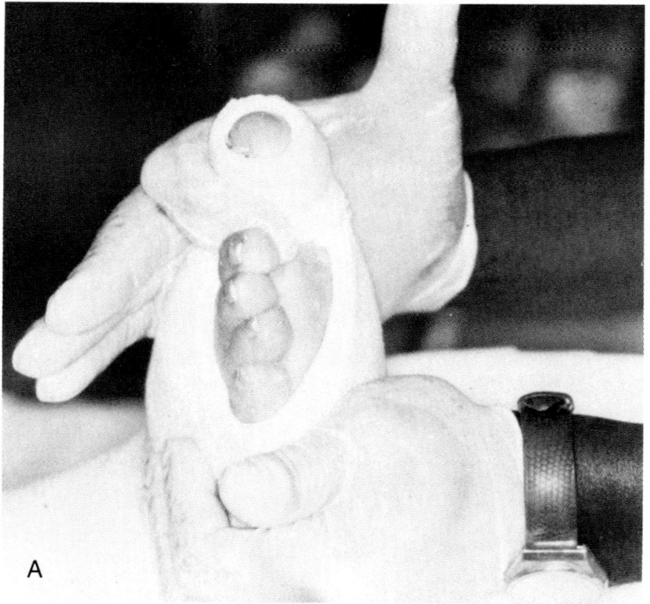

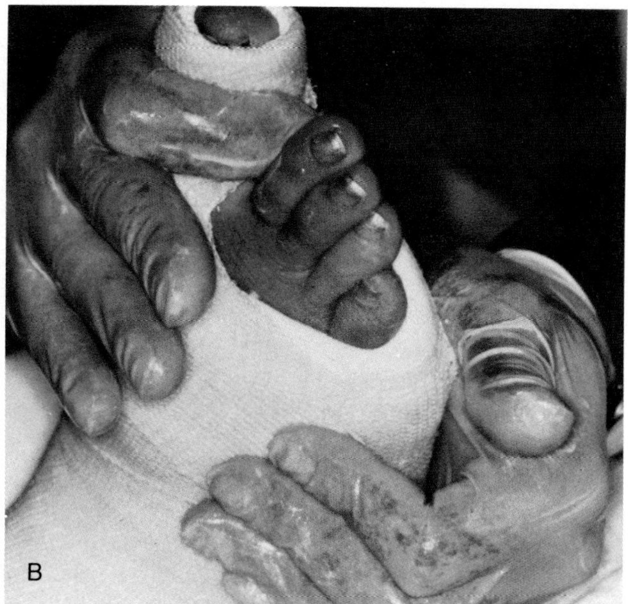

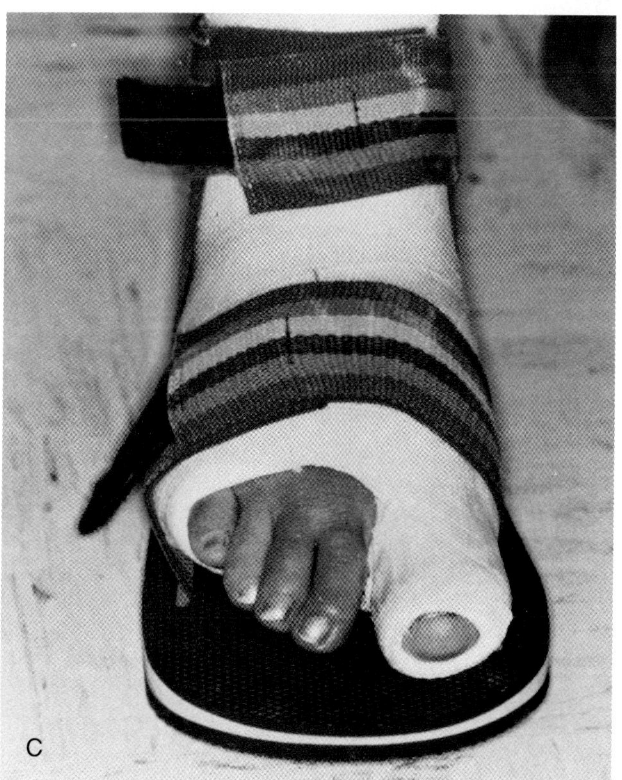

Fig. 8–17. *A, B,* A fiberglass short-leg great toe spica cast has been applied, and the cast technician is using his thumb and index finger to mold the cast around the great toe and to maintain good alignment between the great toe and lesser toes. *C,* Anterior view of the finished cast in a cast sandal.

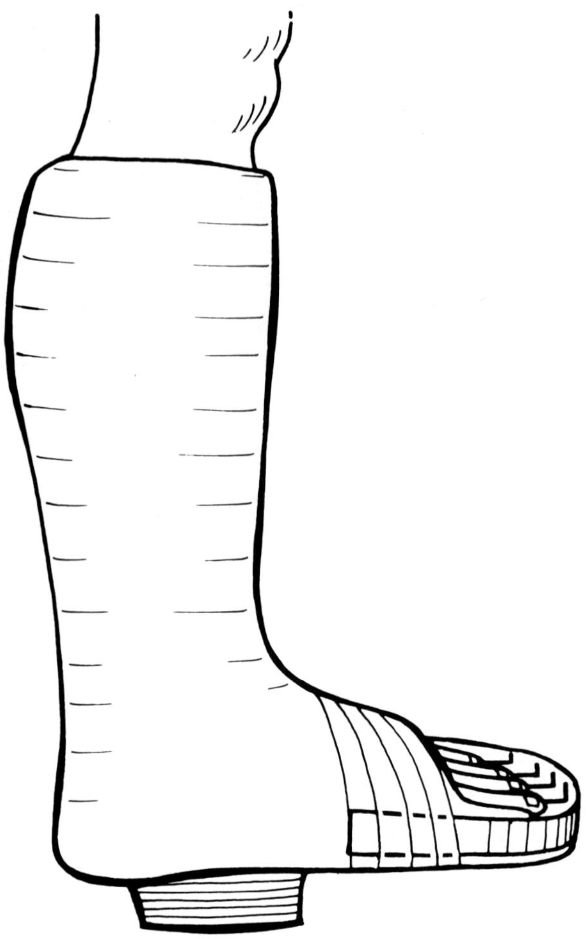

Fig. 8– 18. A short-leg great toe spica cast with a toe guard to protect the K-wires protruding from the toes.

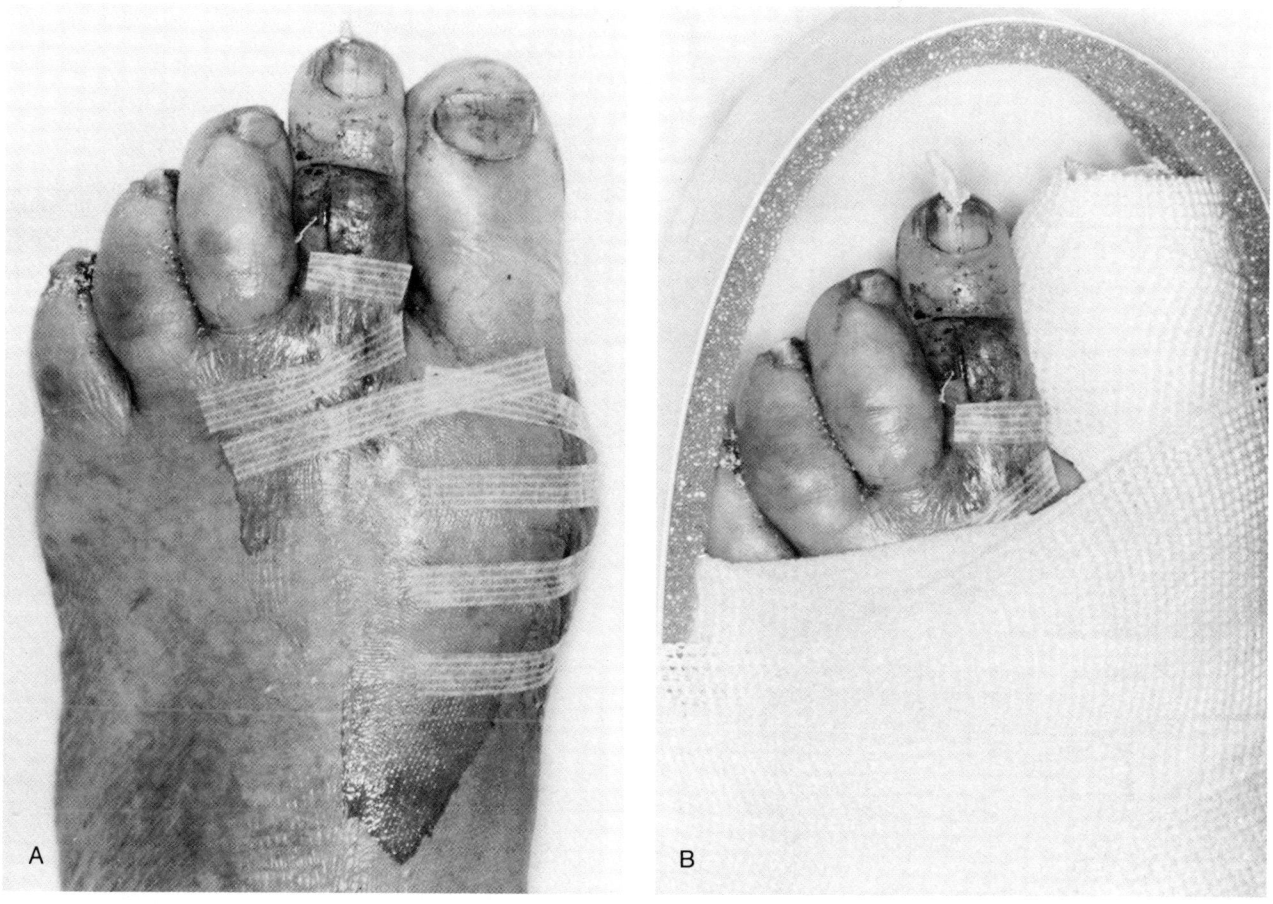

Fig. 8–19. *A*, Two weeks after a Mitchell's bunionectomy of the great toe and a hammertoe correction of the second toe. *B*, A short-leg great toe spica cast with a toe guard has been applied to the same foot.

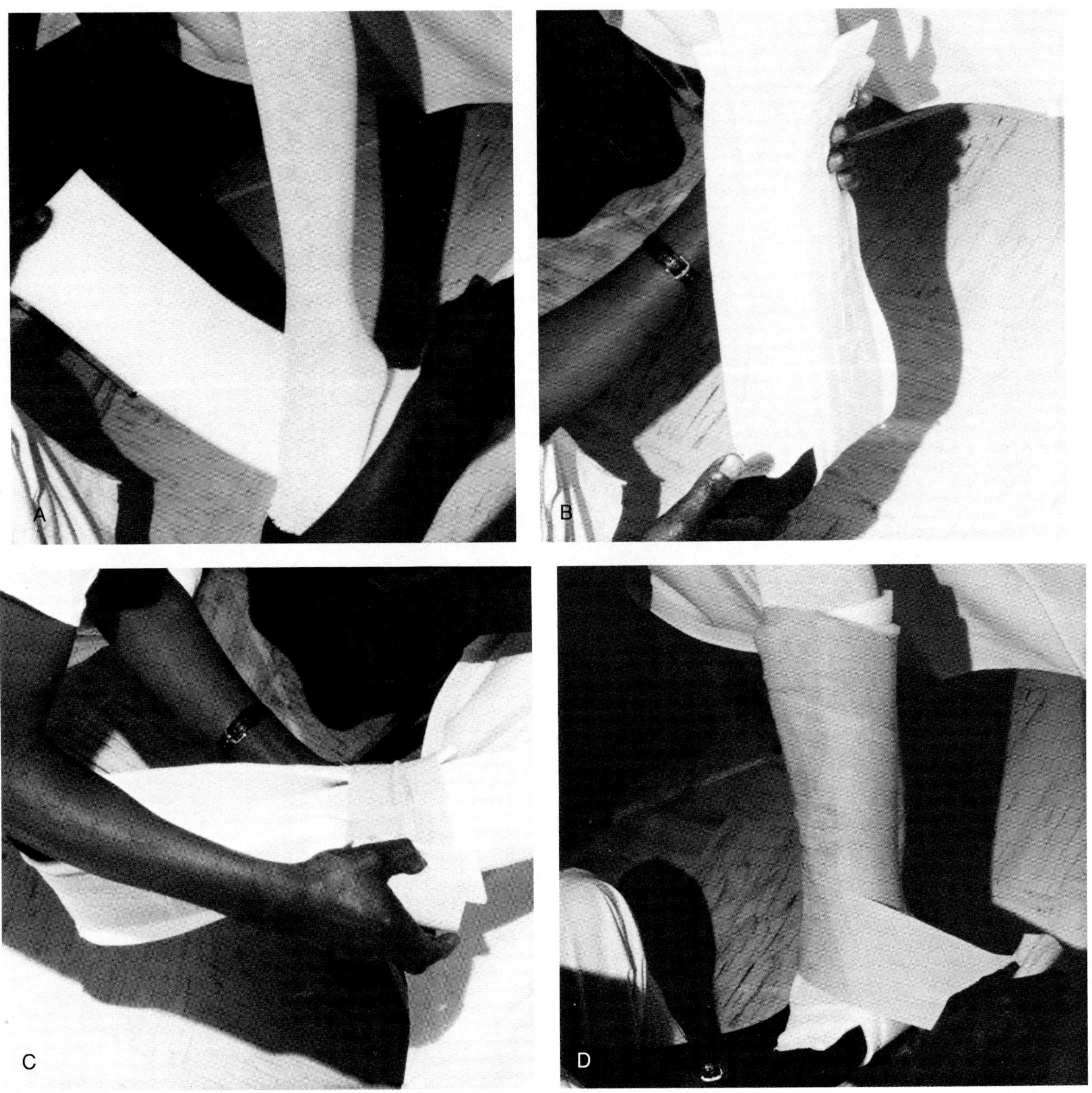

Fig. 8–20. The making of a fiberglass short-leg inversion-eversion splint. *A*, *B*, Application of a 4″ stockinet and a padded fiberglass splint to the lower leg. *C*, *D*, Application of a roll of 4″ Ace bandage to bind the splint to the lower leg.

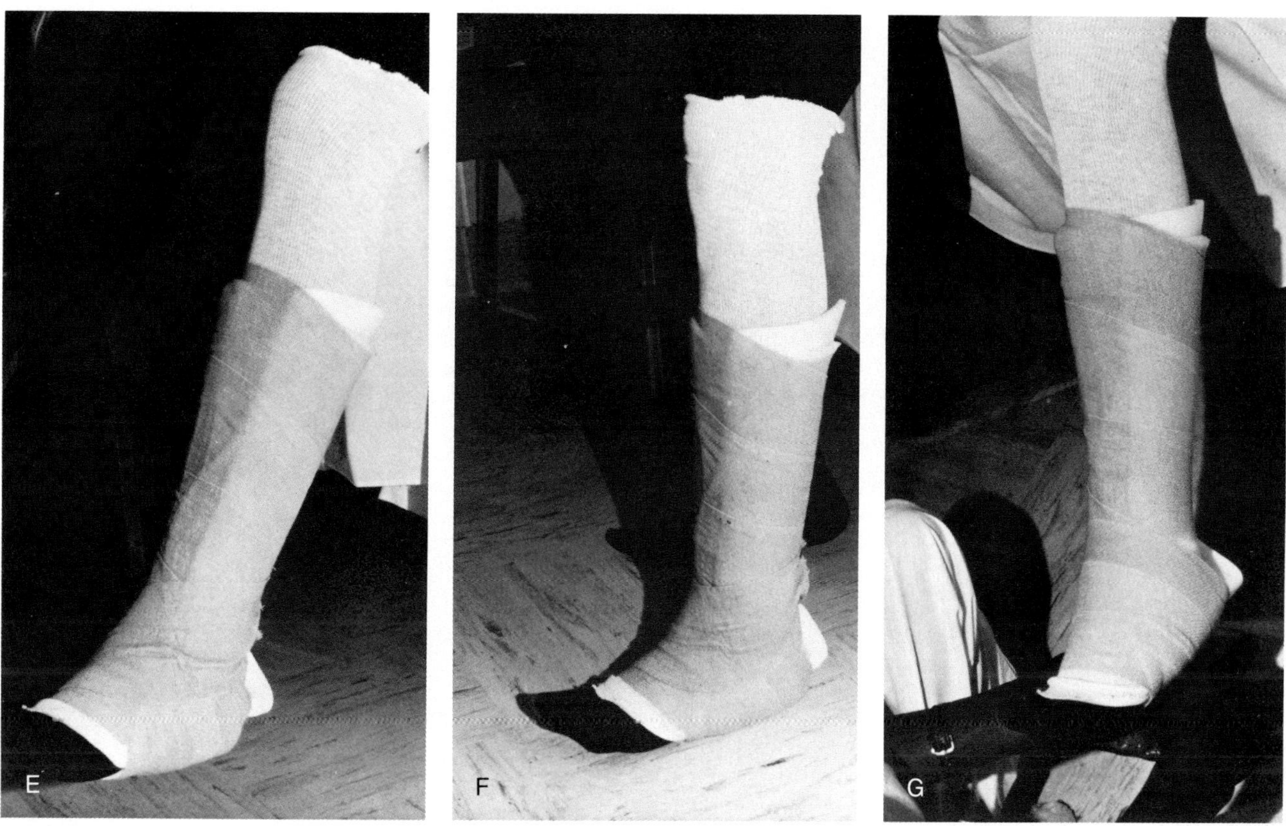

Fig. 8–20 (cont.). *E*, Splint held in place with Ace bandage. *F, G*, The patient is asked to put full weight on the splint, and the splint is carefully molded to fit the contour of the lower leg.

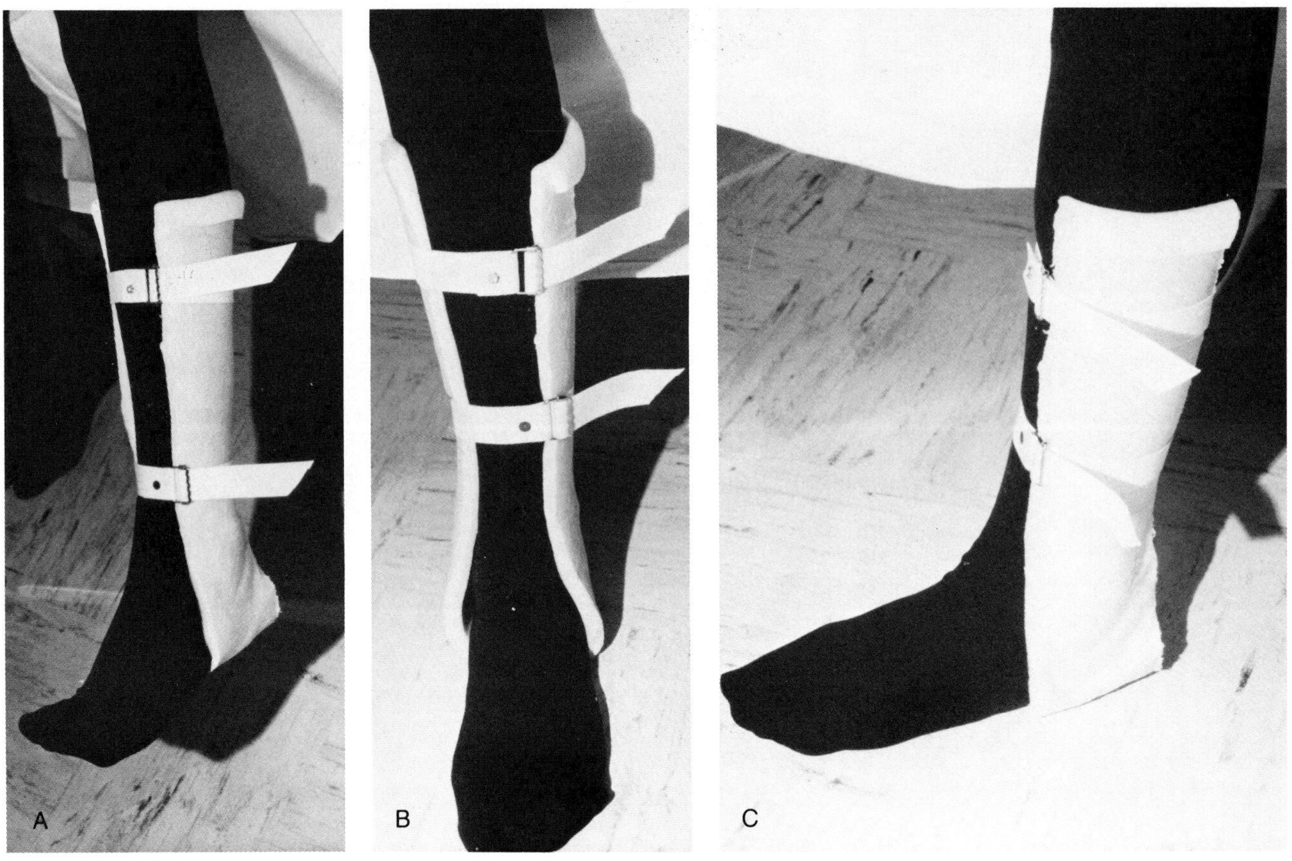

Fig. 8–21. Oblique (*A*), anterior (*B*), and lateral (*C*) views of a removable fiberglass short-leg inversion-eversion splint with two attached webbings and buckles.

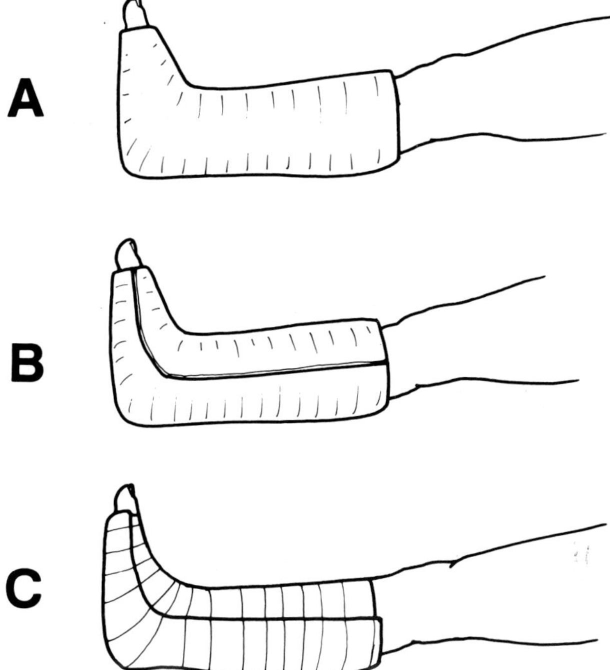

Fig. 8–22. Making of a posterior short-leg splint. *A*, A short-leg cast. *B*, The short-leg cast has been bivalved. *C*, The top half of the cast has been discarded. The bottom half has been lined with moleskin and reapplied to the lower leg and is held in place with an Ace bandage.

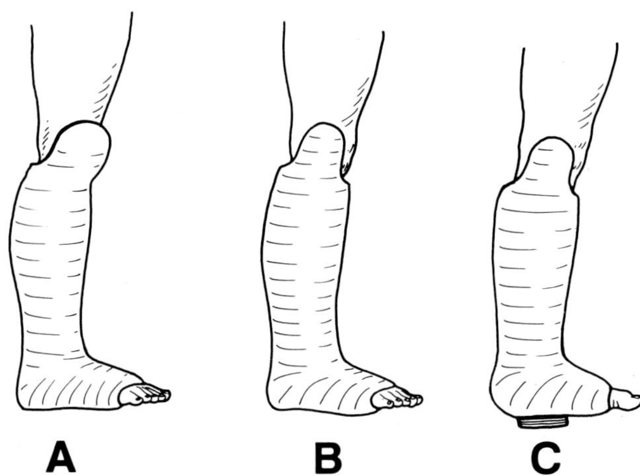

Fig. 8–23. Two main types of PTB cast. *A*, A PTB cast with a transverse indentation at the level of the patellar tendon and the anterosuperior aspect of the cast going over the patella. *B*, A PTB cast with its anterosuperior aspect terminated at the level of the patellar tendon and its two supracondylar flanges radiating upward and then backward and downward from a circular notch over the patellar tendon. *C*, A PTB cast with an infrapatellar notch fitted with a cast cushion.

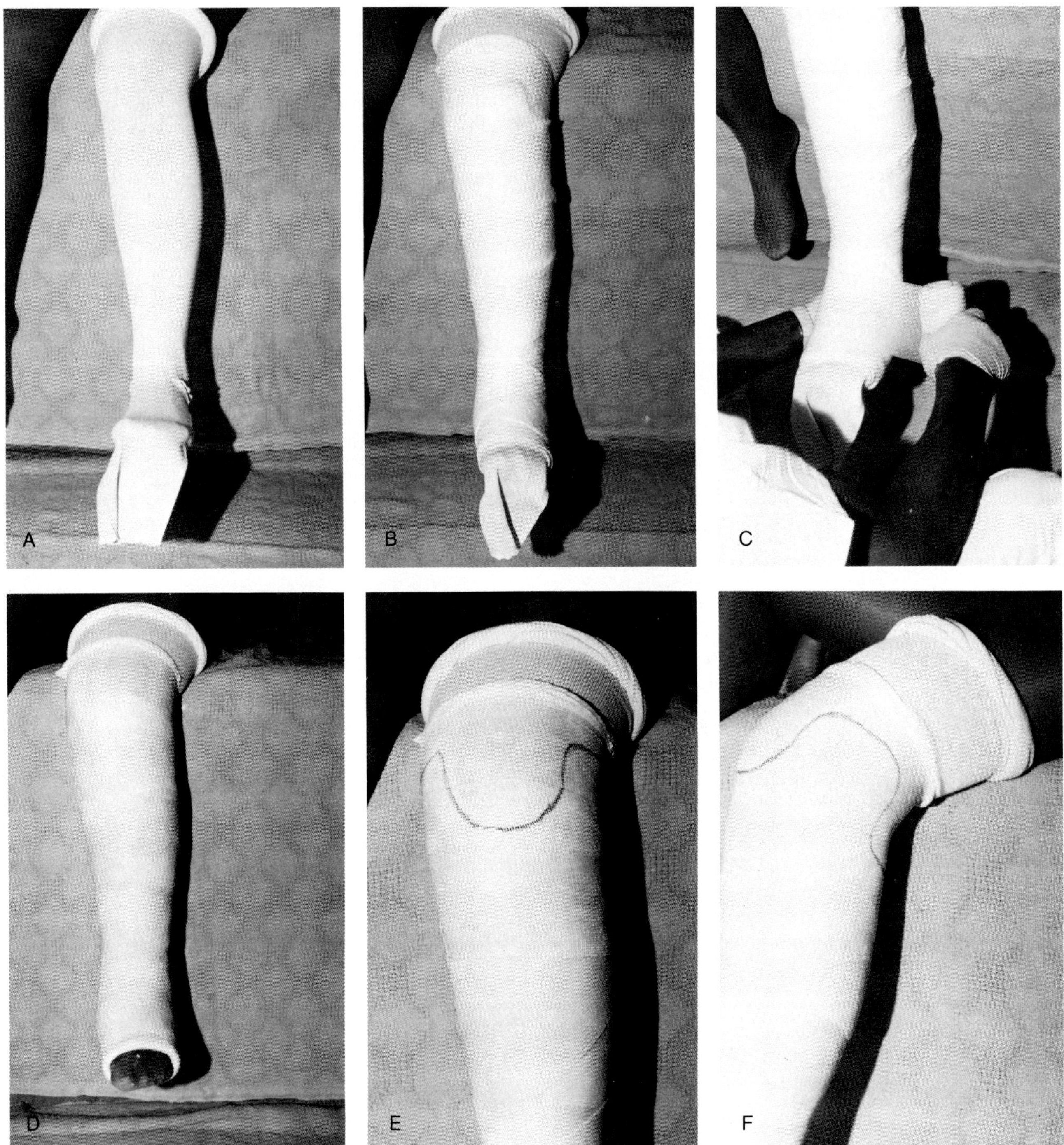

Fig. 8–24. The making of a fiberglass PTB cast. *A*, A 4″ stockinet has been applied to the leg from the toes to the mid-thigh region. *B*, 4″ Webril bandages have been applied to the leg from the bases of the toes to the mid-thigh region. *C*, *D*, Fiberglass bandages have been applied to the leg, indentations have been made over the patellar tendon and below the popliteal crease, and the cast has been molded around the medial and lateral femoral condyles. *E*, *F*, The upper end of the cast has been marked with a wax pencil.

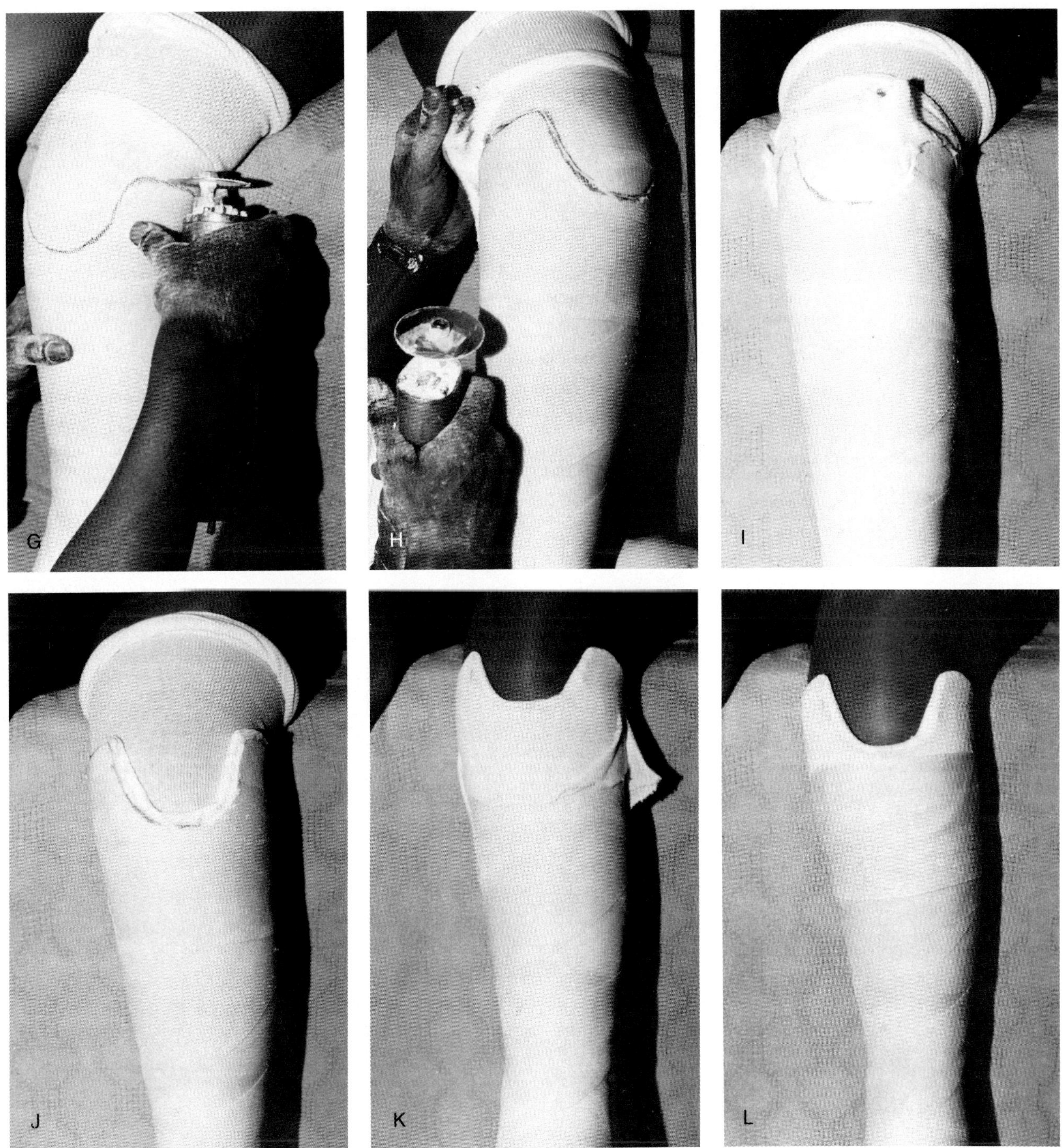

Fig. 8–24 (cont.). *G, H, I,* The redundant material above the upper margins of the cast is removed with a cast saw. *J, K, L,* The 2 stockinet ends are pulled tightly over the proximal and distal ends of the cast, and a roll of 3″ fiberglass bandage is used to go over the whole cast to finish it.

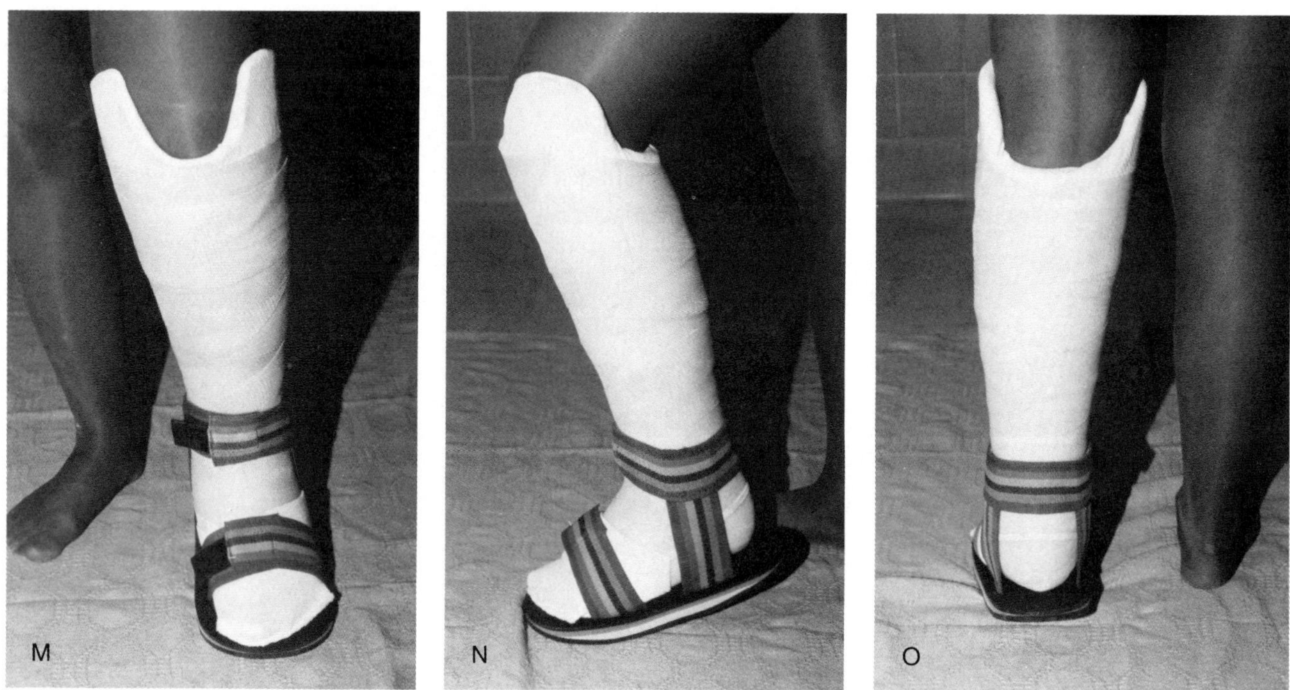

Fig. 8–24 (cont.). *M, N, O,* Anterior, lateral, and posterior views of the finished PTB cast and its cast sandal.

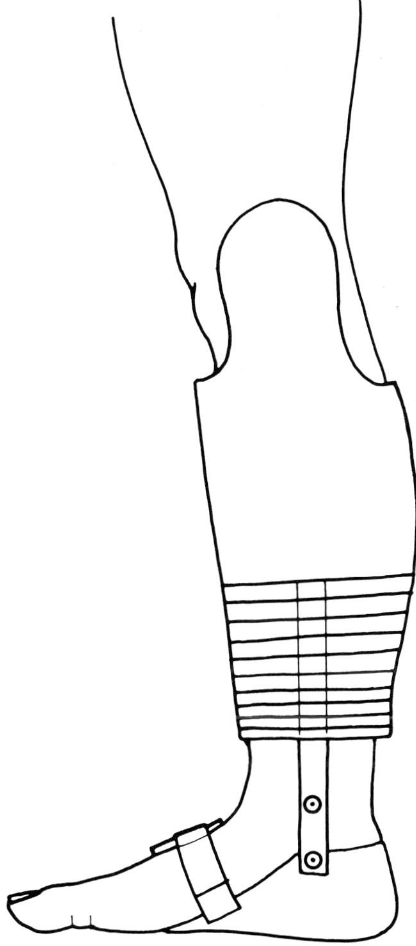

Fig. 8–25. A PTB cast with a heel cup and two ankle hinges.

CHAPTER 9. LONG-LEG CASTS, CAST-BRACES, AND SPLINTS

LONG-LEG CAST

A long-leg cast is illustrated in Fig. 9-1.

Indications

A long-leg cast is used for fractures and dislocations of the knee and ankle joints and for fractures of the tibia, fibula, and the distal end of the femur. As a rule, when an unstable fracture is below the knee, the short-leg portion of the cast should be applied first to stabilize the fracture before extending the cast to the upper thigh region (Fig. 9-2). If the fracture is above the knee joint, a long-leg cylinder cast should be applied first to stabilize the fracture before adding the foot part of the cast to the long-leg cast (Fig. 9-3).

Cast Materials Needed

Plaster Long-Leg Cast

4″ stockinet

5 rolls of 4″ Webril

2 5″ × 30″ plaster splints

5 rolls of 6″ plaster bandage

Fiberglass Long-Leg Cast

4″ stockinet

5 rolls of 4″ Webril

6 rolls of 5″ fiberglass bandage

Patient's Position

A long-leg cast is best applied with the patient in a supine position, the leg supported by a leg stand.

Technique for Applying a Plaster Long-Leg Cast

Stockinet

A 4″ stockinet is applied to the leg from the groin to the toes (Fig. 9-4A).

Webril

Four rolls of 4″ Webril bandage are wrapped around the leg from the upper thigh to the ankle (Fig. 9-4B).

Plaster Bandage

Two rolls of 6″ plaster bandage are applied from the upper thigh to the ankle (Fig. 9-4C). After 2 5″ × 30″ plaster splints have been applied to the posterior aspect of the whole leg, the upper stockinet end is turned down over the proximal cast end and 2 more rolls of 6″ plaster bandage are used to cover the whole cast down to the ankle (Fig. 9-4D).

Webril and Plaster Bandage for the Foot Region

After the transverse stockinet crease in front of the ankle has been removed, the foot and ankle are covered with the 5th roll of 4″ Webril bandage. Then the 5th roll of 6″ plaster bandage is used to cover the foot and ankle to complete the long-leg cast (Fig. 9-4E–I).

Technique for Applying a Fiberglass Long-Leg Cast

The technique for applying a fiberglass long-leg cast is similar to that for applying a plaster long-leg cast except that splints are omitted and 6 rolls of 5″ fiberglass bandage are used instead of 5 rolls of 6″ plaster bandage (Fig. 9-5).

Bivalving a Long-Leg Cast

A long-leg cast can be bivalved easily by longitudinally splitting a long-leg cast along its medial and lateral aspects with a cast saw, cutting the underlying Webril and stockinet, lining the margins of the bivalved cast with moleskin, reapplying the bivalved cast to the injured leg, and holding the bivalved cast together with Velcro straps or webbings and buckles (Fig. 9-6).

LONG-LEG WALKING CAST

A long-leg walking cast is made either by attaching a cast cushion to the bottom of a long-leg cast (Fig. 9-7) or by putting a long-leg cast into a cast sandal. A detailed description of how to apply a cast cushion to the bottom of a cast has been given in the section of Chapter 8 dealing with the short-leg walking cast.

LONG-LEG SPLINT

A long-leg splint can be made easily by bivalving a long-leg cast, discarding the top half of the cast, lining the bottom half of the cast with moleskin, reapplying the fully lined bottom half of the cast to the injured leg, and holding it in place with an Ace bandage (Figs. 9-8, 9-9).

LONG-LEG CYLINDER CAST

A long-leg cylinder cast is illustrated in Fig. 9-10.

Indications

A long-leg cylinder cast is used for patellar fractures and injuries of the knee region.

Cast Materials Needed

Plaster Long-Leg Cylinder Cast

4″ stockinet

3 rolls of 4″ Webril

2 rolls of 6″ plaster bandage

2 5″ × 30″ plaster splints

Fiberglass Long-Leg Cylinder Cast

4″ stockinet

3 rolls of 4″ Webril

2 rolls of 5″ fiberglass bandage

Patient's Position

The patient is placed in a supine position with the heel resting on a foot stand to support the whole leg.

Technique for Applying a Fiberglass Long-Leg Cylinder Cast

Stockinet

A 4″ stockinet is applied from the foot to the upper end of the thigh (Fig. 9-11A). Tincture of benzoin or other skin adhesive should be applied to the stockinet to make it stick to the underlying skin to prevent sliding of the cast.

Webril

Three rolls of 4″ Webril bandage are wrapped around the leg from the upper thigh to the malleolar region (Fig. 9-11B).

Fiberglass Bandage

One roll of 5″ fiberglass bandage is applied to the leg from the upper thigh to the supramalleolar region. The 2 stockinet ends are folded down over the proximal and distal cast ends, and another roll of 5″ fiberglass bandage is used to cover the whole cast. While the cast is still soft, both hands should be used to mold the mid-portion of the cast to fit the contour of the underlying patella and medial and lateral femoral condyles (Fig. 9-11C,D,E). For an obese patient with a sausage-shaped leg, the cylinder cast should be suspended from a waist belt in order to prevent skin irritation from slippage of the cast. The cast should be suspended by means of a 2″ webbing with a buckle, 1 end attached to the anterosuperior aspect of the cast and the other to the waist belt (Fig. 9-12).

Technique for Applying a Plaster Long-Leg Cylinder Cast

The technique for applying a plaster long-leg cylinder cast is similar to that for applying a fiberglass long-leg cylinder cast except that 2 rolls of 6″ plaster bandage and 2 5″ × 30″ plaster splints are used instead of the 2 rolls of 5″ fiberglass bandage. The 2 plaster splints are applied to the anterior and posterior aspects of the leg and are sandwiched between the 2 rolls of 6″ plaster bandage.

Bivalving a Long-Leg Cylinder Cast

A long-leg cylinder cast can best be bivalved by splitting the cast longitudinally along its medial and lateral aspects. Two triangular projections should be built into the bivalving cuts, 1 at thigh level on one side and the other at calf level on the other side, so that the 2 halves will not slide when they are put together. The margins of the cast should be lined with moleskin. The cast can then be reapplied to the injured leg and held in place by means of Velcro straps or webbings and buckles (Fig. 9-13).

LONG-LEG CAST-BRACE WITH KNEE HINGES

The basic steps in making a long-leg cast-brace with knee hinges are shown in Fig. 9-14.

Indications

A long-leg cast-brace with knee hinges is used for fractures of the tibia, fibula, and the distal end of the femur and for fractures and dislocations of the ankle.

Cast Materials Needed

Plaster Long-Leg Cast-Brace with Knee Hinges

4″ stockinet

5 rolls of 4″ Webril

2 5″ × 30″ plaster splints

5 rolls of 6″ plaster bandage

2 rolls of 4″ plaster bandage

2 polycentric knee hinges

Fiberglass Long-Leg Cast-Brace with Knee Hinges

4″ stockinet

5 rolls of 4″ Webril

6 rolls of 5″ fiberglass bandage

2 rolls of 4″ fiberglass bandage

2 polycentric knee hinges

Patient's Position

The patient's position is the same as for a long-leg cast.

Technique for Applying a Fiberglass Long-Leg Cast-Brace with Knee Hinges

Two 4″ transverse cuts, perpendicular to the longitudinal axes of the femur and tibia, and about 4″ from the center of the femoral condyles, are made in the medial and lateral aspects of the knee region of a long-leg cast (Fig. 9-15A,B). After the centers of 2 polycentric knee hinges have been placed over the centers of the femoral condyles with a fracture-brace alignment fixture, 2 rolls of 4″ fiberglass bandage are used to fix the 2 knee hinges to the distal femoral and proximal tibial portions of the cast (Fig. 9-15C–F). The knee section of the cast between the 4 transverse cuts is removed by linking these cuts circumferentially and by splitting the knee section of the cast longitudinally (Fig. 9-15G,H,I). After the exposed Webril in the knee region has been removed (Fig. 9-15J), a cast sandal can be applied to allow weight-bearing (Fig. 9-15K,L).

Technique for Applying a Plaster Long-Leg Cast-Brace with Knee Hinges

The technique for applying a plaster long-leg cast-brace with knee hinges is similar to that for applying a fiberglass long-leg cast-brace with knee hinges. After the knee section of the cast has been marked on the cast with 4 transverse cuts, the 2 polycentric knee hinges are fixed to the knee region with 2 rolls of 4″ plaster bandage. After the knee section of the cast and its underlying Webril have been removed, a cast cushion can be applied to the bottom of the foot portion of the cast to allow weight-bearing.

LONG-LEG CYLINDER CAST-BRACE WITH KNEE HINGES

Long-leg cylinder cast-braces with knee hinges allow flexion and extension of the knee but restrict varus and valgus as well as rotational stresses on the knee and are therefore useful in treating mild to moderate injuries of the knee. The construction of this cast begins with application of a regular long-leg cylinder cast; the 2 polycentric knee hinges are then installed by removing the knee section of the cast and fixing the 2 knee hinges to the cast by means of 2 rolls of 4″ plaster or fiberglass bandage (Fig. 9-16). When this cast-brace is used for an obese patient, a suspender should be used to attach the anterosuperior aspect of the cast to a waist belt (Fig. 9-17). If the need arises, a long-leg cylinder cast-brace can be bivalved by splitting it longitudinally along the midlines of its anterior and posterior surfaces (Fig. 9-18).

LONG-LEG CAST-BRACE WITH KNEE AND ANKLE HINGES

A long-leg cast-brace with knee and ankle hinges can be constructed by first making a long-leg cylinder cast-brace with knee hinges and then adding a heel cup with ankle hinges to the distal portion of the cast-brace (Fig. 9-19).

LONG-LEG CAST-BRACE WITH A MOLDED QUADRILATERAL SOCKET AND HEEL CUP AND ANKLE HINGES

Indications

A long-leg cast-brace with a molded quadrilateral socket and heel cup and ankle hinges is used for femoral fractures and for fractures and fusion of the knee joint. I currently use this cast for limb salvage operations of the knee region in which the femur and/or tibia and the surrounding muscles have to be excised en bloc and autogenous bone grafts have to be used to bridge the gap created by the resection. This cast allows partial weight-bearing a few days after the operation and protects the bone grafts during the many months required to incorporate them into the host bones.

Cast Materials Needed

Plaster Long-Leg Cast-Brace with a Molded Quadrilateral Socket and Heel Cup and Ankle Hinges

4″ stockinet

5 rolls of 4″ Webril

2 5″ × 30″ plaster splints

5 rolls of 6″ plaster bandage

1 roll of 3″ plaster bandage

1 heel cup with 2 attached ankle hinges

Fiberglass Long-Leg Cast-Brace with a Molded Quadrilateral Socket and Heel Cup and Ankle Hinges

4″ stockinet

5 rolls of 4″ Webril

6 rolls of 5″ fiberglass bandage

1 roll of 3″ fiberglass bandage

1 heel cup with 2 attached ankle hinges

Patient's Position

The whole long-leg portion of the cast can be applied easily with the patient in a recumbent position with the heel supported by a leg stand. However, the quadrilateral socket portion of the cast is best applied with the patient in a standing position so that accurate molding can be performed over the greater trochanter, ischial tuberosity, and femoral triangle.

Technique for Applying a Fiberglass Long-Leg Cast-Brace with a Molded Quadrilateral Socket and Heel Cup and Ankle Hinges

Stockinet

A 4″ stockinet is applied from the foot to the end of the upper thigh, where the medial aspect of the stockinet is cut longitudinally to allow the remainder of the stockinet to be pulled tightly upward to the lower abdominal region, where it can be held by the patient or taped to the iliac crest region with adhesive tape (Fig. 9-20A,B).

Webril

Four rolls of 4″ Webril are applied from the ankle to the upper end of the thigh, where 3 or 4 strips of Webril are applied from the anterior perineal crease, along the inguinal ligament to the top of the greater trochanter. Another 3 or 4 strips of 4″ Webril are applied from the top of the greater trochanter, obliquely across the lower part of the buttock to the ischial tuberosity and the posterior perineal crease (Fig. 9-20C).

Fiberglass Bandage

Five rolls of 5″ fiberglass bandage are applied to the leg from the supramalleolar region to the end of the thigh, and the sixth roll is used to wrap around the upper thigh, groin, and lower gluteal areas by going from the anterior perineal crease along the inguinal ligament to the top of the greater trochanter, where the fiberglass bandage proceeds in an oblique and downward direction to the ischial tuberosity and the posterior perineal crease. At least 4 layers of fiberlass bandage should be applied to the base of the thigh in order to make the quadrilateral socket strong enough for prolonged use. While the cast is still soft, the thumb should be used to make a large, shallow indentation over the femoral triangle. The upper end of the cast should also be molded carefully around the greater trochanter and ischial tuberosity (Fig. 9-10D,E). A heel cup can then be applied to the foot. A roll of 3″ fiberglass bandage is used to fix the ankle hinges to the distal end of the cast (Fig. 9-20F,G,H).

Technique for Applying a Plaster Long-Leg Cast-Brace with a Molded Quadrilateral Socket and Heel Cup and Ankle Hinges

Application of a plaster long-leg cast-brace with a molded quadrilateral socket and heel cup and ankle hinges is similar to that of its fiberglass counterpart except that 2 5″ × 30″ plaster splints and 5 rolls of 6″ plaster bandage replace the 6 rolls of 5″ fiberglass bandage in making the cast and a 3″ plaster bandage is used to fix the ankle hinges and heel cup to the distal end of the cast.

LONG-LEG CAST WITH A MOLDED QUADRILATERAL SOCKET

A long-leg cast with a molded quadrilateral socket is applied in the same manner as the long-leg cast-brace with a molded quadrilateral socket and heel cup and ankle hinges except that the Webril and plaster or fiberglass bandage extend to the bases of the toes (Fig. 9-21).

LONG-LEG CAST-BRACE WITH A MOLDED QUADRILATERAL SOCKET AND KNEE HINGES

A long-leg cast-brace with a molded quadrilateral socket and knee hinges is used primarily in treating femoral fractures. It is made by first applying a long-leg cast with a molded quadrilateral socket and then installing two polycentric knee hinges (Fig. 9-22).

LONG-LEG CAST-BRACE WITH A MOLDED QUADRILATERAL SOCKET AND KNEE AND ANKLE HINGES

A long-leg cast-brace with a molded quadrilateral socket and knee and ankle hinges allows knee and ankle motion and is used mainly in treating femoral fractures. It can be made by first applying a long-leg cast with a molded quadrilateral socket and then installing the two polycentric knee hinges and the two ankle hinges and heel cup (Fig. 9-23).

QUADRICEPS-TENDON-BEARING (QTB) THIGH CAST WITH A QUADRILATERAL SOCKET AND FEMORAL CONDYLAR FLANGES

Indications

A QTB thigh cast with a quadrilateral socket and femoral condylar flanges is used mainly for treating femoral fractures after these fractures have produced enough fracture callus to become partially stabilized (Fig. 9-24). In addition, this cast can be used in treating unstable, comminuted, and segmental femoral fractures by incorporating Steinmann pins into it (Fig. 9-25).

Cast Materials Needed

Plaster QTB Thigh Cast with a Quadrilateral Socket and Femoral Condylar Flanges

4″ stockinet

3 rolls of 4″ Webril

2 5″ × 30″ plaster splints

2 rolls of 6″ plaster bandage

Fiberglass QTB Thigh Cast with a Quadrilateral Socket and Femoral Condylar Flanges

4″ stockinet

3 rolls of 4″ Webril

2 rolls of 5″ fiberglass bandage

1 roll of 4″ fiberglass bandage

Patient's Position

The thigh portion of the cast can be applied with the patient either supine or standing, but the quadrilateral socket is best applied with the patient in a standing position in order to get a snug fit at the base of the thigh.

Technique for Applying a QTB Thigh Cast with a Molded Quadrilateral Socket and Femoral Condylar Flanges

Stockinet

A 4″ stockinet is applied from the proximal tibial region to the base of the thigh, where the stockinet is split longitudinally along its medial aspect so that the anterior, lateral, and posterior aspects of the stockinet can be pulled tightly upward to cover the lower abdominal, iliac, and gluteal regions. This proximal stockinet end can be held up by the patient or taped to the body with adhesive tape. Tincture of benzoin or other skin adhesive should be applied to the whole stockinet to make it stick to the underlying skin.

Webril

Three rolls of 4″ Webril are applied to the thigh from the proximal tibial region to the base of the thigh. To make the base of the quadrilateral socket fit the pelvic bones snugly, 3 strips of 4″ Webril should be applied obliquely to the groin area starting from the anterior half of the perineal crease and following the inguinal ligament to the top of the greater trochanter. Another 3 strips of 4″ Webril are applied from the top of the greater trochanter going obliquely in a downward, medial direction across the lower portion of the gluteal region to the ischial tuberosity and then the posterior half of the perineal crease to overlap the ends of the anterior Webril strips (Fig. 9-26A,B).

Fiberglass Bandage

The 2 rolls of 5″ fiberglass bandage should be wrapped evenly around the thigh from the level of the proximal tibia to the base of the thigh, where the bandage should closely and evenly follow the perineal crease, the inguinal ligament, the top of the greater trochanter, the inferior gluteal region, and the ischial tuberosity back to the perineal crease; 3 or 4 layers of bandage are required to produce a strong, smooth upper end for the quadrilateral socket. While the fiberglass is still soft, 3 shallow indentations should be made in the cast in order that the upper end of the cast fit snugly: 1 over the femoral triangle, another behind the greater trochanter, and the 3rd immediately below the ischial tuberosity. The distal end of the cast should be carefully molded around the patella and the medial and lateral femoral condyles.

A cast saw is used to cut the distal end of the cast around the superior pole and the medial and lateral borders of the patella and the medial and lateral femoral condyles and along a transverse line about 2 inches above the popliteal crease. A liberal amount of plastic adhesive is applied to the femoral condylar flanges and the adjacent distal portion of the cast, and the distal end of the stockinet is split longitudinally and then tightly pulled over the distal cast end to stick to the femoral condylar flanges and the adjacent distal portion of the cast. The opposite stockinet end is folded down over the proximal end of the cast, and a roll of 4″ fiberglass bandage is used to fix the 2 stockinet ends to the cast (Fig. 9-26C–F).

OUTRIGGER LONG-LEG CAST

An outrigger long-leg cast is illustrated in Fig. 9-27.

Indications

I invented the outrigger long-leg cast to take care of severe and extensive injuries of the soft tissues and bones of the lower leg caused by automobile and motorcycle accidents, shotgun blasts at close range, and high-power rifle bullets. The cast keeps the leg elevated, holds the fracture site in good alignment, and provides unobstructed access to the open wound. The whole tibial section of the cast can be removed if the need arises, and a wide felt or canvas sling can be used to support the lower leg by attaching the sling to the superior outrigger bar.

Cast Materials Needed

4″ stockinet

5 rolls of 4″ Webril

8 5″ × 30″ plaster splints

5 rolls of 6″ plaster bandage

3 rolls of 3″ plaster bandage

Patient's Position

The cast is applied with the patient in a supine position.

Technique for Applying an Outrigger Long-Leg Cast

The first step is to apply a standard plaster long-leg cast (Fig. 9-28A). Next, 2 5″ × 30″ plaster splints are rolled into a rope with both hands, and the 2 ends of this plaster rope are attached to the dorsum of the foot portion of the cast and the anterior aspect of the distal thigh portion of the cast by means of 3 or 4 wrappings of 3″ plaster bandage. While this plaster rope is still soft, it can be molded into the shape of a C-clamp with 2 short vertical sections and a long horizontal section (Fig. 9-28B,C). When this superior outrigger bar has hardened, a leg stand is placed under the heel portion of the cast to elevate the whole leg, and 2 more plaster ropes of similar construction are attached, from the lateral aspect of the heel portion of the cast to the lateral aspect of the upper thigh portion of the cast and from the medial aspect of the heel portion of the cast to the medial aspect of the upper thigh portion of the cast. While these 2 plaster ropes are being hardened, their bottom parts are spread apart and made parallel to the surface of the casting table. The ends of these 2 bottom outriggers are fixed to the heel and upper thigh portions of the long-leg cast with 3″ plaster bandages (Fig. 9-28D). After the whole cast is completely set, a large window (or the whole tibial section of the cast) can be removed to give access to an open wound (Fig. 9-28E).

CAST WEDGING

Cast wedging is a useful method of correcting fracture angulations. The transverse cut through the cast should pass through the point where the two longitudinal axes of the two major fracture fragments intersect. There are four major ways of wedging a cast:

Opening Wedging. Opening wedging produces tension on the concave side of the fracture and compression on the convex side, where the plaster may buckle inward to cause skin necrosis (Fig. 9-29).

Closing Wedging. Closing wedging creates some tension on the concave side of the fracture and a significant amount of compression on the convex side, where the sharp plaster edges can dig into the underlying skin to produce ulceration (Fig. 9-30).

Combined Opening/Closing Wedging. Combined opening/closing wedging can be used to correct severe fracture angulation and may reduce the chance of producing pressure skin necrosis on the convex side of the fracture (Fig. 9-31).

Circumferential Wedging. Circumferential wedging is the method I prefer for correcting angular or rotational deformities of fractures. The cast is cut circumferentially, and by applying traction to both sides of the fracture, shortening, angulation, and malrotation of the fracture can be corrected easily by applying various correcting forces to the fracture site (Fig. 9-32A,B,C). The configuration of the fracture site can be checked with an image intensifier. When a satisfactory fracture reduction has been achieved, a roll of 4″ plaster bandage is used to repair the transected cast. To eliminate skin necrosis caused by the displaced edges of the transected cast, a 4″ × 4″ plaster window should be cut out of the 2 sides of the cast containing the step-off cast edges, and 2 pieces of 4″ × 4″ felt should be placed into these 2 windows. A 4″ plaster bandage should be used to cover these 2 felt pads and the adjacent cast to make the cast strong and free of pressure points (Fig. 9-32D,E,F).

In any kind of cast wedging, it is possible that a pressure point will be created on the convex side of the fracture. Therefore, in order to avoid the unpleasant occurrence of pressure skin necrosis, it is a good idea to take out a 4″ × 4″ piece of cast material from the convex side of the fracture on a routine basis (Fig. 9-33).

Many open and comminuted fractures require meticulous debridement and washing of the fracture sites under direct vision. This requirement provides one with a golden opportunity to achieve an anatomical reduction that can be maintained easily with transfixing K-wires. Several Steinmann pins can then be driven through the major bone fragments of the fracture, and these Steinmann pins can be incorporated into a cast to stabilize the fracture. After the fracture reduction has been securely obtained through the use of Steinmann pins and a cast, the K-wires can be withdrawn from the fracture sites (Fig. 9-34).

CORRECTION OF JOINT CONTRACTURE BY MEANS OF CAST WEDGING

Cast wedging is a good method for correcting joint contracture because correcting forces can be distributed to the whole leg through the cast; the joint contracture can be corrected without causing abnormally high pressure points on any portion of the leg except the joint itself. As a rule, cast wedging is most commonly employed in correcting a flexion contracture of the knee. I usually use a double Y-shaped cut through about 75% of the circumference of the cast in the knee joint region so that the cut edges of the cast will not cause a pressure problem (Fig. 9-35A). While the cut edges are separated with a cast spreader, a cast wedge is inserted into the open space (Fig. 9-35B, C). By gradually increasing the width of the inserted cast wedge, more and more correction of the flexion contracture of the knee can be obtained over time.

Another method for correcting a flexion contracture of the knee is to attach a turnbuckle device to the cast on the posterior aspect of the knee joint. By turning the turnbuckle to increase its length, the flexion contracture of the knee is proportionally corrected. The size of the turnbuckle required to correct the flexion contracture is also proportional to the severity of the flexion contracture (Fig. 9-36).

WINDOWING A CAST

One may window a cast either to provide pressure relief or to facilitate inspection and treatment of an open wound. As a rule, in order to prevent the development of cast window edema (which may lead to serious skin necrosis), the rectangular plaster removed from a window has to be put back into the window after a piece of felt has been placed in the window. After the window in the cast is properly covered, an Ace bandage is commonly wrapped around the windowed portion of the cast (Fig. 9-37).

Before a large window is removed from a cast, a 5″ × 30″ splint and a roll of 6″ plaster bandage should be applied to the part of the cast exactly opposite to the cast window so that the cast will not break after the cast window has been made (Fig. 9-38).

CAST SLEEVING

Cast sleeving is a casting technique by which a cast greatly weakened by a large cast window can be protected from breakage, yet an open wound under the cast window can be treated with ease at frequent intervals. As in any other windowed cast, a felt pad is usually placed in the window, followed by the original plaster piece. A roll of 6″ Webril bandage is used to wrap the windowed portion of the cast to a level of about 1 or 2 inches beyond the proximal and distal margins of the cast window. Next, a roll of 6″ plaster bandage is used to cover all the Webril and to extend about 1 inch beyond the proximal and distal margins of the Webril bandage (Fig. 9-39). Whenever the wound has to be inspected or treated, the plaster sleeve can be removed easily by splitting it longitudinally; the cast window soon comes into view after the overlying Webril bandage has been removed.

BIBLIOGRAPHY

Allum, R.L., and Mowbray, M.A.S.: A retrospective review of the healing of fractures of the shaft of the tibia with special reference to the mechanism of injury. Injury, *11*:304, 1980.

Anderson, L.D., Hutchins, W.C., Wright, M.D., and Disney, J.M.: Fractures of the tibia and fibula treated by casts and transfixing pins. Clin. Orthop., *105*:179, 1974.

Apley, A.G.: Fractures of the tibial plateau. Orthop. Clin. North Am., *10*:61, 1979.

Barquet, A.: Posterior dislocation of the ulna at the elbow with associated fracture of the distal shaft. Injury, *15*:390, 1984.

Bassett, C.A., Mitchell, S.N., and Gaston, S.R.: Treatment of ununited tibial diaphyseal fractures with pulsing electromagnetic fields, J. Bone Joint Surg. [Am.], *63*:511, 1981.

Bassett, F.H., Beck, J.L., and Weiker, G.: A modified cast brace: Its use in non-operative and postoperative management of serious knee ligament injuries. Am. J. Sports Med., *8*:63, 1980.

Beach, R.B.: Management of a femur fracture using a patellar tendon bearing cast-brace. Phys. Ther., *57*:655, 1977.

Bergquist, R.J.: Brace conversion: Long leg to short leg. Phys. Ther., *53*:1071, 1973.

Blair, W.F., and Pontarelli, W.R.: Ambulatory dynamic patellar traction for patellar reconstruction. Clin. Orthop., *169*:145, 1982.

Borgen, D., and Sprague, B.L.: Treatment of distal femoral fractures with early weight-bearing. A preliminary report. Clin. Orthop., *111*:156, 1975.

Bowes, D., and Hohl, M.: Tibial condylar fractures. Evaluation of treatment and outlook. Clin. Orthop., *171*:104, 1982.

Bowker, P., Pratt, D.J., McLauchlan, J., and Wardlaw, D.: Early weight-bearing treatment of femoral shaft fractures using a cast-brace: A preliminary biomechanical study. J. Bioeng., *2*:463, 1978.

Brau, E.A.: Open fractures: Fundamentals of management. Postgrad. Med., *39*:11, 1966.

Brighton, C.T., et al.: A multi-center study of the treatment of non-union with constant direct current. J. Bone Joint Surg. [Am.], *63*:2, 1981.

Brown, G.A., and Sprague, B.L.: Cast brace treatment of plateau and bicondylar fractures of the proximal tibia. Clin. Orthop., *119*:184, 1976.

Brown, P.E., and Preston, E.T.: Ambulatory treatment of femoral shaft fractures with cast brace. J. Trauma, *15:*860, 1975.
Brown, P.W., and Urgan, J.G.: Early weight-bearing treatment of open fractures of tibia. An end-result study of 63 cases. J. Bone Joint Surg. [Am.], *51:*59, 1969.
Cetti, R., Christensen, S.E., and Corfitzen, M.T.: Ruptured fibular ankle ligament. Plaster or pliton brace: Br. J. Sports Med., *18:*104, 1984.
Chacha, P.B., Ahmed, M., and Daruwalla, J.S.: Vascular pedicle graft of the ipsilateral fibula for non-union of the tibia with a large defect. An experimental and clinical study. J. Bone Joint Surg. [Br.], *63:*244, 1981.
Charnley, J., and Lowe, H.G.: A study of the end-results of compression arthrodesis of the knee. J. Bone Joint Surg. [Br.], *40:*633, 1958.
Connolly, J.F., Dehne, E., and LaFollette, B.: Closed reduction and early cast-brace ambulation in the treatment of femoral fractures. II. Results in one hundred and forty-three fractures. J. Bone Joint Surg. [Am.], *55:*1581, 1973.
Connolly, J.F., Dehne, E., and LaFollette, B.: Closed revision and early cast brace ambulation in the treatment of femoral shaft fractures. J. Bone Joint Surg. [Am.], *60:*112, 1978.
Connolly, J.F., and King, P.: Closed reduction and early cast-brace ambulation in the treatment of femoral fractures. 1. An in vivo quantitative analysis of immobilization in skeletal traction and a cast-brace. J. Bone Joint Surg. [Am.], *55:*1559, 1973.
Crotwell, W.H., III.: The thigh-lacer: Ambulatory non-operative treatment of femoral shaft fractures. J. Bone Joint Surg. [Am.], *60:*112, 1978.
Daniel, E., and Rice, T.: Valgus-varus stability in the hinged cast used for controlled mobilization of the knee. J. Bone Joint Surg. [Am.], *61:*135, 1979.
Dehne, E.: Ambulatory treatment of the fractured tibia. Clin. Orthop., *105:*192, 1974.
DeLee, J.C.: Ipsilateral fracture of the femur and tibia treated in a quadrilateral cast brace. Clin. Orthop., *142:*115, 1979.
DeLee, J.C., Clanton, T.O., and Rockwood, C.A., Jr.: Closed treatment of subtrochanteric fractures of the femur in a modified cast-brace. J. Bone Joint Surg. [Am.], *63:*773, 1981.
DeLee, J.C., and Stiehl, J.B.: Open tibia fracture with compartment syndrome. Clin. Orthop., *160:*175, 1981.
Dommisse, G.F.: Fractures of the tibial shaft. S. Afr. Med. J., *54:*1021, 1978.
Dowd, G.S.E.: Marginal fractures of the patella. Injury, *14:*287, 1982.
Drennan, D.B., Locher, F.G., and Maylahn, D.J.: Fractures of the tibial plateau. Treatment by closed reduction and spica cast. J. Bone Joint Surg. [Am.], *61:*989, 1979.
Elstrom, J., Pankovich, A.M., Sasson, H., and Rodriguez, J.: The use of tomography in the assessment of fractures of the tibial plateau. J. Bone Joint Surg. [Am.], *58:*551, 1976.
Garland, D.E., Chick, R., Taylor, J., and Salisbury, R.B.: Treatment of proximal-third femur fractures with pins and thigh plaster. Clin. Orthop., *160:*86, 1981.
Gross, R.H., et al.: Cast brace management of the femoral shaft fracture in children and young adults. J. Pediatr. Orthop., *3:*572, 1983.
Guess, V.A.: Plaster cuff-in splints to reduce knee flexion contracture in patients with chronic rheumatoid arthritis. Phys. Ther., *52:*634, 1972.
Guestilo, R.B., Simpson, L., Nixon, R., and Ruiz, A.: Analysis of 511 open fractures. Clin. Orthop., *66:*148, 1969.
Haggmark, T., and Eriksson, E.: Cylinder or mobile cast brace after knee ligament surgery. A clinical analysis and morphologic and enzymatic studies of changes in the quadriceps muscle. Am. J. Sports Med., *7:*48, 1979.
Halpenny, J., and Rorabeck, C.H.: Supracondylar fractures of the femur: Result of treatment of 61 patients. Can. J. Surg., *27:*606, 1984.
Hand, W.L., Hand, C.R., and Dunn, A.W.: Avulsion fractures of the tibial tubercle. J. Bone Joint Surg. [Am.], *53:*1579, 1971.
Hardy, A.E.: Pressure recordings in patients with femoral fractures in cast-braces and suggestions for treatment. J. Bone Joint Surg. [Am.], *61:*365, 1979.
Hardy, A.E.: Shortening and angulation of femoral shaft fractures treated by cast brace application and early ambulation. Clin. Orthop., *168:*139, 1982.
Hardy, A.E.: The treatment of femoral fractures by cast-bracing application and early ambulation. A prospective review of one hundred and six patients. J. Bone Joint Surg. [Am.], *65:*56, 1983.
Hardy, A.E., and Baddeley, S.: Pressure generated in the thigh muscles and under the thigh cast of an uninjured subject wearing a cast-brace. J. Bone Joint Surg. [Am.], *61:*362, 1979.
Hardy, A.E., White, P., and William, J.: The treatment of femoral fractures by cast-brace and early walking: A review of seventy-nine patients. J. Bone Joint Surg. [Br.], *61:*151, 1979.
Harrison, M.H., and Menon, M.P.: Legg-Calve-Perthes disease. The value of roentgenographic measurement in clinical practice with special reference to the broomstick plaster method. J. Bone Joint Surg. [Am.], *48:*1301, 1966.
Hastings, D.E.: The non-operative management of collateral ligament injuries of the knee joint. Clin. Orthop., *147:*22, 1980.

Herndon, J.H., Tolo, V.T., Langue, A.M., and Deffer, P.A.: Management of fractured femora in acute amputees. Results of early ambulation in a cast-brace and pylon. J. Bone Joint Surg. [Am.], *55:*1600, 1973.

Holm, C.L.: Management of humeral shaft fractures. Clin. Orthop., *71:*132, 1970.

Hughes, J.L., Weber, H., Willenegger, H., and Kuner, E.H.: Evaluation of ankle fractures. Clin. Orthop., *138:*111, 1979.

Hughston, J.C., Andrews, J.R., Cross, M.J., and Moschi, A.: Classification of knee ligament instabilities. Part I. The medial compartment and cruciate ligaments. J. Bone Joint Surg. [Am.], *58:*159, 1976.

Hughston, J.C., Andrews, J.R., Cross, M.J., and Moschi, A.: Classification of knee ligament instabilities. Part II. The lateral compartment. J. Bone Joint Surg. [Am.], *58:*173, 1976.

Hohl, M.:Tibial condylar fractures. J. Bone Joint Surg. [Am.], *49:*1455, 1967.

Iwegbu, C.G.: Preliminary results of treatment of fractures of the femur by cast-bracing using the Zaria metal hinge. Injury, *15:*250, 1984.

Karlstrom, G., and Olerud, S.: Percutaneous pin fixation of open tibial fractures. J. Bone Joint Surg. [Am.], *57:*915, 1975.

Key, J.A.: Arthrodesis of the knee with a large central autogenous bone peg. South. Med. J., *30:*524, 1937.

Kolmert, L., Egund, N., and Persson, B.M.: Internal fixation of supracondylar and bicondylar femoral fractures using a new semielastic device. Clin. Orthop., *181:*204, 1983.

Krackow, K.A., and Vetter, W.L.: Knee motion in a long leg cast. Am. J. Sports Med., *9:*233, 1981.

Kriegshauser, L.A., and Bryan, R.S.: Early motion with cast brace after modified Coventry high tibial osteotomy. Clin. Orthop., *195:*168, 1985.

Kumar, R.: Treatment of fracture of the femur in children by a "cast-brace". Int. Surg., *67:*551, 1982.

Lesin, B.E., Mooney, V., and Ashby, M.E.: Cast-bracing for fractures of the femur. A preliminary report of a modified device. J. Bone Joint Surg. [Am.], *59:*917, 1977.

Leung, P.C., Mak, K.H., and Lee, S.Y.: Percutaneous tension band wiring: A new method of internal fixation for mildly displaced patella fracture. J. Trauma, *23:*62, 1983.

McCollough, N.C., III., Vinsant, J.E., and Sarmiento, A.: Functional fracture bracing of long bone fractures of the lower extremity in children. J. Bone Joint Surg. [Am.], *60:*314, 1978.

McDaniel, W.J., and Wilson, F.C.: Trimalleolar fractures of the ankle. An end result study. Clin. Orthop., *122:*37, 1977.

McEachern, A.G., and Plewes, J.L.: Bilateral simultaneous, spontaneous rupture of the quadriceps tendons. Five case reports and a review of the literature. J. Bone Joint Surg. [Br.], *66:*81, 1984.

McLuor, J.B., Ross, P., Landry, G., and David, L.S.: Treatment of femoral fractures with the cast brace. Can J. Surg., *27:*592, 1984.

Matthewson, M.H., and Dandy, D.J.: Osteochondral fractures of the lateral femoral condyle: A result of indirect violence to the knee. J. Bone Joint Surg. [Br.], *60:*199, 1978.

Meggitt, B.F., Juett, D.A., and Dereksmith, S.J.: Cast bracing for fractures of the femoral shaft: A biomechanical and clinical study. J. Bone Joint Surg. [Br.], *63:*12, 1981.

Mital, M.A., and Bonadio, O.: Fractures of the shaft of the femur: Progress in treatment (1961–1971). Experience with conservative traction with ambulatory cast brace treatment in seventy-five patients. Am. J. Surg., *127:*434, 1974.

Mohl, J.H.: The cast brace walking treatment of open and closed femoral fractures. South Med. J., *66:*345, 1973.

Mooney, V., Nickel, V.L., Harvey, J.P., and Snelson, R.: Cast-brace treatment of fractures of the distal part of the femur. J. Bone Joint Surg. [Am.], *52:*1563, 1970.

Moore, T.M.: Fracture-dislocation of the knee. Clin. Orthop., *156:*128, 1981.

Nicholas, J.J., and Ziegler, G.: Cylinder splints: Their use in the treatment of arthritis of the knee. Arch. Phys. Med. Rehabil., *58:*264, 1977.

Nicoll, E.A.: Fractures of the tibial shaft. A survey of 705 cases. J. Bone Joint Surg. [Br.], *46:*373, 1964.

O'Donoghue, D.H.: An analysis of end results of surgical treatment of major injuries to the ligaments of the knee. J. Bone Joint Surg. [Am.], *37:*1, 1955.

Prather, J.L., Nusynowitz, M.L., and Snowdy, H.A.: Scintigraphic findings in stress fractures. J. Bone Joint Surg. [Am.], *59:*869, 1977.

Pryce, J.C.: Cast-bracing. Principles, indications, and applications. Phys. Ther., *57:*21, 1977.

Putti, V.: Arthrodesis for tuberculosis of the knee and of the shoulder. Chir. Org. Movimento, *18:*217, 1933.

Roberts, J.M.: Fractures of the condyles of the tibia. J. Bone Joint Surg. [Am.], *50:*1505, 1968.

Rorabeck, C.H., and Bobechko, W.P.: Acute dislocation of the patella with osteochondral fracture: A review of eighteen cases. J. Bone Joint Surg. [Br.], *58:*237, 1976.

Rothwell, A.G.: Closed Kuntscher nailing for comminuted femoral shaft fractures. J. Bone Joint Surg. [Br.], *64*:1276, 1982.
Sarmiento, A.: Functional bracing of tibial and femoral shaft fractures. Clin. Orthop., *82*:2, 1972.
Schulak, D.J., Duyar, A., Schlicke, L.H., and Gradisar, I.A.: A theoretical analysis of cast wedging with practical applications. Clin. Orthop., *130*:239, 1978.
Schulak, D.J., and Gunn, D.R.: Fractures of tibial plateaus. A review of the literature. Clin. Orthop., *109*:166, 1975.
Scotland, T., and Wardlaw, D.: The use of cast-bracing as treatment for fractures of tibial plateau. J. Bone Joint Surg. [Br.], *63*:575, 1981.
Scudese, V.A.: Femoral shaft fractures. Percutaneous multiple pin fixation, thigh cylinder plaster cast and early weight bearing. Clin. Orthop., *77*:164, 1971.
Seinsheimer, F., 3rd: Fractures of the distal femur. Clin. Orthop., *153*:169, 1980.
Sisto, D.J., Lachiewicz, P.F., and Insall, J.N.: Treatment of supracondylar fractures following prosthetic arthroplasty of the knee. Clin. Orthop., *196*:265, 1985.
Spak, I.: Humeral shaft fractures—treatment with a simple hand sling. Acta Orthop. Scand., *49*:234, 1978.
Suman, R.K.: Treatment of fractures of the femoral shaft with early cast bracing. Injury, *13*:239, 1981.
Suman, R.K.: Functional bracing in lower limb fractures. Ital. J. Orthop. Traumatol., *9*:201, 1983.
Thomas, T.L., and Meggitt, B.F.: A comparative study of methods for treating fractures of the distal half of the femur. J. Bone Joint Surg. [Br.], *63*:3, 1981.
Thomason, P.A., and Linson, M.A.: Isolated dislocation of the proximal tibiofibular joint. J. Trauma, *26*:192, 1986.
Vaughan-Lane, T., and Meggitt, B.F.: New cast material and improved functional design for lower femoral fracture bracing. Prosthet. Orthot. Int., *4*:145, 1980.
Wang, G.J., Baugher, W.H., Reger, S.I., and Stamp, W.G.: Early ischial weight-bearing cast brace for femoral fractures. South. Med. J., *73*:698, 1980.
Wardlaw, D.: The cast brace treatment of femoral shaft fractures. J. Bone Joint Surg. [Br.], *59*:411, 1977.
Wardlaw, D.: Cast bracing in practice: A two-year study in Aberdeen. Injury, *12*:213, 1980.
Wardlaw, D., McLauchlan, J., Pratt, D.J., and Bowker, P.: A biomechanical study of cast-brace treatment of femoral shaft fractures. J. Bone Joint Surg. [Br.], *63*:7, 1981.
Weiss, A.B.: Cast bracing for femoral shaft fractures, South. Med. J., *69*:326, 1976.
Whitesides, T.E., Jr., Harada, H., and Morimoto, K.: Compartment syndromes and role of fasciectomy, its parameters and techniques. American Academy of Orthopaedic Surgeons Instructional Course Lectures, *26*:179, 1977.
Zaricznyj, B.: Avulsion fracture of the tibial eminence: Treatment by open reduction and pinning. J. Bone Joint Surg. [Am.], *59*:1111, 1977.

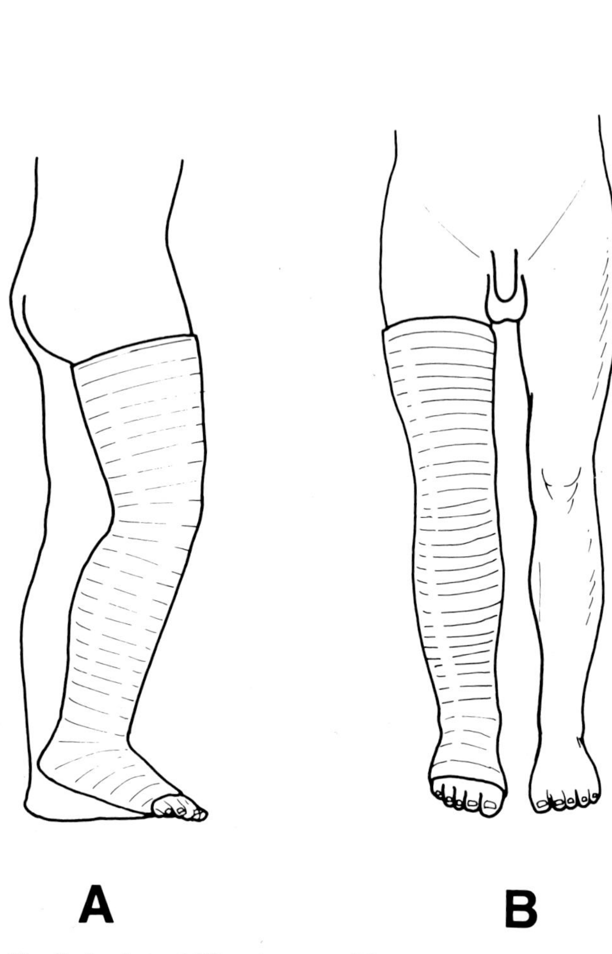

Fig. 9–1. Lateral (*A*) and anterior (*B*) views of a long-leg cast.

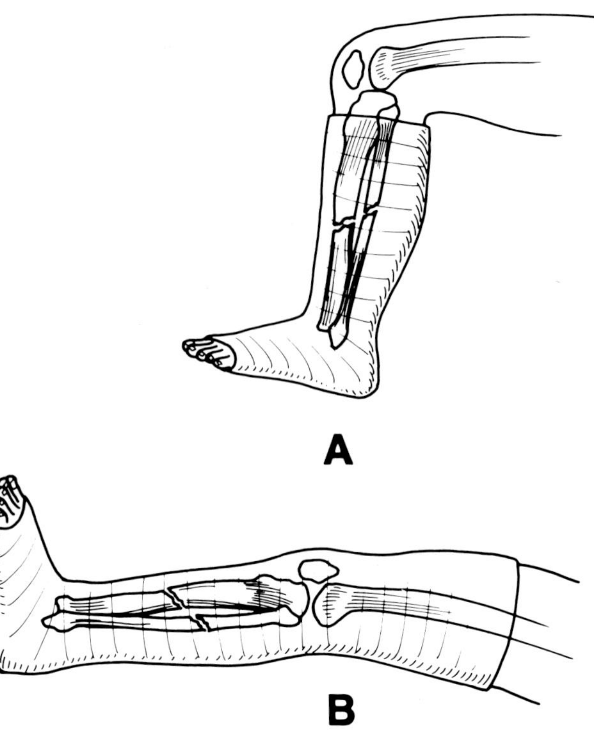

Fig. 9–2. In treatment of an unstable tibial and fibular fracture with a long-leg cast, a short-leg cast should be applied first to stabilize the tibial and fibular fracture (*A*) before cast is extended to the upper thigh (*B*).

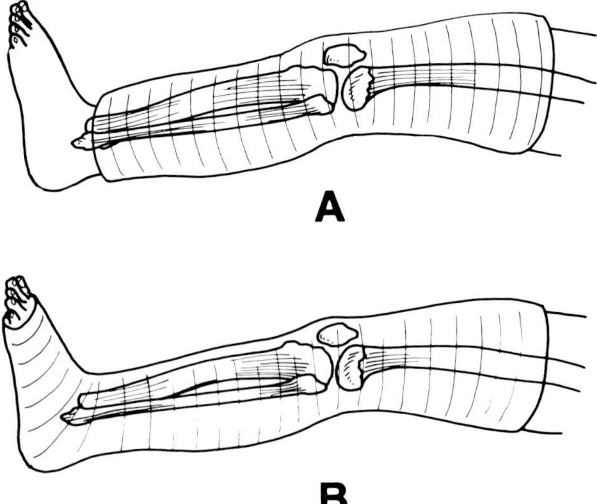

Fig. 9–3. In treatment of a supracondylar femoral fracture with a long-leg cast, a long-leg cylinder cast should be applied first to stabilize the fracture (*A*) before the foot portion is added (*B*).

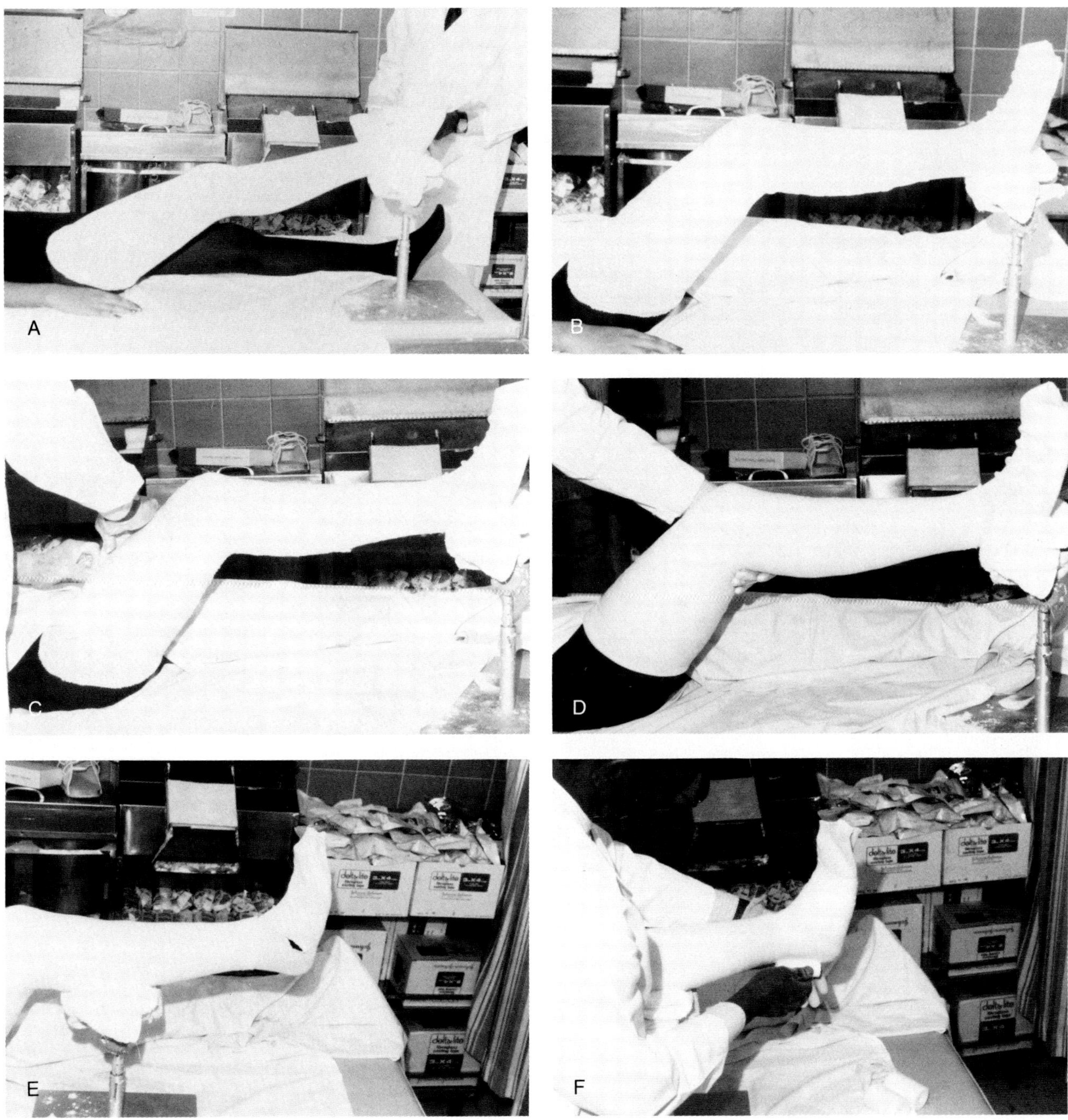

Fig. 9–4. Plaster long-leg cast. *A*, A 4″ stockinet has been applied to the leg from the groin to the toes. *B*, Four rolls of 4″ Webril bandage have been applied to the leg from the upper thigh to the ankle. *C*, Two rolls of 6″ plaster bandage have been applied to the leg from the upper thigh to the ankle. *D*, After 2 5″ × 30″ plaster splints have been applied to the posterior aspect of the cast and the upper end of the stockinet has been turned over the proximal end of the cast, 2 more rolls of 6″ plaster bandage are used to cover the cast down to the ankle. *E*, The stockinet crease in front of the ankle has been removed. *F*, 4″ Webril bandage is used to pad the foot and ankle.

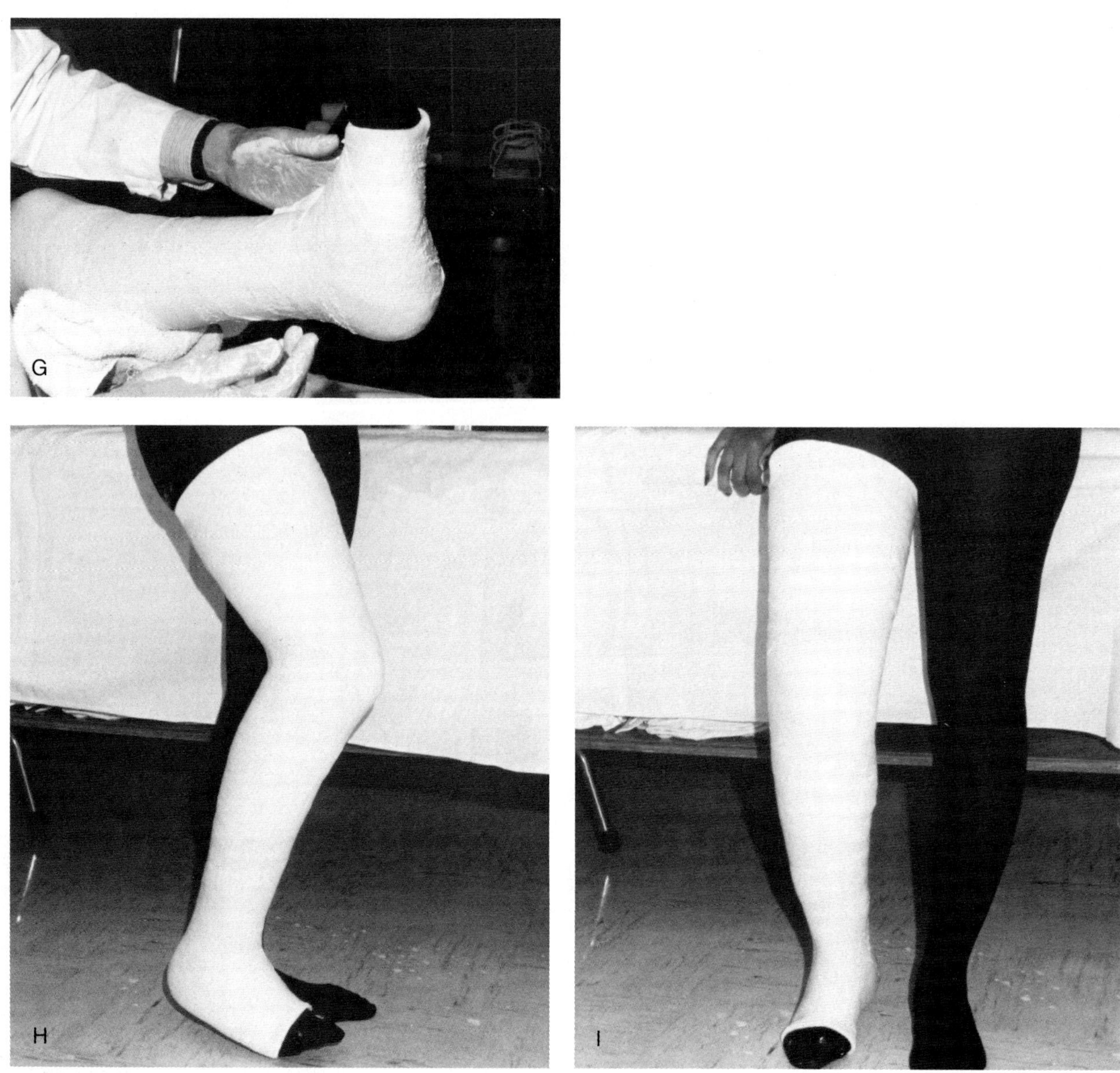

Fig. Fig. 9–4 (cont.). *G,* A roll of 6″ plaster bandage is used to cover the foot and ankle region. *H,I,* Lateral and anterior views of the finished cast.

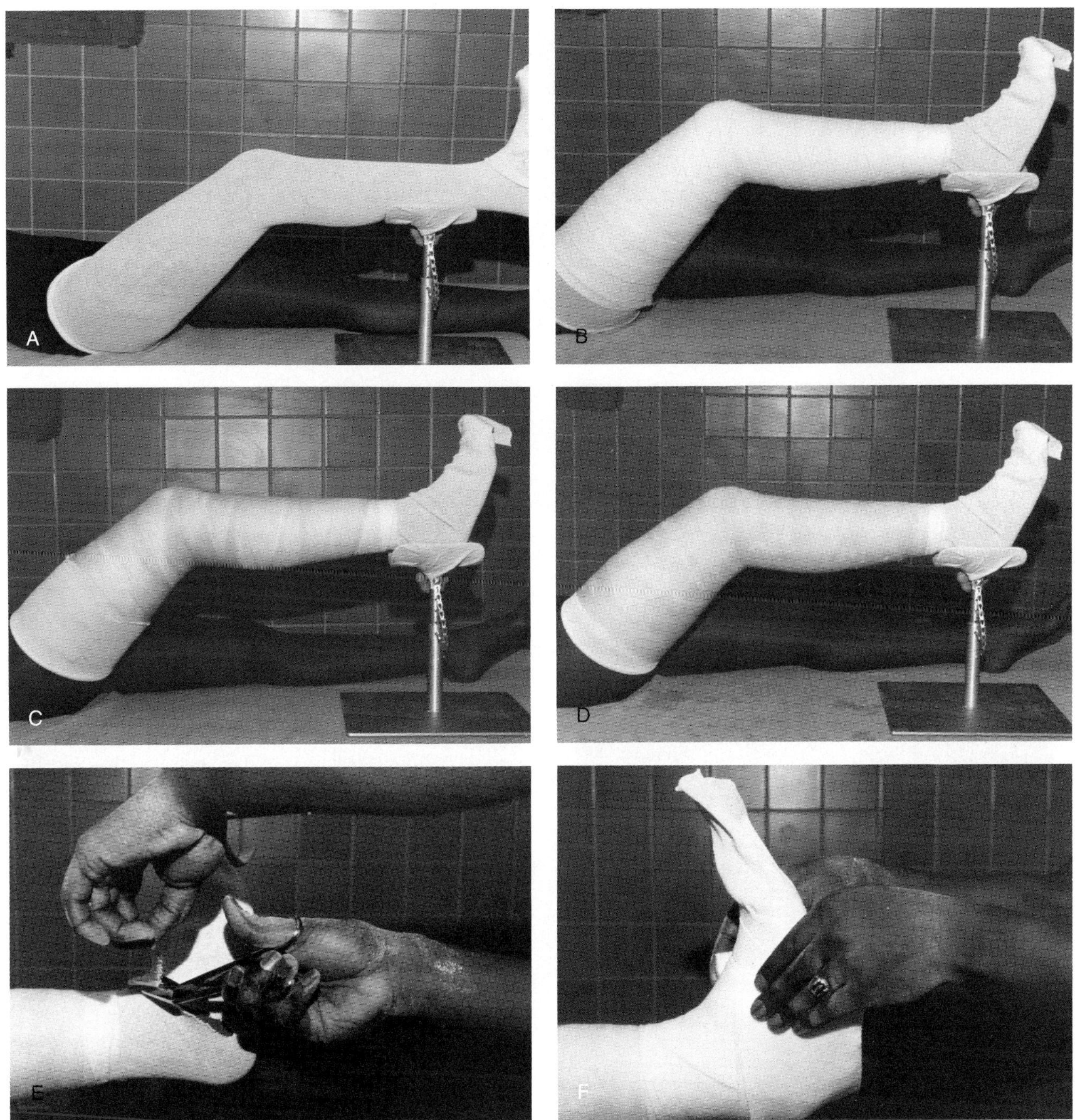

Fig. 9–5. The making of a fiberglass long-leg cast. *A*, A 4″ stockinet has been applied to the whole leg. *B*, Four rolls of 4″ Webril bandage have been applied to the leg. *C*, The leg has been wrapped from the upper thigh to the ankle with 3 rolls of 5″ fiberglass bandage, and the upper end of the stockinet has been turned down over the proximal end of the cast. *D*, Another 2 rolls of 5″ fiberglass bandage have been applied to the cast all the way down to the ankle. *E*, Removing the stockinet wrinkle in front of the ankle joint. *F*, After 4″ Webril has been applied to the ankle region in an overlapping figure-8 fashion, several strips of Webril are applied to the back of the heel.

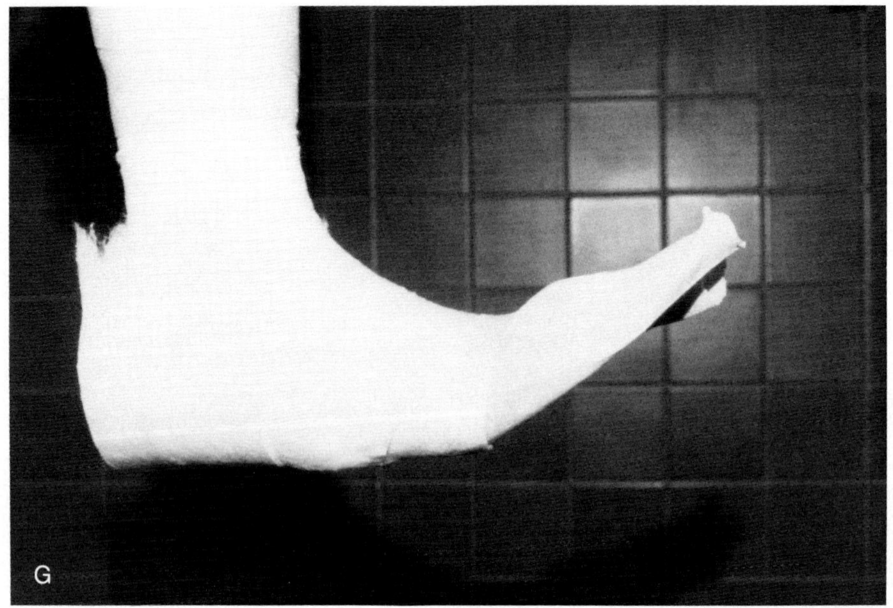

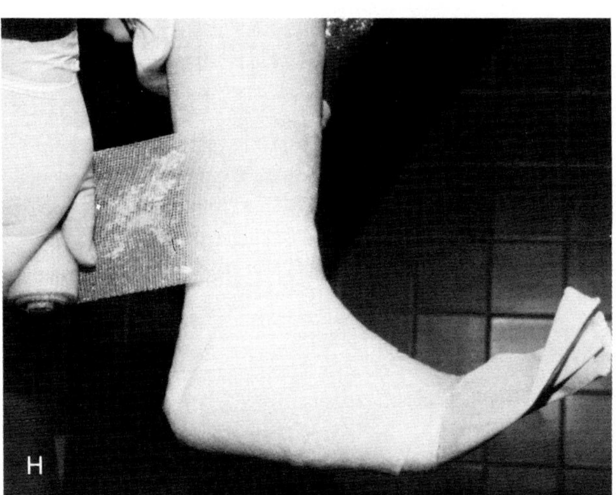

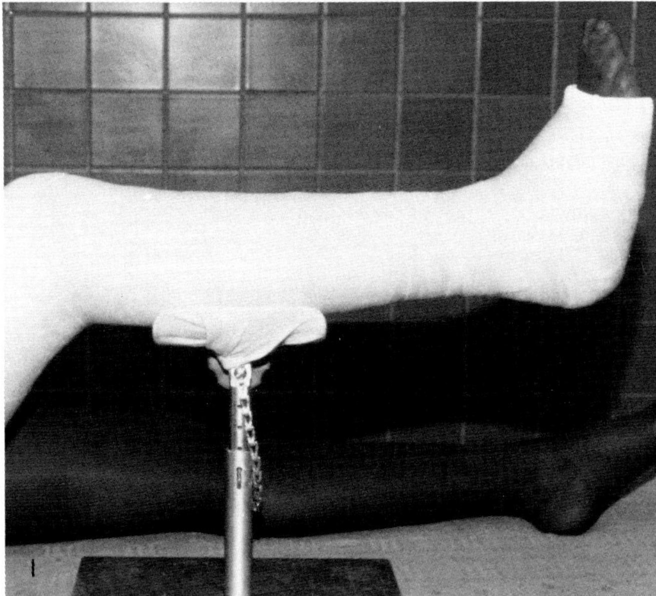

Fig. 9–5 (cont.). *G*, Another several strips of Webril are applied to the heel region, at a right angle to the first ones. The redundant Webril margins behind and below the heel should be removed. *H*, Applying the 6th roll of 5″ fiberglass bandage around the foot and ankle to finish the cast. *I*, The completed cast.

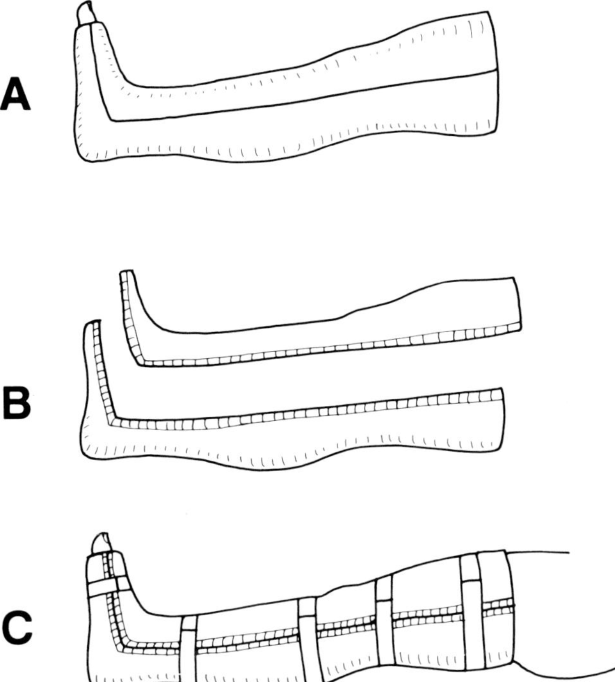

Fig. 9–6. Bivalving a long-leg cast. *A*, The cast is split along its medial and lateral aspects. *B*, The margins of the bivalved long-leg cast are lined with moleskin. *C*, The bivalved cast has been reapplied to the leg and is held in place with Velcro straps or webbings and buckles.

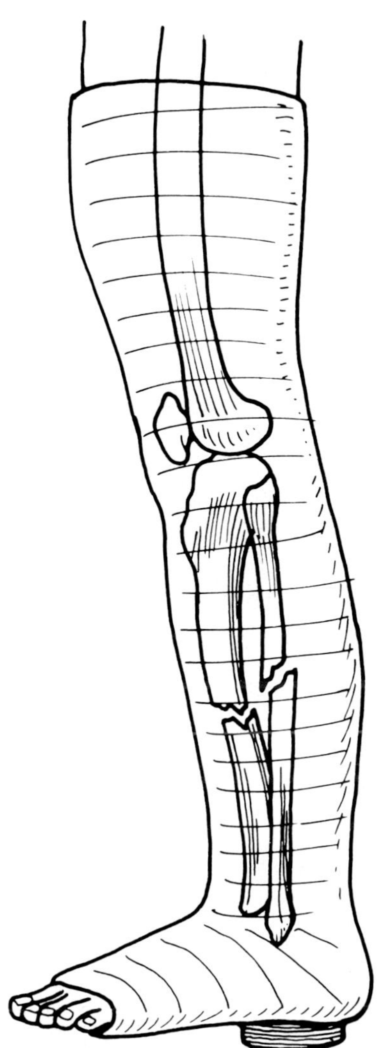

Fig. 9–7. Lateral view of a long-leg walking cast.

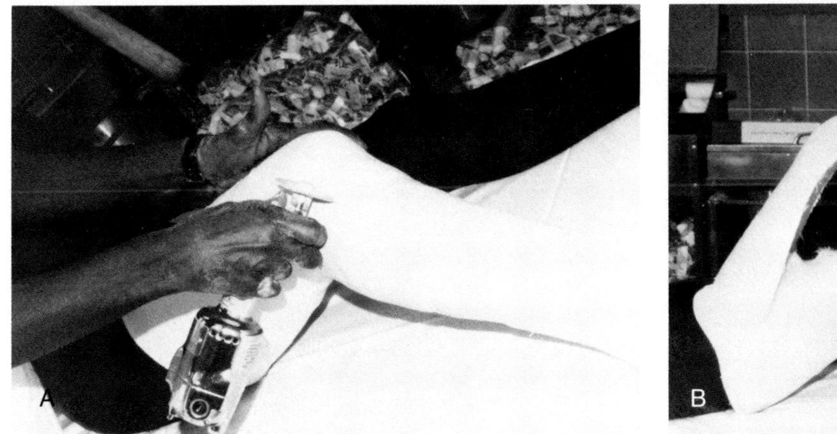

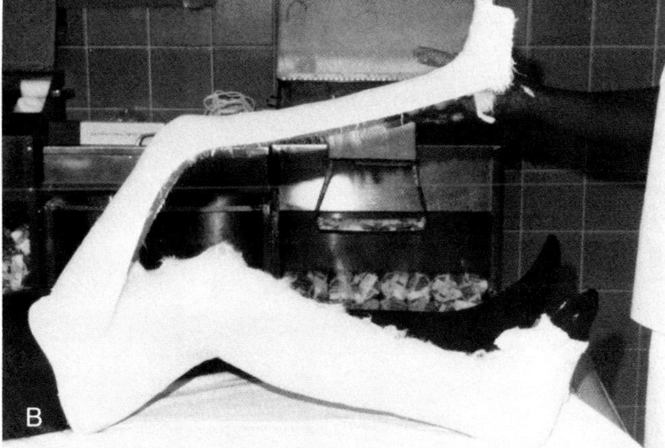

Fig. 9–8. The making of a posterior long-leg splint. *A*, The entire long-leg cast is being split along its medial and lateral aspects. *B*, The anterior half of the bivalved long-leg cast is being removed.

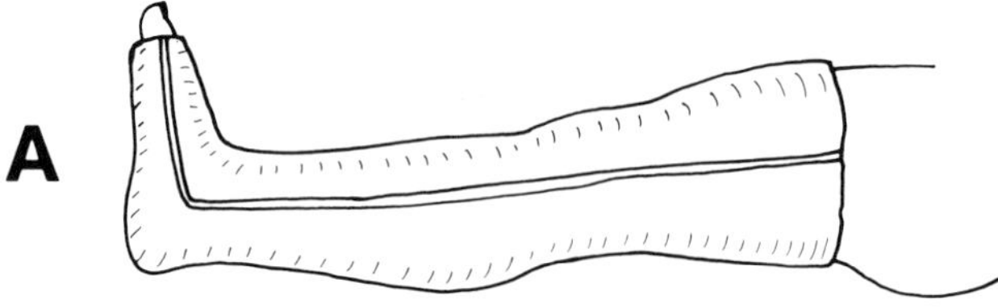

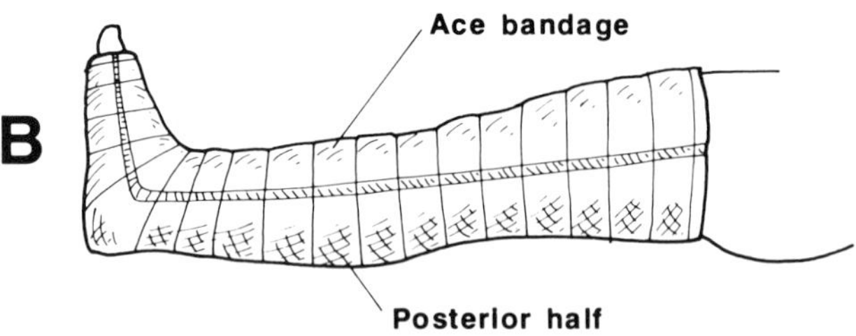

Fig. 9–9. *A*, The long-leg cast has been split along its medial and lateral aspects. *B*, The anterior half of the bivalved long-leg cast has been discarded, the margins of the posterior half of the cast have been lined, the posterior half has been reapplied to the injured leg, and the finished splint is held in place with an Ace bandage.

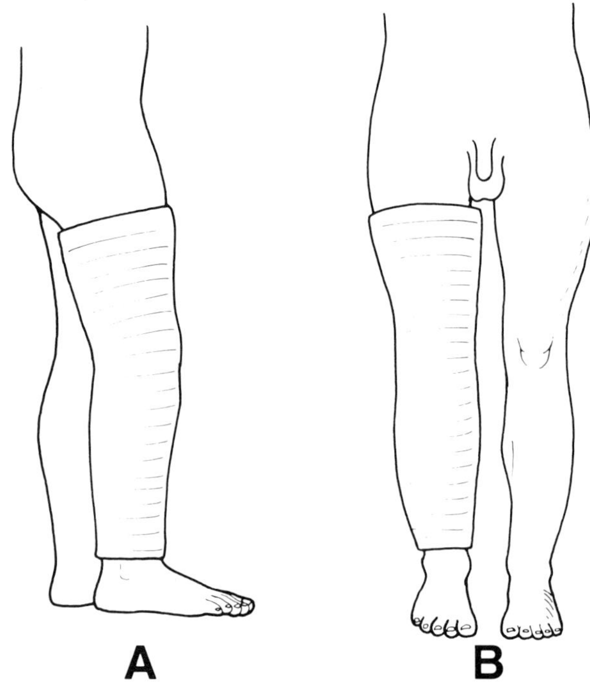

Fig. 9–10. Lateral (*A*) and anterior (*B*) views of a long-leg cylinder cast.

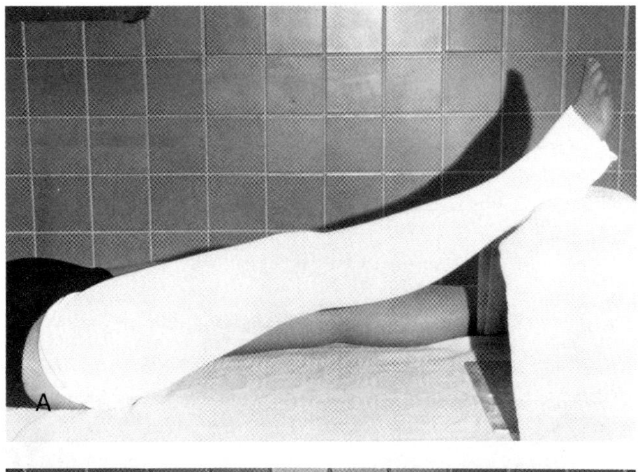

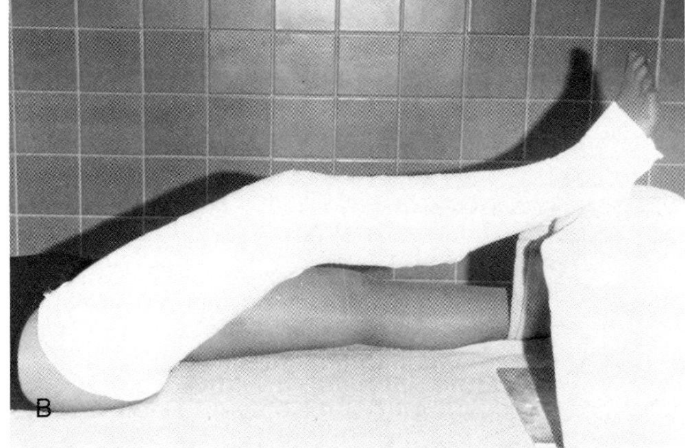

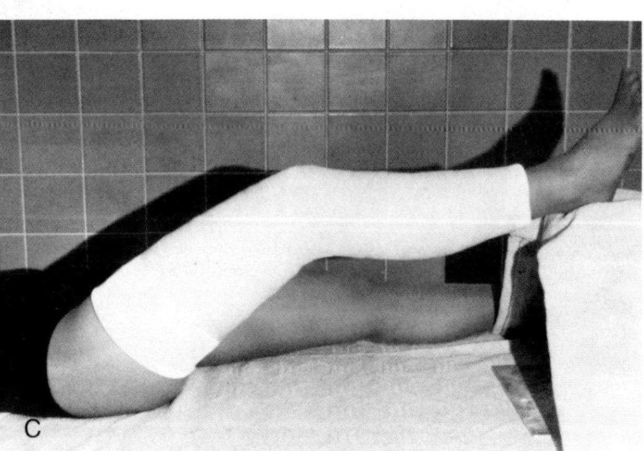

Fig. 9–11. The making of a fiberglass long-leg cylinder cast. *A*, A 4″ stockinet has been applied from the foot to the upper thigh. *B*, Three rolls of 4″ Webril have been applied to the leg from the upper thigh to the malleolar region. *C*, One roll of 5″ fiberglass bandage has been applied to the leg from the upper thigh to the supramalleolar region, and the 2 stockinet ends have been turned down over the 2 cast ends.

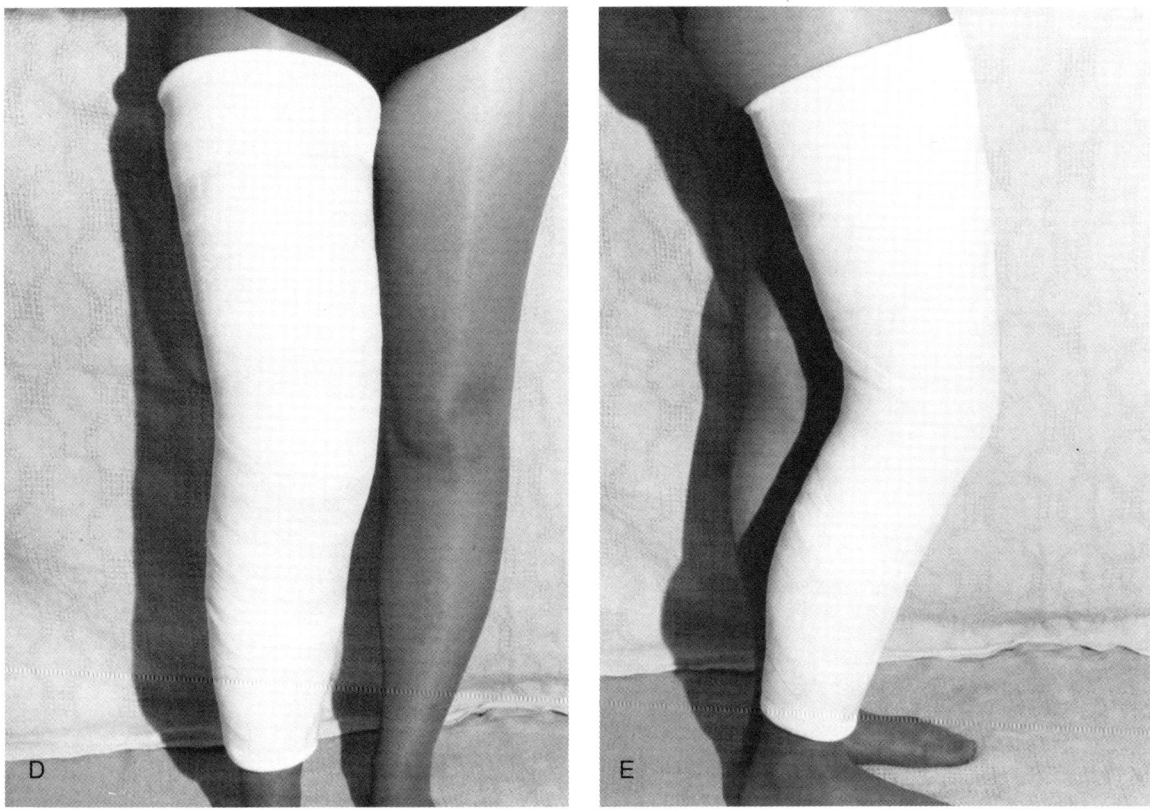

Fig. 9–11 (cont.). *D,E,* Anterior and lateral views of the finished cast after the 2nd roll of 5″ fiberglass bandage has been wrapped around the whole cast.

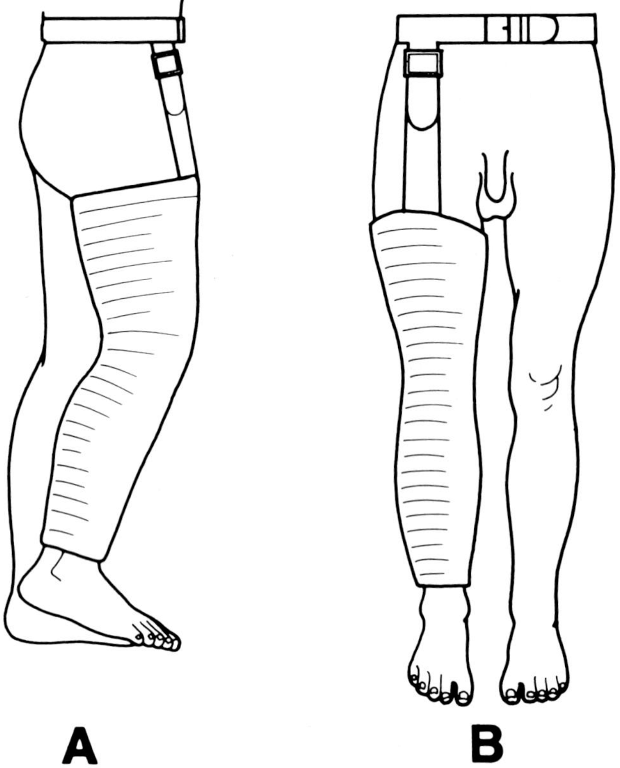

Fig. 9–12. Lateral (*A*) and anterior (*B*) views of a cylinder cast with an anterior suspender, which is attached to a waist belt for support. The suspender is useful for obese patients, who usually have a hard time wearing cylinder casts.

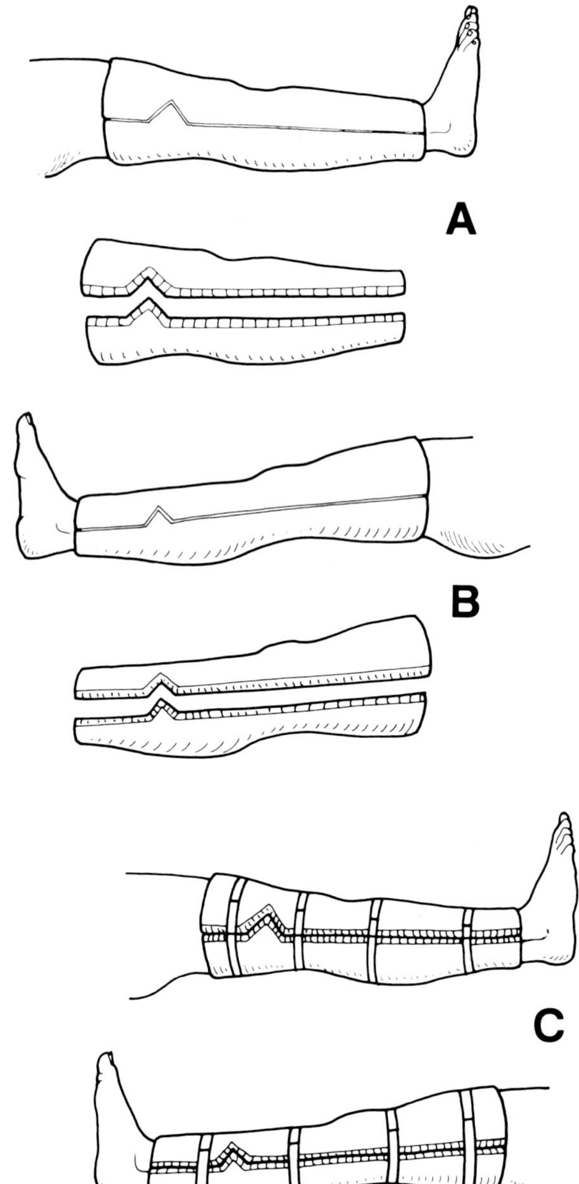

Fig. 9–13. Bivalving a long-leg cylinder cast. *A*, Longitudinally splitting the lateral aspect of the cast and lining the lateral cast margins with moleskin. *B*, Longitudinally splitting the medial aspect of the cast and lining the medial cast margins with moleskin. *C*, Reapplying the bivalved cast to the leg and holding it in place with Velcro straps or webbings and buckles.

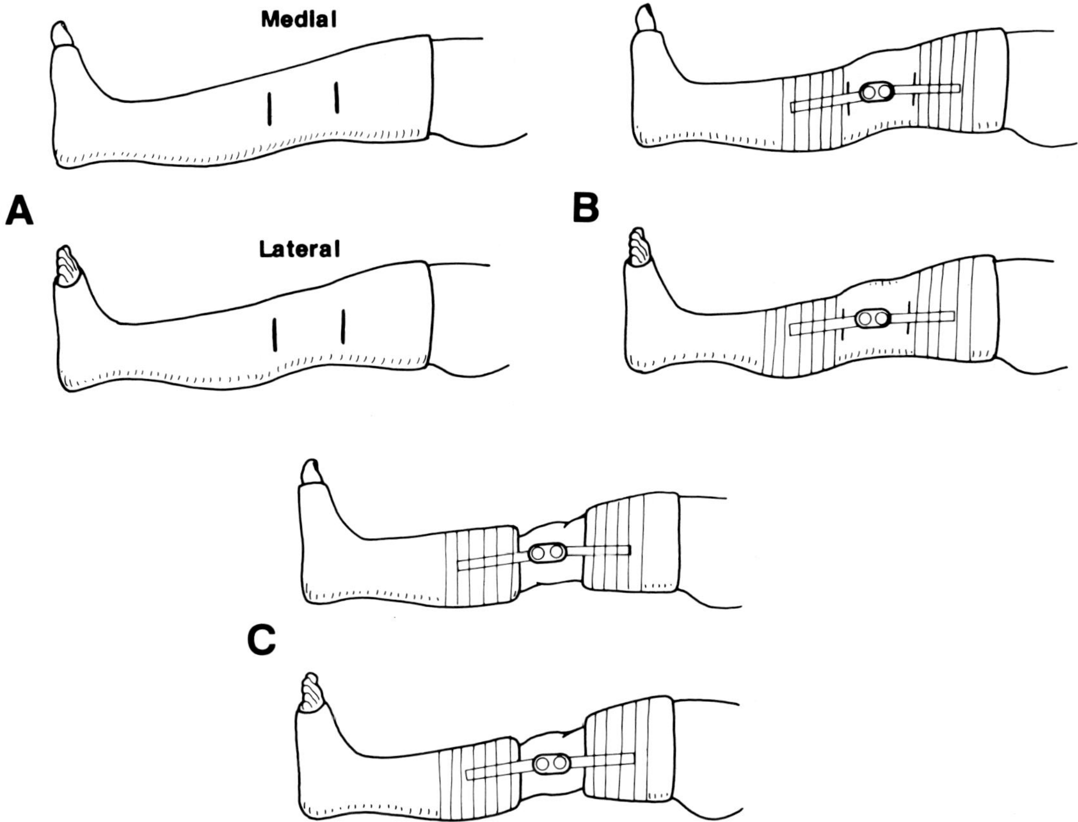

Fig. 9–14. The making of a long-leg cast-brace with knee hinges. *A*, Transverse cuts are made above and below the knee joint on both the medial and lateral aspects of the knee. *B*, Two polycentric knee hinges are fixed to the medial and lateral aspects of the knee. *C*, The section of the cast between the four transverse cuts is removed.

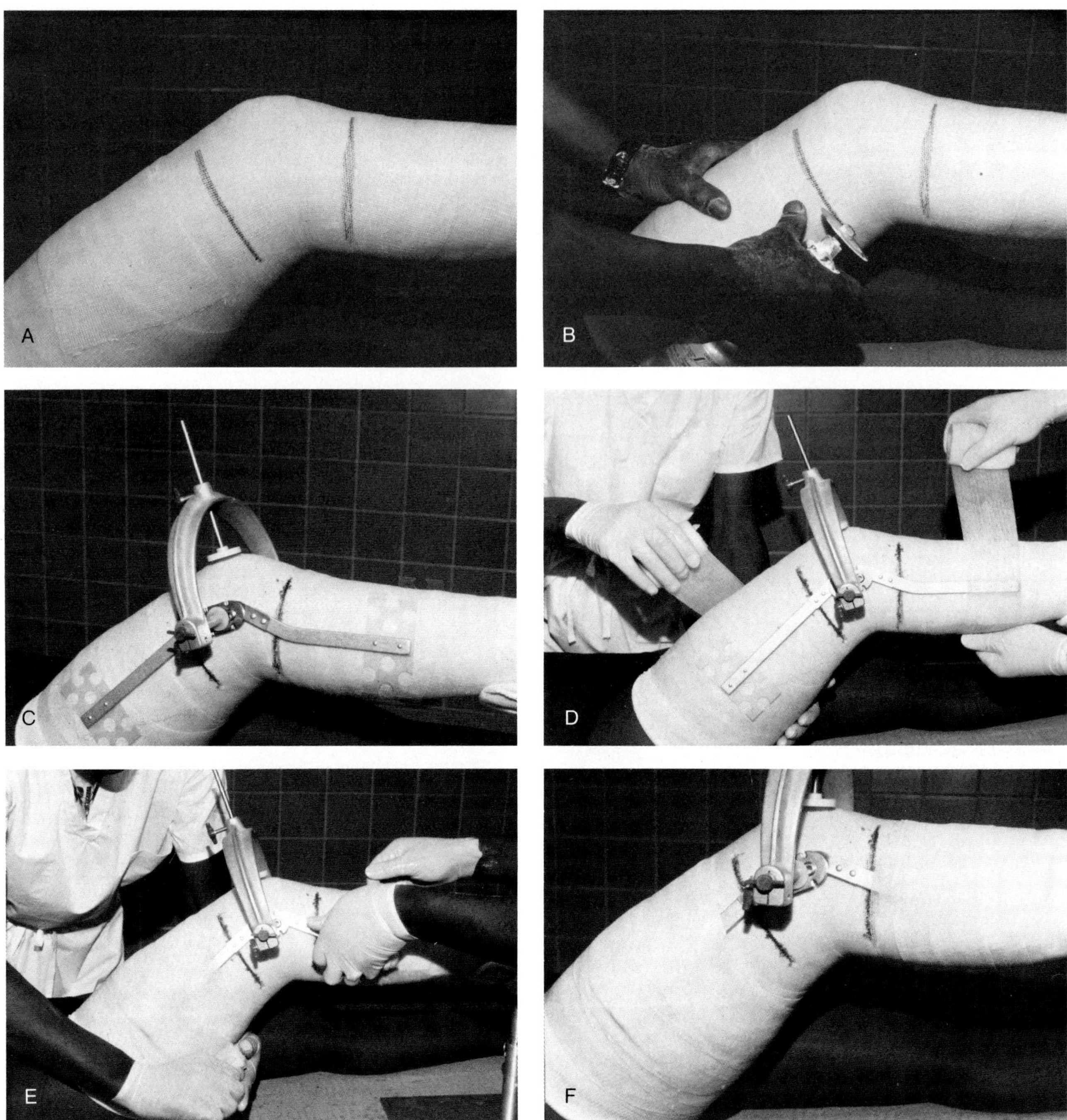

Fig. 9–15. The making of a fiberglass long-leg cast-brace with knee hinges. *A,B,* Two transverse cuts are made in the cast about 4″ from the center of the femoral condyles on the medial and lateral aspects of the knee region. *C–F,* After the two polycentric knee hinges have been aligned correctly with the knee joint with a fracture-brace alignment fixture, 2 rolls of 4″ fiberglass bandage are used to fix the knee hinges to the cast immediately above and below the knee joint.

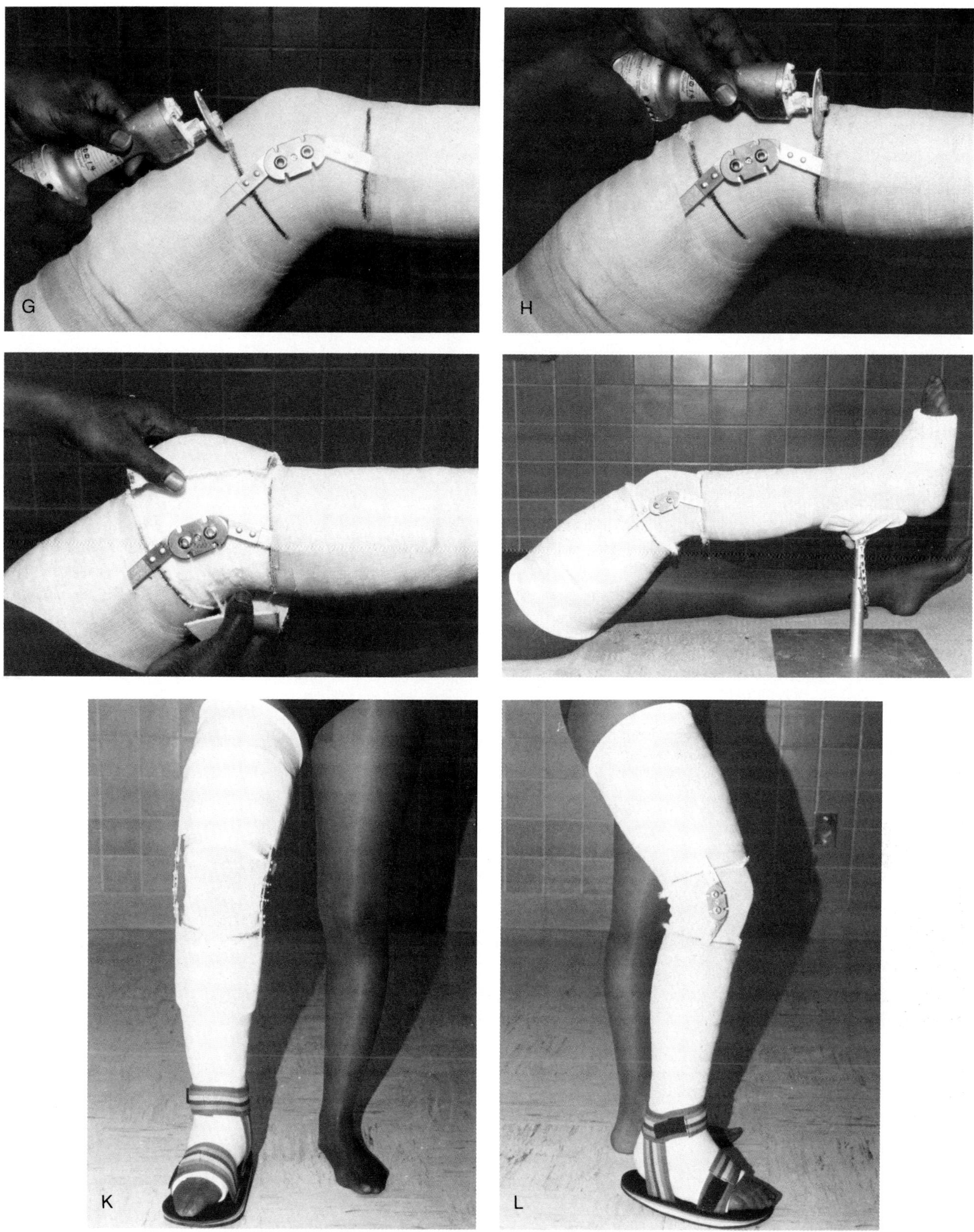

Fig. 9–15 (cont.). *G,H,I,* The knee section of the cast is removed by linking the transverse cuts and longitudinally splitting the isolated knee section of the cast. *J,* The Webril in the knee region has been removed. *K,L,* Anterior and lateral views of the finished cast-brace, with cast sandal.

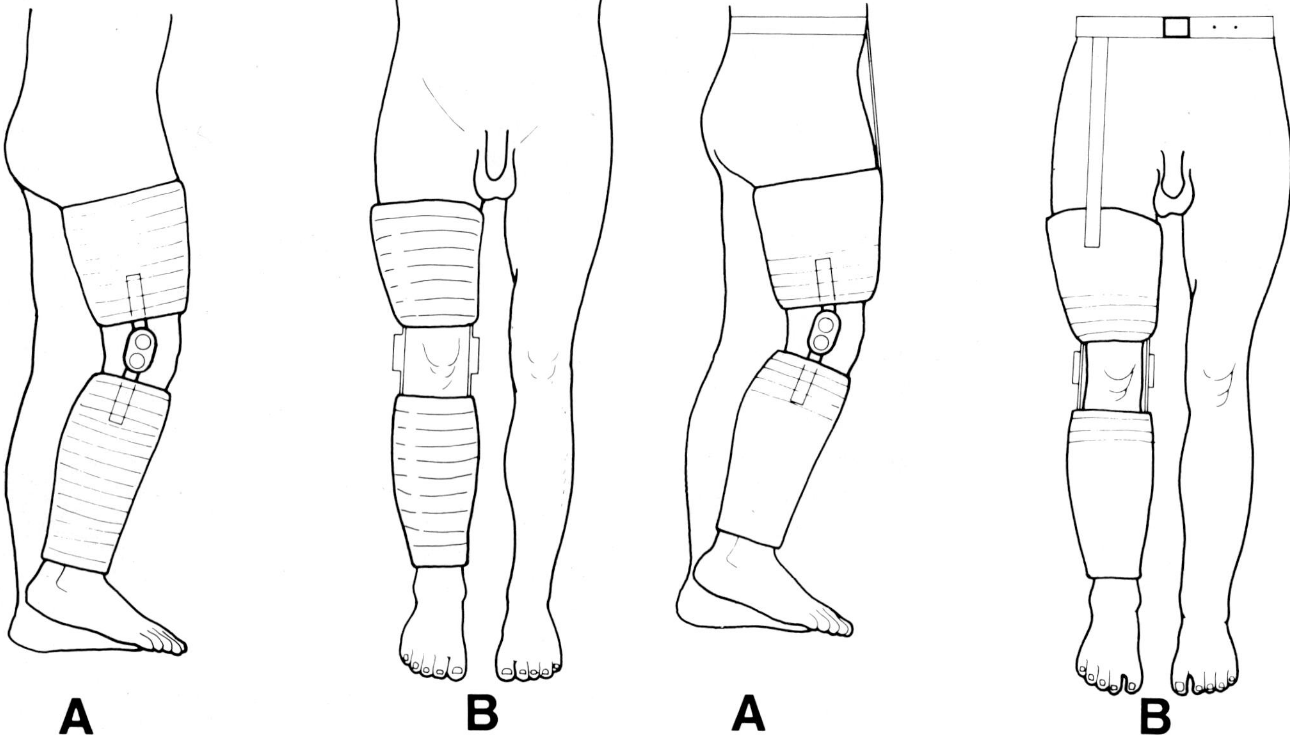

Fig. 9–16. Lateral (*A*) and anterior (*B*) views of a long-leg cylinder cast-brace.

Fig. 9–17. Lateral (*A*) and anterior (*B*) views of a long-leg cylinder cast-brace with a suspender attached to the waist belt and to the anterosuperior aspect of the cast.

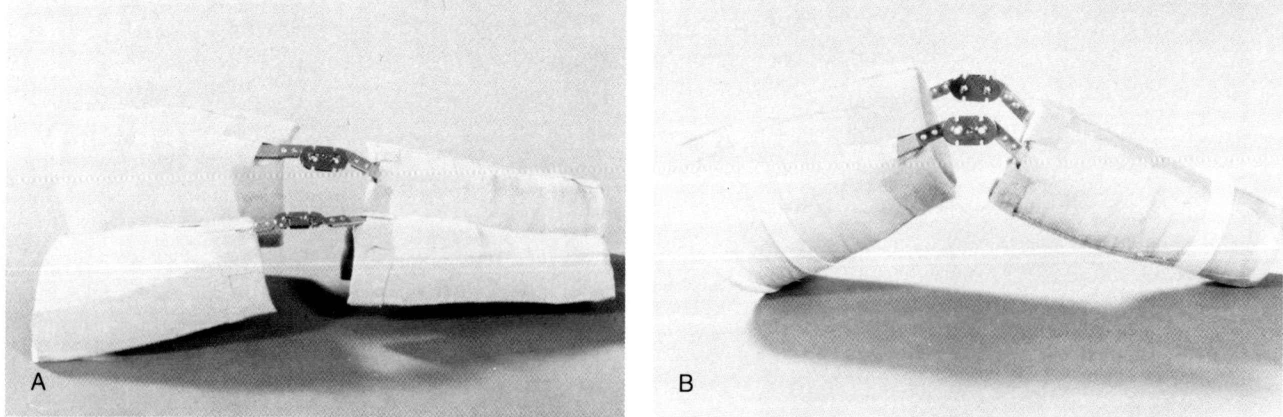

Fig. 9–18. *A,B,* A bivalved long-leg cylinder cast brace, which can be reapplied to the injured leg by holding the two halves together with Velcro straps or webbings and buckles.

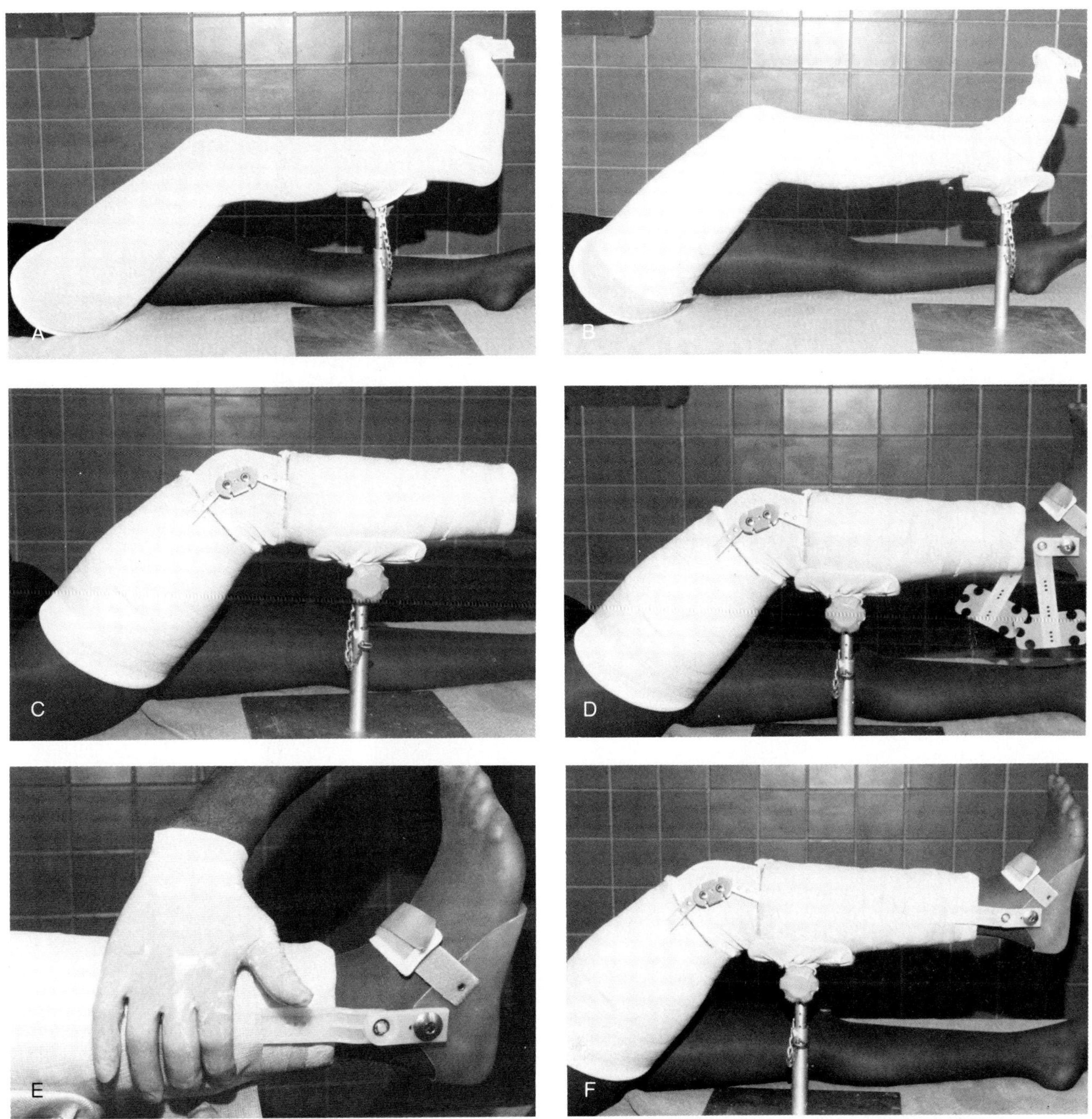

Fig. 9–19. The making of a long-leg cast-brace with knee and ankle hinges. *A*, A 4″ stockinet has been applied from the groin to the toes. *B*, 4″ Webril has been wrapped around the leg from the upper thigh to the ankle. *C*, A long-leg cylinder cast has been made and then converted to a long-leg cylinder cast-brace with knee hinges. *D,E,F*, A heel cup with 2 ankle hinges is attached to the distal portion of the cast with a roll of 3″ plaster or fiberglass bandage.

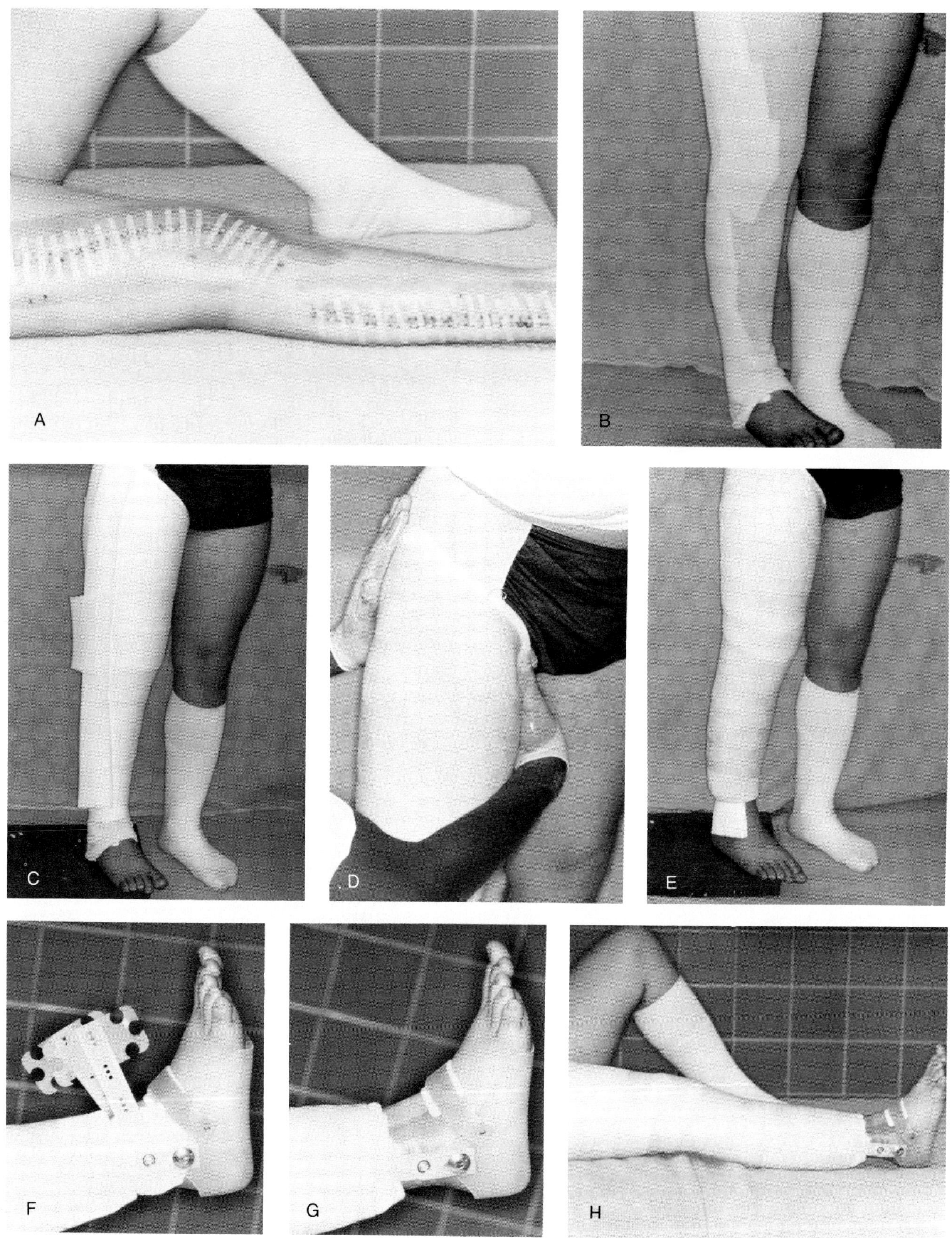

(Legend on Facing Page)

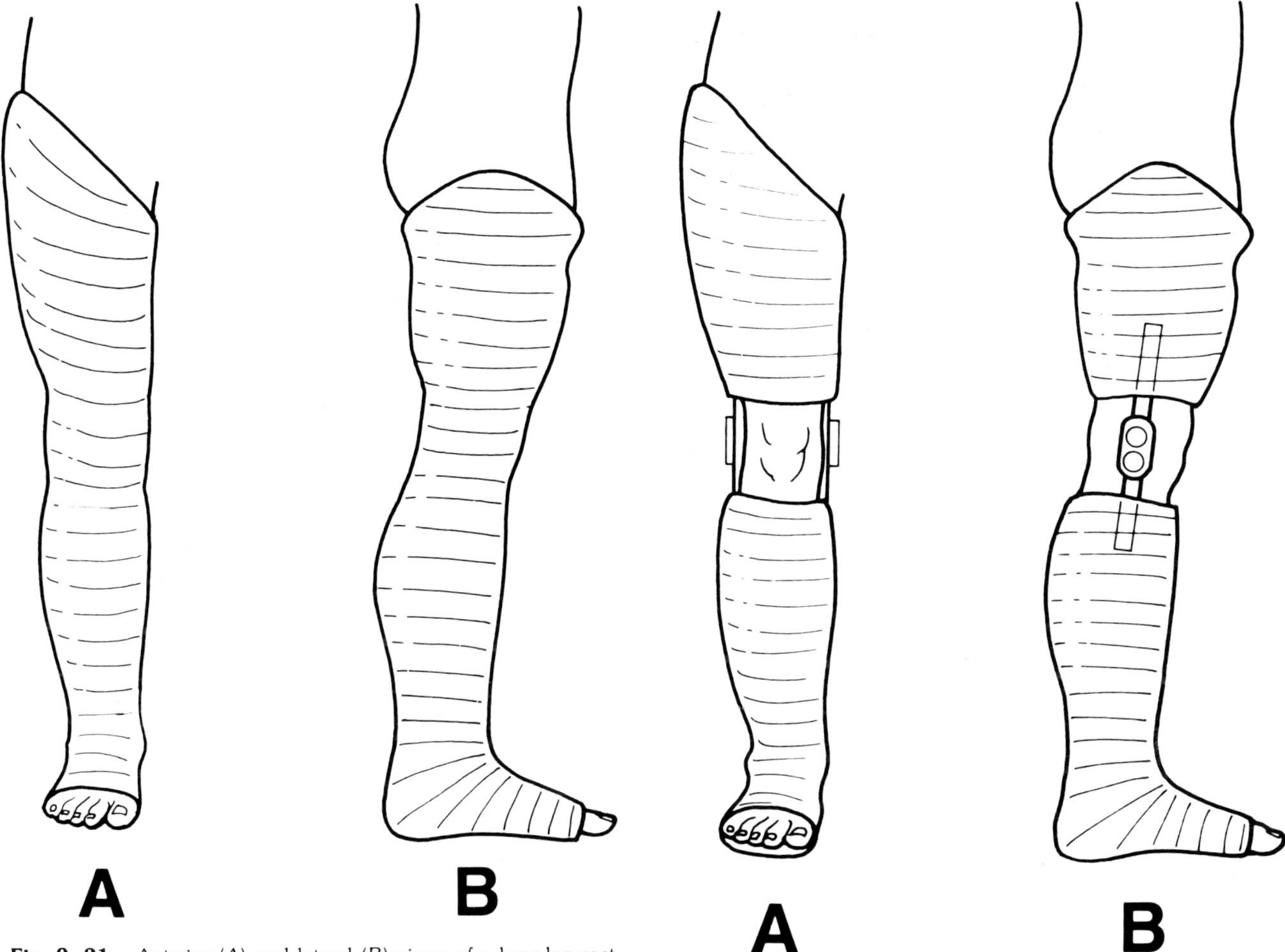

Fig. 9–21. Anterior (*A*) and lateral (*B*) views of a long-leg cast with a molded quadrilateral socket.

Fig. 9–22. Anterior (*A*) and lateral (*B*) views of a long-leg cast-brace with a molded quadrilateral socket and knee hinges.

Fig. 9–20. The making of a fiberglass long-leg cast-brace with heelcup and ankle hinges. *A*, This 20-year-old white male underwent en bloc resection of his right distal femur and the overlying quadriceps muscle for a distal femoral sarcoma with extraosseous tumor extension. The bony gap was bridged with autogenous bone grafts and stabilized with an internal metallic device. *B*, A 4″ stockinet has been applied from the foot to the end of the thigh; the stockinet has been cut longitudinally in the perineal region to allow the rest of the upper stockinet ends to be pulled up to the iliac crest region. *C*, Four rolls of 4″ Webril have been applied to the whole leg. Six to 8 strips of 4″ Webril are used to cover the groin and gluteal area in an oblique fashion in preparation for the application of a molded quadrilateral socket. *D*, *E*, Six rolls of 5″ fiberglass bandage are applied to the leg from the supramalleolar region to the base of the thigh. The upper end of the cast has an indentation over the femoral triangle and is molded closely around the greater trochanter and the ischial tuberosity to produce a quadrilateral configuration. *F,G,H*, The heel cup is applied to the foot, and its 2 ankle hinges are fixed to the distal end of the cast.

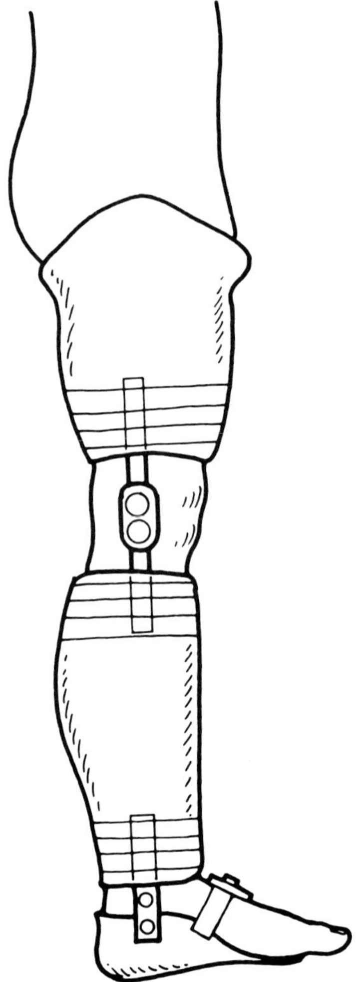

Fig. 9–23. A long-leg cast-brace with a molded quadrilateral socket and knee and ankle hinges.

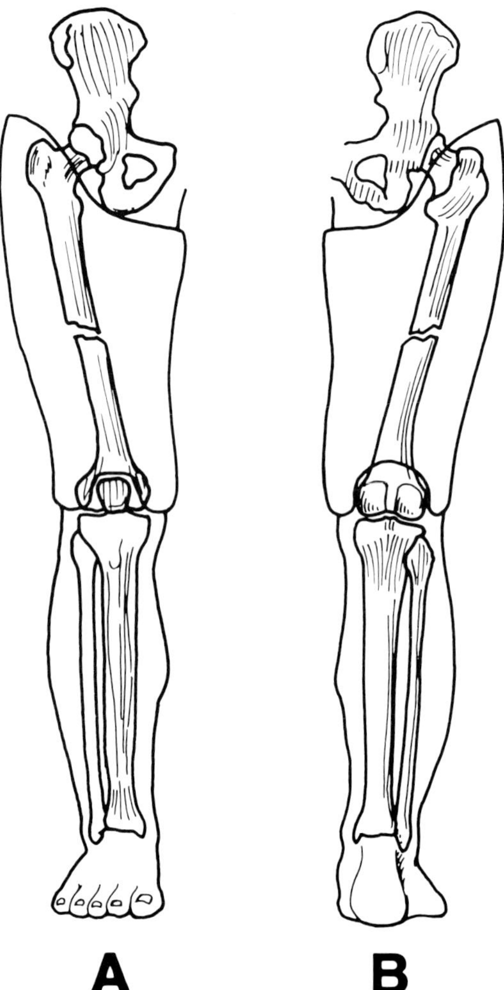

Fig. 9–24. Anterior (*A*) and posterior (*B*) views of a lower extremity showing the use of a thigh cast with quadrilateral socket for the treatment of femoral fractures.

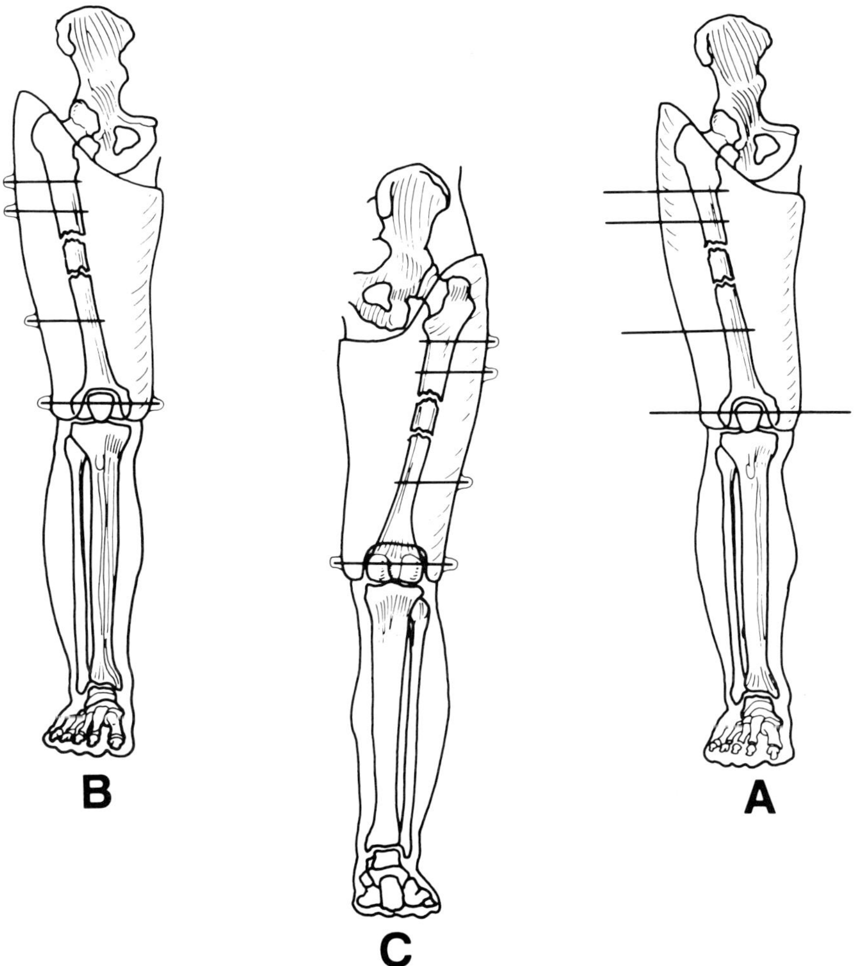

Fig. 9–25. Use of a thigh cast with a molded quadrilateral socket in treating a segmental femoral fracture. The Steinmann pins inserted into the femur (*A*) are incorporated into the cast (*B*,*C*).

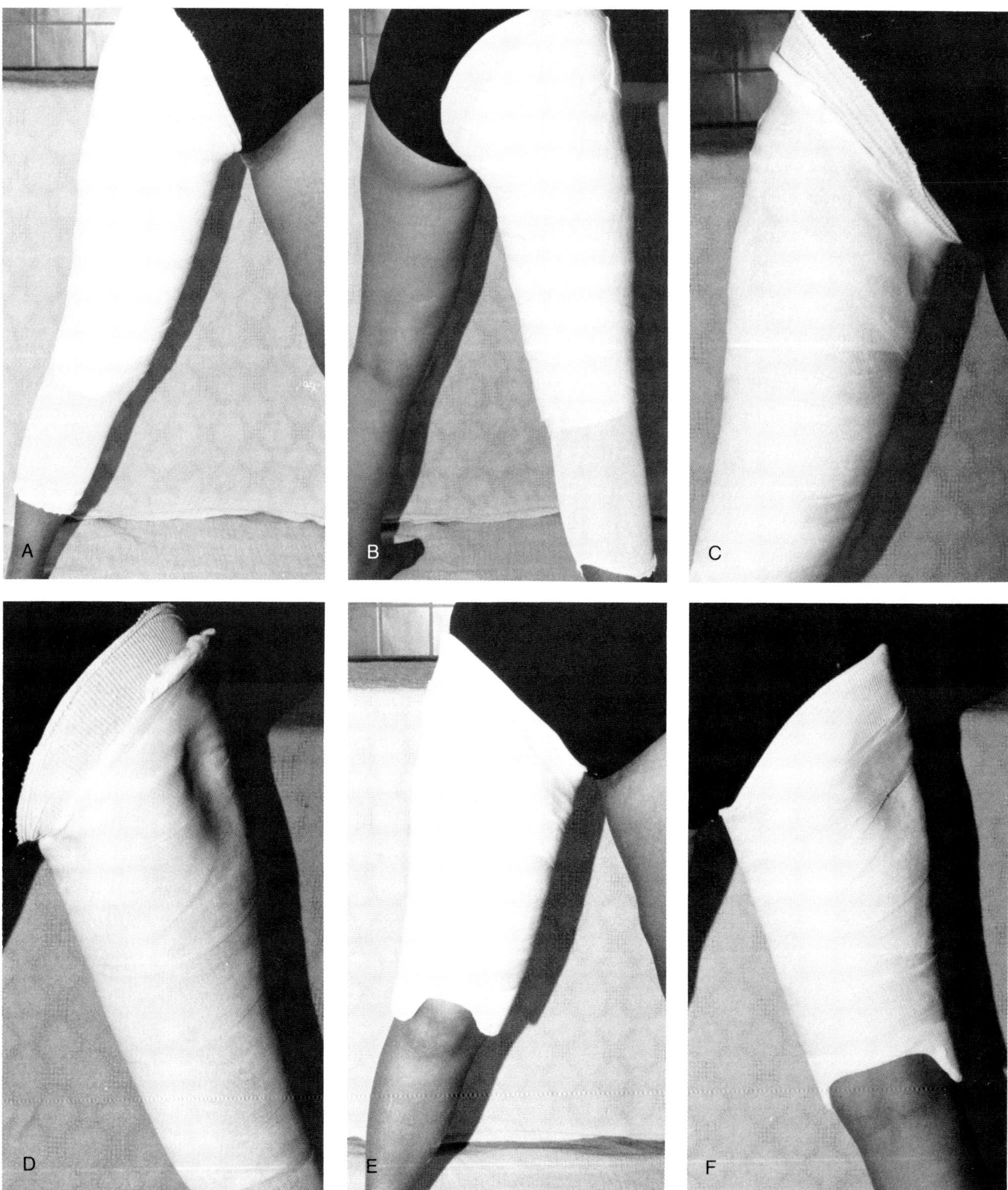

Fig. 9–26. The making of a fiberglass QTB thigh cast with molded quadrilateral socket and femoral condylar flanges. *A,B,* Three rolls of 4″ Webril have been wrapped evenly around the thigh from the knee to the base of the thigh over the 4″ stockinet. *C,D,* Two rolls of 5″ fiberglass bandage have been applied to the leg from the knee to the base of the thigh. Note the shallow indentations in the cast over the femoral triangle, behind the greater trochanter, and immediately below the ischial tuberosity to stabilize the upper end of the cast to the base of the thigh. *E,F,* After the 2 femoral condylar flanges and the suprapatellar and suprapopliteal notches have been carved out from the distal end of the cast, the proximal and distal ends of the stockinet are folded down over the cast ends and secured to the thigh cast with a roll of 4″ fiberglass bandage.

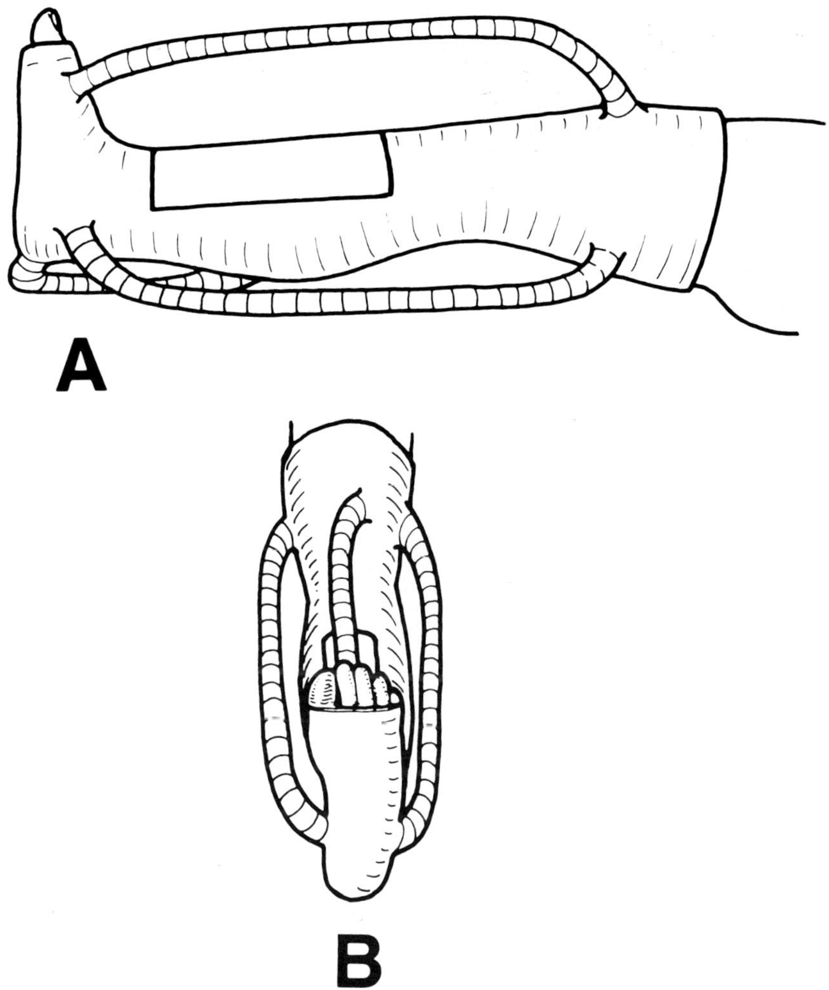

Fig. 9–27. Medial (*A*) and anterior (*B*) views of an outrigger long-leg cast with a window in the tibial region.

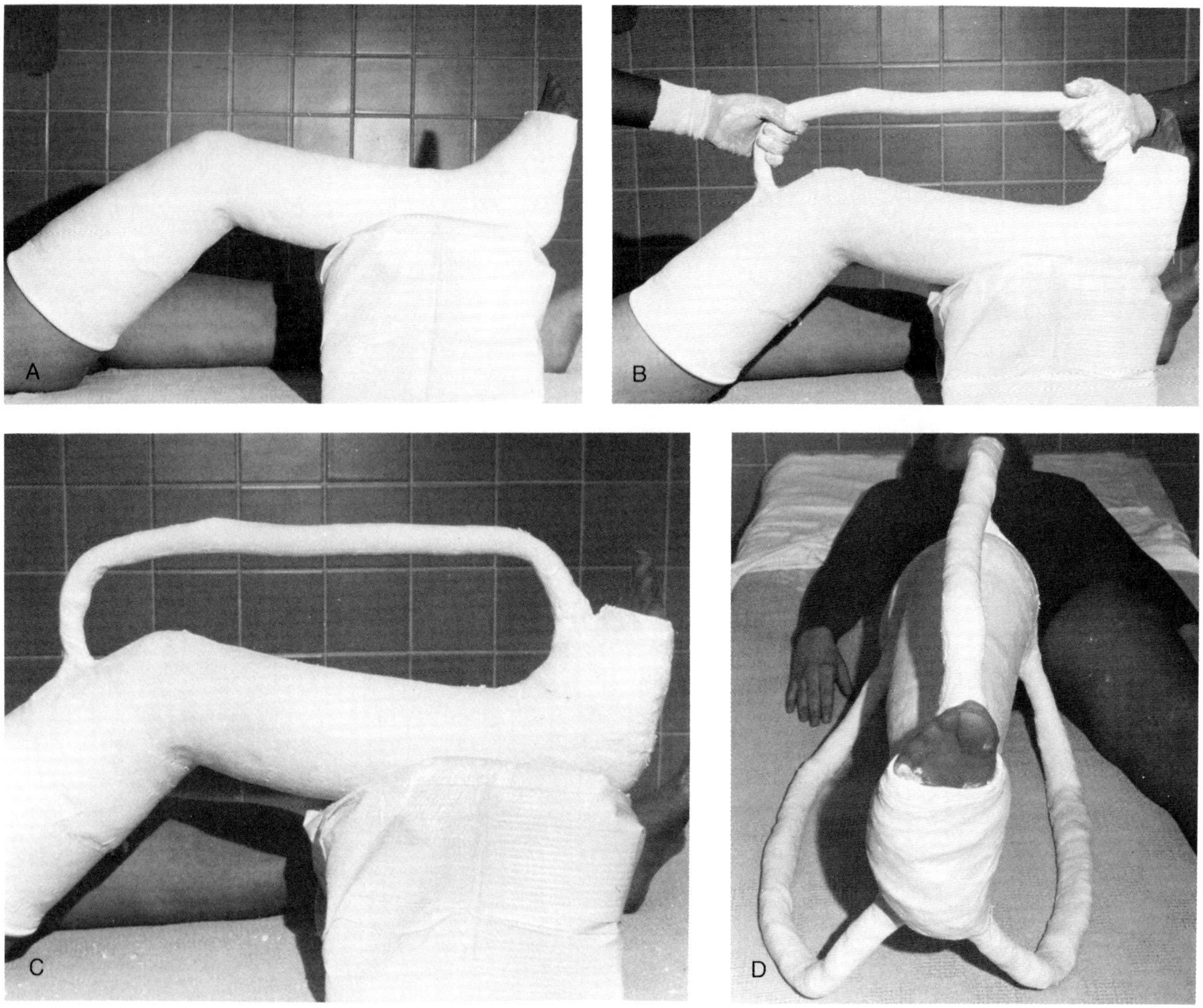

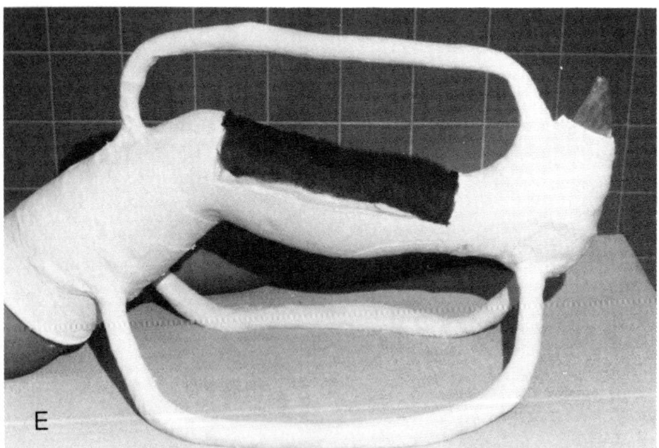

Fig. 9–28. The making of an outrigger long-leg cast. *A*, Lateral view of a standard long-leg cast. *B*, The superior outrigger bar has been attached to the cast, and two cast technicians hold the outrigger bar in an upright position while the plaster is setting. *C*, The finished superior outrigger bar. *D*, The two bottom outrigger bars have been attached to the medial and lateral aspects of the cast. *E*, A large window has been removed from the upper half of the tibial portion of the finished outrigger cast.

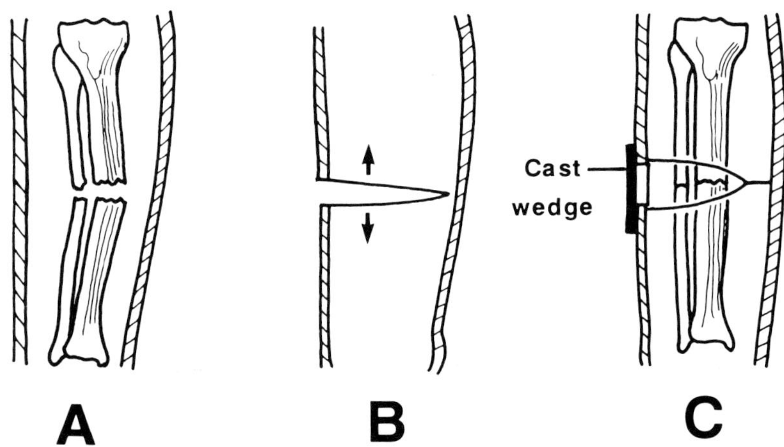

Fig. 9–29. Opening wedging of a leg cast. *A*, Fracture angulation. *B*, A circumferential cut through the cast, followed by manual reduction of fracture angulation. *C*, Cast wedge in place.

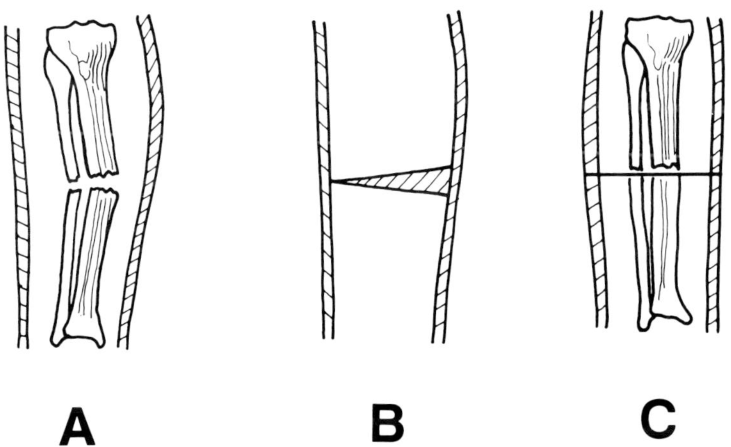

Fig. 9–30. Closing wedging of a leg cast. *A*, Fracture angulation. *B*, Section of cast to be removed. *C*, Edges of cast are reunited after manual reduction of fracture angulation.

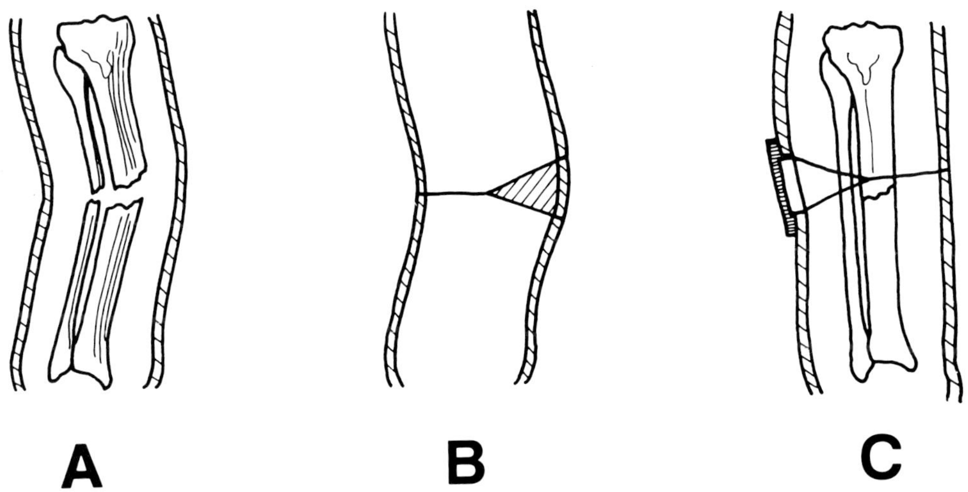

Fig. 9–31. Combined opening/closing wedging of a leg cast. *A*, Severely angulated fracture. *B*, Cast cut as for closing wedging, but cutout portion extends only halfway through cast. *C*, Wedge inserted on side opposite cutout portion, angulation corrected.

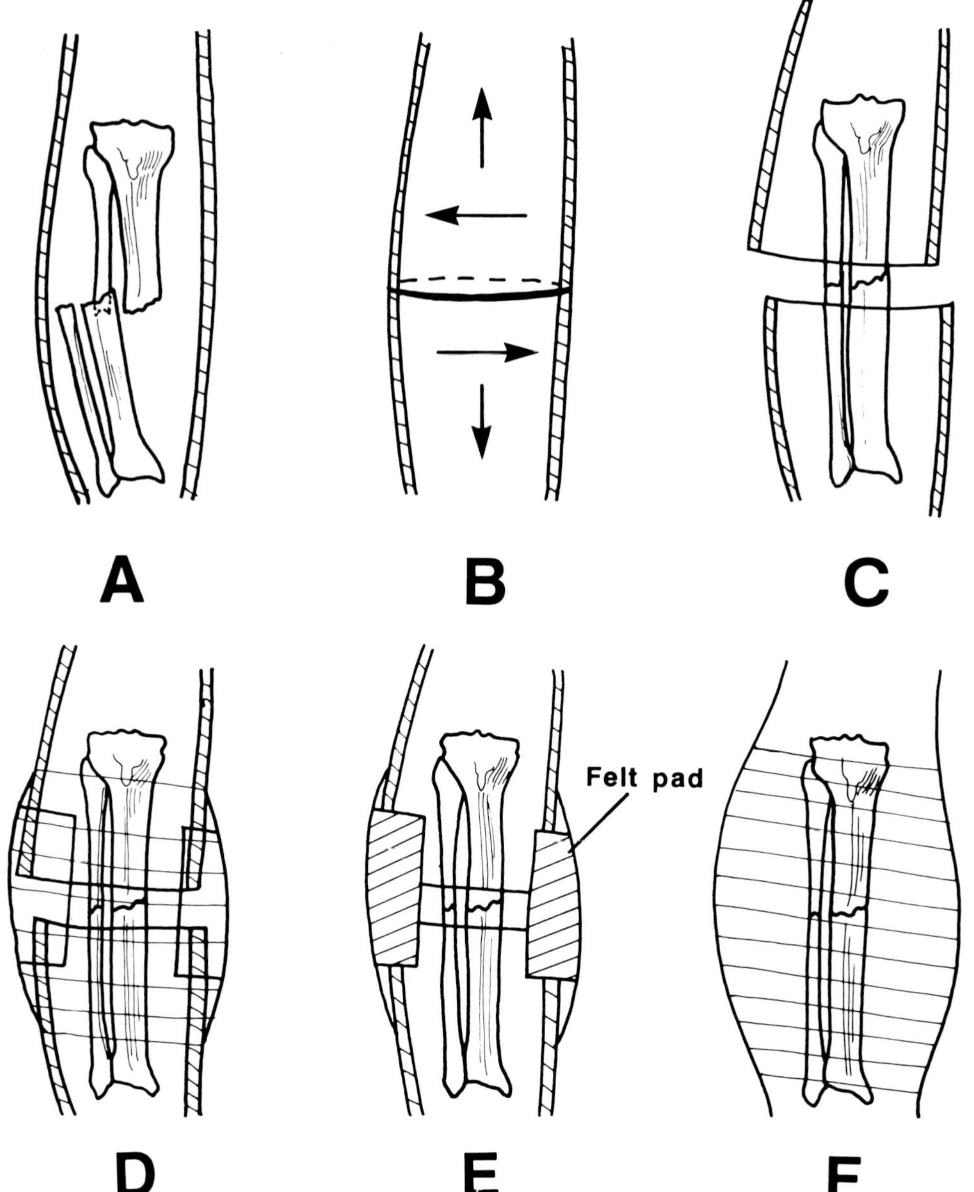

Fig. 9–32. Circumferential wedging of a cast. *A*, A markedly angulated and displaced fracture. *B*, A circumferential cut through the cast followed by traction and manual reduction of the fracture displacement. *C*, An anatomically reduced fracture in association with 2 malaligned cast parts. *D*, A 4″ × 4″ section of cast material has been removed from both sides of the cast where a step-off of the 2 cut cast edges is present. *E*, The 2 4″ × 4″ cast windows have been filled with 2 pieces of 4″ × 4″ felt. *F*, The 2 pieces of felt have been bound into the cast with a roll of 4″ plaster bandage.

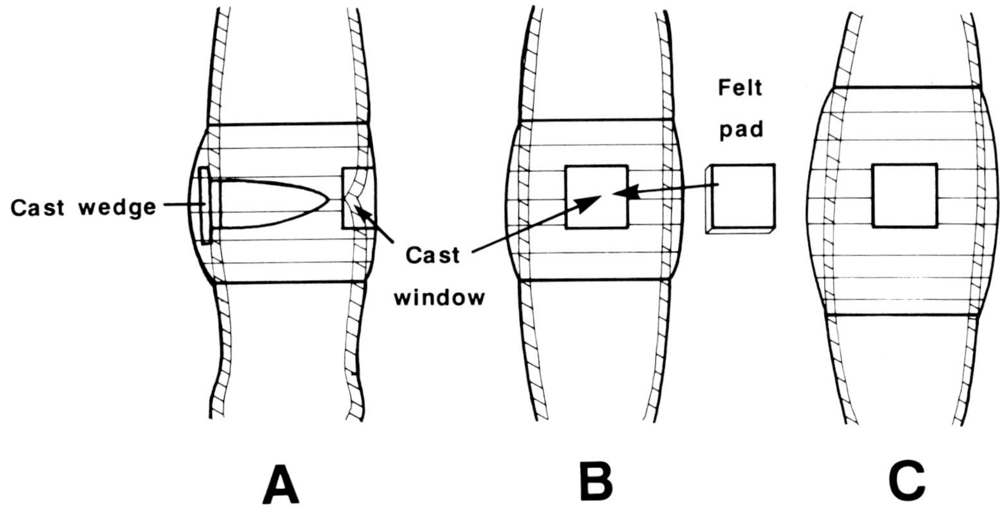

Fig. 9–33. Prevention of development of skin ulceration following a cast wedging. *A*, An opening wedging of the cast, with resulting inward buckling of the cast edges on the convex side of the fracture. *B*, A 4″ × 4″ section of cast material is removed from the convex side of the fracture, and the cast window is filled with a 4″ × 4″ felt pad. *C*, The felt pad is bound into the cast with a roll of 4″ plaster bandage.

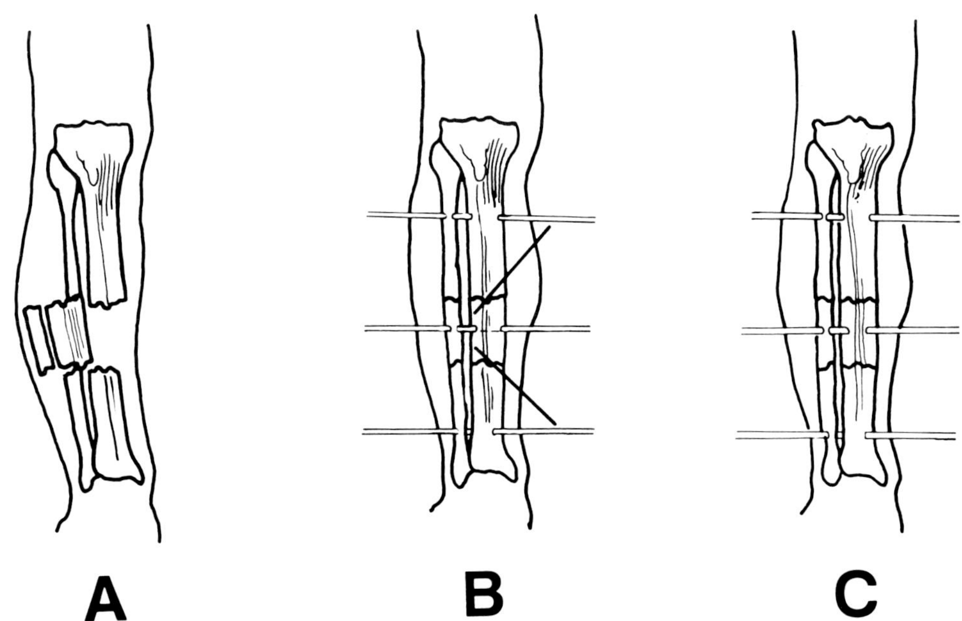

Fig. 9–34. Pin-and-plaster method of treating a compound and comminuted fracture. *A*, A compound and comminuted fracture. *B*, The fracture sites have been reduced and fragments have been fixed in place with small K-wires. Steinmann pins have been inserted through the major fragments of the fracture, and the Steinmann pins have been incorporated into a cast to stabilize the fracture reduction. *C*, The K-wires have been removed from the fracture sites.

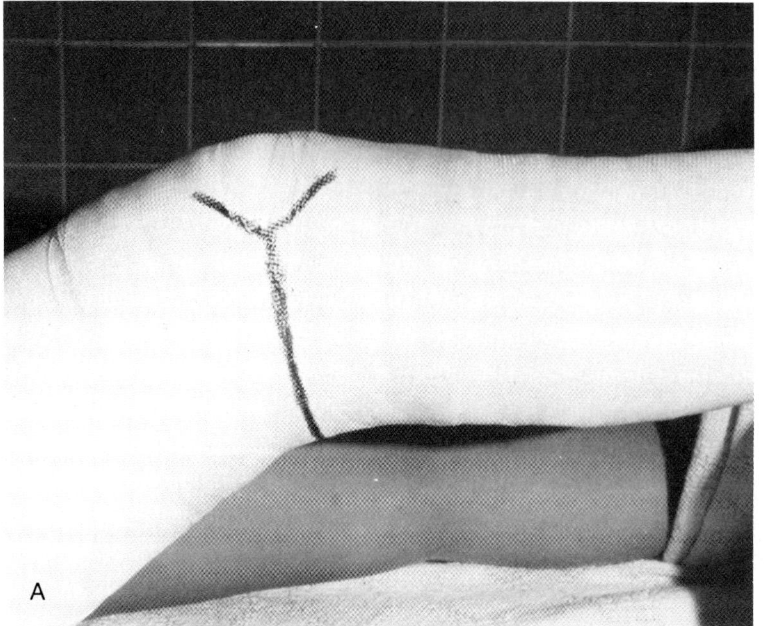

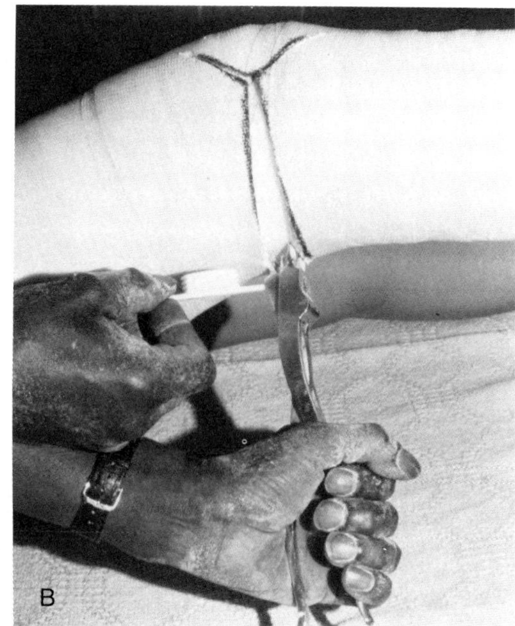

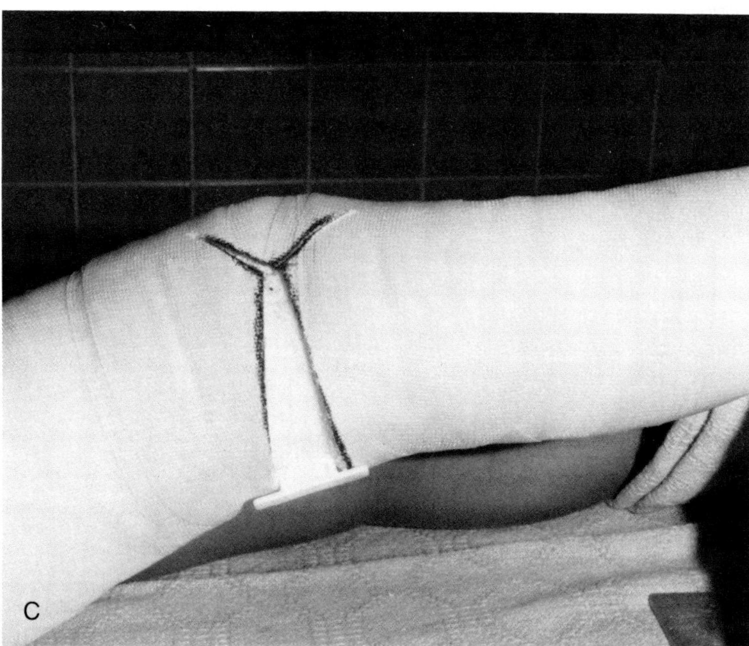

Fig. 9–35 Correction of a flexion contracture of the knee by means of cast wedges. *A*, Making a double Y-shaped cut through about 75% of the circumference of the cast in the knee joint region. *B*, Separating the 2 cut edges with a cast spreader. *C*, Inserting a cast wedge between the 2 cut edges of the cast to achieve some correction of the flexion contracture of the knee.

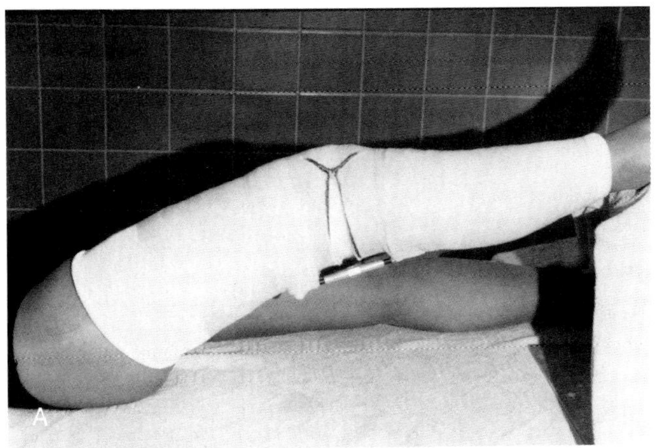

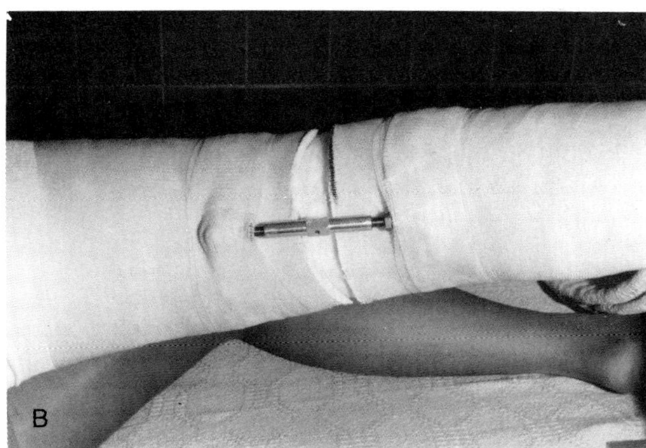

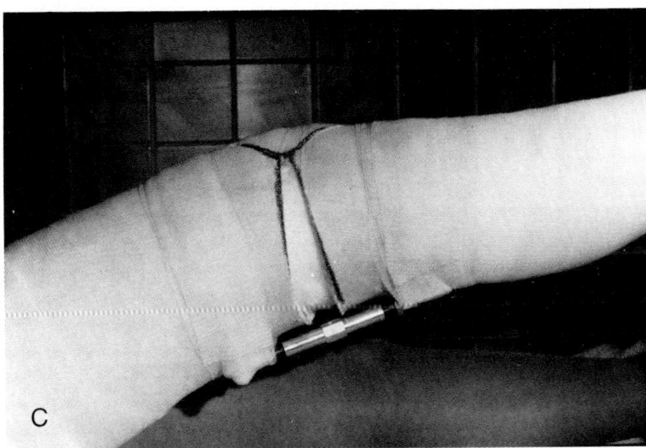

Fig. 9–36. Use of a turnbuckle to correct a flexion contracture of the knee. *A*, Turnbuckle attached to the posterior aspect of the cast directly behind the knee joint. *B*, Posterior view of the turnbuckle. *C*, Lateral view of the turnbuckle.

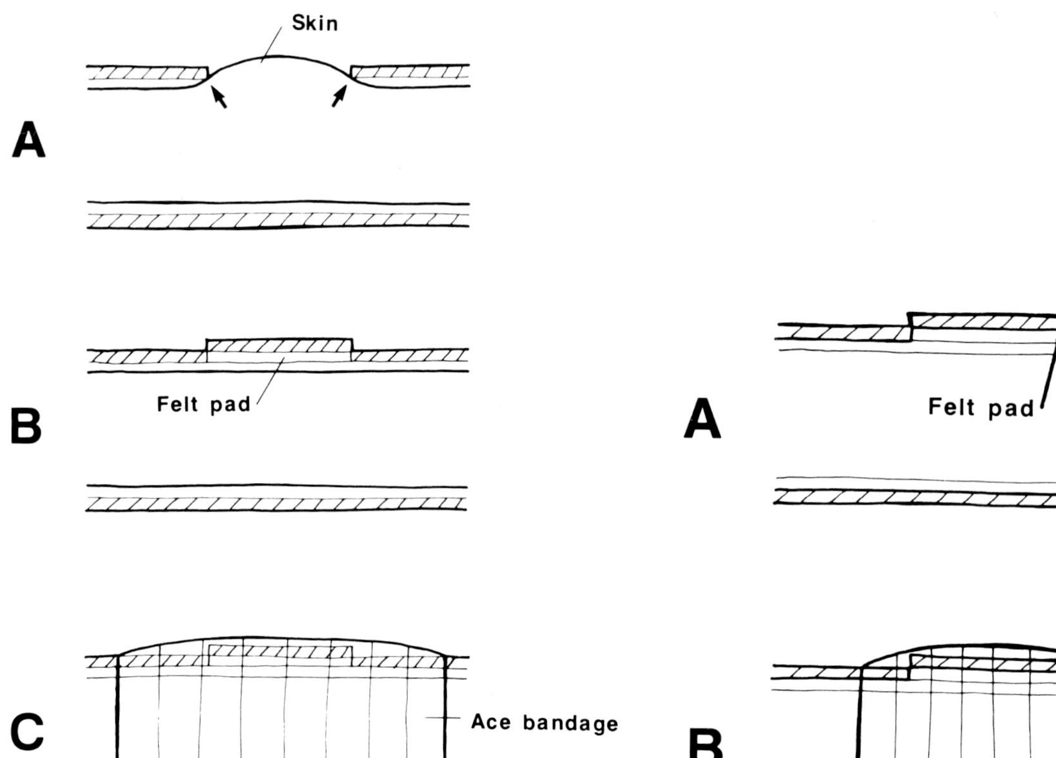

Fig. 9–37. Windowing a cast. *A*, Cast-window edema. Arrows indicate the common sites of skin necrosis. *B,C*, A felt pad is placed in the window with the original plaster on top of it and is bound to the cast with an Ace bandage.

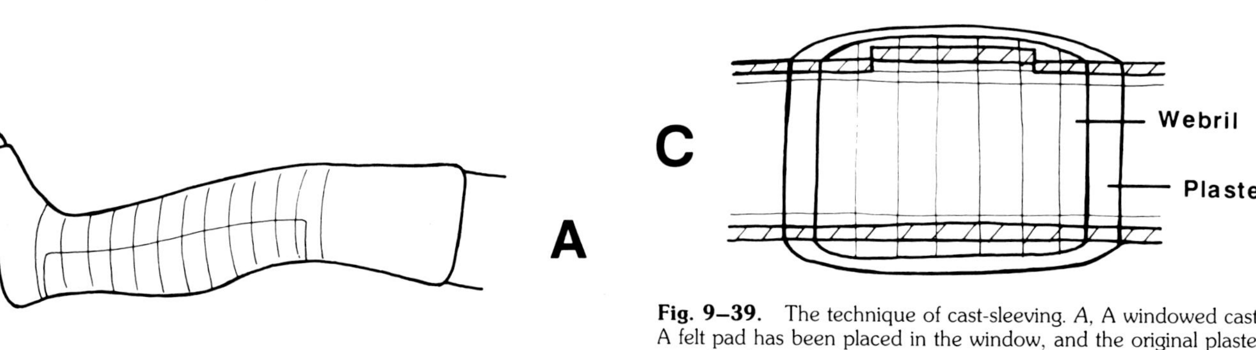

Fig. 9–38. Reinforcement of a cast before windowing the cast. *A*, A 5″ × 30″ plaster splint is placed behind the cast and bound to the cast with a roll of 6″ plaster bandage. *B*, A large window is created in front of the incorporated plaster splint.

Fig. 9–39. The technique of cast-sleeving. *A*, A windowed cast. A felt pad has been placed in the window, and the original plaster piece has been placed over the pad. *B*, A roll of 6″ Webril bandage has been applied to the windowed portion of the cast. The bandage extends 1 to 2 inches beyond the proximal and distal margins of the cast window. *C*, A roll of 6″ plaster bandage has been applied over the Webril. Its proximal and distal margins extend about 1″ beyond those of the Webril bandage.

CHAPTER 10. HIP SPICA CASTS

THE FIVE MAIN HIP SPICA CASTS

Double (Bilateral) Hip Spica Cast. A double (bilateral) hip spica cast (Fig. 10-1) extends from about 3″ below the nipple line to the metatarsal heads of both legs. It is used to treat bilateral femoral fractures and various combinations of femoral, pelvic, and tibial fractures.

One and One-Half Hip Spica Cast. A $1^1/_2$ hip spica cast (Fig. 10-2) extends from about 3″ below the nipple line to the metatarsal heads on one side, and to about 2″ above the superior pole of the patella on the other. It is used to treat different combinations of femoral and pelvic fractures.

Single (Unilateral) Hip Spica Cast. A single (unilateral) hip spica cast (Fig. 10-3) extends from about 3″ below the nipple line to the metatarsal heads on one side, and to the level of the greater trochanter on the other. It is typically used to treat femoral fractures.

Double (Bilateral) Pantaloon Hip Spica Cast. A double (bilateral) pantaloon hip spica cast (Fig. 10-4) extends from a line about 3″ below the nipple line to a point about 2″ above the superior pole of the patella on both legs. It is typically used to treat lumbar spine and pelvic fractures.

Single (Unilateral) Pantaloon Hip Spica Cast. A single (unilateral) pantaloon hip spica cast (Fig. 10-5) extends from about 3″ below the nipple line to a point about 2″ above the superior pole of the patella on one side, and to the level of the greater trochanter on the other. It is typically used to treat lumbar spine injuries.

DOUBLE (BILATERAL) HIP SPICA CAST

Cast Materials Needed

Plaster Double Hip Spica Cast

1 10″ or 12″ body stockinet

2 4″ leg stockinets

5 rolls of 6″ Webril

15 rolls of 4″ Webril

13 rolls of 6″ plaster bandage

7 rolls of 4″ plaster bandage

2 boxes of 5″ × 30″ plaster splints (10 splints per box)

5 felt pads (for upper medial thighs, anterior iliac crests, and sacrococcygeal region)

1 wooden bar approximately 18″ in length

Fiberglass Double Hip Spica Cast

1 10″ or 12″ body stockinet

2 4″ leg stockinets

5 rolls of 6″ Webril

15 rolls of 4″ Webril

9 rolls of 5″ fiberglass bandage

7 rolls of 4″ fiberglass bandage

5 felt pads (for upper medial thighs, anterior iliac crests, and sacrococcygeal region)

1 wooden bar approximately 18″ in length

Patient's Position

The patient is placed in a supine position on a fracture table with the upper back supported by the upper end of the fracture table, the sacrococcygeal area by a small padded seat, and both feet by two foot rests or cloth slings.

Technique for Applying A Fiberglass Double Hip Spica Cast

Stockinette

Before the patient is placed on a fracture table, a 10″ or 12″ stockinet is applied to the body from the upper chest to the mid-thigh level, and 4″ stockinets are applied to both legs from the toes to the upper thighs. Next, the body stockinet is split longitudinally between the legs, and the leg stockinets are rolled up over the upper thighs to cover the ends of the body stockinet (Fig. 10-6A–D).

Webril

Five rolls of 6″ Webril bandage are applied to the body from about 3″ below the nipple line to the level of the greater trochanters. Then 4 rolls of 4″ Webril bandage are applied to each leg from the upper thigh to the ankle. To produce even Webril coverage over the junction between the body and thighs, 3 rolls of 4″ Webril are applied to these transitional areas in an overlapping figure-8 fashion in the following sequence: pubic symphysis→greater trochanter→gluteal fold→perineal crease→inguinal ligament→anterior superior iliac spine→lower part of sacrum→opposite anterior superior iliac spine→inguinal ligament→perineal crease→gluteal fold→greater trochanter→pubic symphysis (Fig. 10-6E,F,G).

Fiberglass Bandage

After felt pads have been applied to the upper medial aspects of the thighs, the anterior iliac crests, and the sacrococcygeal region, 5 rolls of 5″ fiberglass bandage are applied to the body portion of the cast and 4 rolls of 5″ fiberglass bandage are applied to each leg from the base of the thigh to the ankle (Fig. 10-6H,I,J). Both of the patient's legs should then be suspended with cloth slings so that 2 rolls of 4″ Webril bandage can be applied from the ankle to the metatarsal head region of each foot and 2 rolls of 4″ fiberglass bandage can be applied to the ankles and feet (Fig. 10-6K,L).

A wooden bar approximately 18″ in length is fixed to the anterior aspect of the cast in the vicinity of the knee joint by means of 2 rolls of 4″ fiberglass bandage, which should also cover the wooden bar (Fig. 10-6M,N). The perineal area of the cast should be trimmed in a circular manner as high as the pubic symphysis anteriorly, and as high as the lower sacrum posteriorly, to provide room for personal hygienic care (Fig. 10-6O–R). The stockinet in the perineal area is pulled tightly over the cast margins of the perineal opening and fixed to the adjacent cast surface with a roll of 4″ fiberglass bandage. To minimize the chance of development of cast syndrome or other gastrointestinal distress, a round hole 6″ to 8″ in diameter can be cut out of the epigastric portion of the cast (Fig. 10-6S).

Technique for Applying a Plaster Double Hip Spica Cast

The stockinets, Webril bandages, and felt pads are applied as for a fiberglass double hip spica cast. After all the padding materials have been applied, 2 rolls of 6″ plaster bandage are wrapped around the body from a level 3″ below the nipple line to the level of the greater trochanters, and 2 rolls of 6″ plaster bandage are applied to each leg from the base of the thigh to the ankle. 5″ × 30″ plaster splints are applied transversely to the anterior and posterior aspects of the body, overlapping each other about 25% of their width. In addition, 3 5″ × 30″ plaster splints are applied to each leg, the 1st from the buttock to the posterior aspect of the lower leg, the 2nd from the anterior iliac crest to the anterior aspect of the lower leg, and the 3rd on top of the felt pads over the upper medial aspects of the thighs. Both ends of this splint should go upward and laterally toward the greater trochanters so that it reinforces the 2 thigh and body junctions of the cast. The upper end of the body stockinet is folded down over the proximal cast end, and 2 rolls of 6″ plaster bandage are used to cover and finish the body portion of the cast down to the level of the greater trochanters.

The junction between legs and body is covered with 1 roll of 6″ plaster bandage in a figure-8 manner (Fig. 10-6F). Next, 2 rolls of 6″ plaster bandage are used to wrap each leg from the upper thigh to the ankle. Two rolls of 4″ Webril bandage are wrapped from the ankle to the metatarsal heads of each leg. For each leg, 1 roll of 4″ plaster bandage is applied from the ankle to the metatarsal heads, the distal end of the 4″ stockinet is folded down over the cast end, and another roll of 4″ plaster is applied over the ankle and foot region to finish the cast.

An 18″ wooden bar is usually applied to the anterior aspect of the knee region of both legs to strengthen the cast; 2 rolls of 4″ plaster bandage are used to fix the wooden bar to the legs. After the perineal region of the cast has been trimmed, the stockinet is folded down over the cast margins of the perineal opening and fixed to the adjacent portion of the cast with a roll of 4″ plaster bandage.

ONE AND ONE-HALF HIP SPICA CAST

A $1^1/_2$ hip spica cast differs from the double hip spica cast in that one leg of the cast ends about 2″ above the superior pole of the patella. Thus, in a plaster $1^1/_2$ hip spica cast, 4 rolls of 4″ Webril bandage, 2 rolls of 6″ plaster bandage, and 2 rolls of 4″ plaster bandage are eliminated from the materials used for a plaster double hip spica cast. Similarly, in a fiberglass $1^1/_2$ hip spica cast, 4 rolls of 4″ Webril bandage, 2 rolls of 5″ fiberglass bandage, and 2 rolls of 4″ fiberglass bandage are omitted from the materials used for a fiberglass double hip spica cast (Fig. 10-7A–G).

SINGLE HIP SPICA CAST

A single hip spica cast can be differentiated from a double hip spica cast by the absence of cast materials on one leg. In covering the junction between the leg and the body, only 2 rolls of 4″ Webril bandage are needed; they are wrapped around the hip in an asymmetrical figure-8 manner (Fig. 10-8). In a plaster single hip spica cast, 7 rolls of 4″ Webril bandage, 4 rolls of 6″ plaster bandage, and 4 rolls of 4″ plaster bandage are omitted from the materials used for double hip spica cast; in a fiberglass single hip spica cast, 7 rolls of 4″ Webril bandage, 4 rolls of 5″ fiberglass bandage, and 4 rolls of 4″ fiberglass bandage are excluded from the materials used for a fiberglass double hip spica cast (Fig. 10-9).

DOUBLE PANTALOON HIP SPICA CAST

A double pantaloon hip spica cast can be distinguished from a double hip spica cast by the termination of the distal cast ends just above the knee joints. Therefore, in making a plaster double pantaloon hip spica cast, 8 rolls of 4″ Webril bandage, 4 rolls of 6″ plaster bandage, and 4 rolls of 4″ plaster bandage are omitted from the materials used for a double hip spica cast. In making a fiberglass double pantaloon hip spica cast, 8 rolls of 4″ Webril bandage, 4 rolls of 5″ fiberglass bandage, and 4 rolls of 4″ fiberglass bandage are eliminated from the materials used for a double hip spica cast. Because the 2 leg extensions of the cast end above the knee joints, only 2 short 4″ leg stockinets are used. The ends of the wooden bar are fixed to the cast slightly above the knees (Figs. 10-10, 10-11).

SINGLE PANTALOON HIP SPICA CAST

A single pantaloon hip spica cast (Fig. 10-12) differs from a double hip spica cast in the absence of cast materials from one leg and termination of the cast just above the opposite knee joint. In comparison with a plaster double hip spica cast, a single pantaloon hip spica cast saves 10 rolls of 4″ Webril bandage, 6 rolls of 6″ plaster bandage, 6 rolls of 4″ plaster bandage, and a wooden bar. In comparison with a fiberglass double hip spica cast, a single pantaloon hip spica cast saves 10 rolls of 4″ Webril bandage, 6 rolls of 5″ fiberglass bandage, 6 rolls of 4″ fiberglass bandage, and a wooden bar. Furthermore, a single pantaloon hip spica cast uses only a short 4″ leg stockinet instead of the 2 long 4″ leg stockinets routinely used in a double hip spica cast (Fig. 10-13).

SINGLE HIP SPICA CAST WITH KNEE HINGES

A single hip spica cast with knee hinges (Fig. 10-14) is used mainly for treating femoral fractures. It allows knee motion while immobilizing femoral fractures, especially those in which significant fracture callus has formed. The first step in making this cast-brace is to apply a single hip spica cast. The two polycentric knee hinges can then be installed by using the technique described in Chapter 9 for a long-leg cast-brace with knee hinges.

SINGLE HIP SPICA CAST WITH UNILATERAL HIP HINGE

A single hip spica cast with a hip hinge (Fig. 10-15) allows a limited range of hip motion and is useful in treating femoral fractures. Although this cast can be made by first applying a single hip spica cast and then installing the hip hinge, a much better and easier way to do it is to apply a wide waistband and a long-leg cast and then link them with the hip hinge (Fig. 10-16). The materials for the waistband include 10″ or 12″ stockinet, 6″ Webril bandages, 6″ plaster bandages, 5″ × 30″ plaster splints, and 5″ fiberglass bandages, which can be used in different combinations. The materials for the long-leg cast have been listed in Chapter 9.

SINGLE HIP SPICA CAST WITH UNILATERAL HIP HINGE AND TWO POLYCENTRIC KNEE HINGES

A single hip spica cast with a hip hinge and two polycentric knee hinges (Fig. 10-17) is made by first applying a wide waistband and a long-leg cast. The hip hinge is then used to link the waistband and the long-leg cast, and finally the two polycentric knee hinges are installed.

SINGLE HIP SPICA CAST WITH UNILATERAL HIP HINGE, TWO POLYCENTRIC KNEE HINGES, AND A HEEL CUP WITH TWO ANKLE HINGES

A single hip spica cast with a hip hinge, two polycentric knee hinges, and a heel cup with two ankle hinges (Fig. 10-18) is made by first applying a waistband and a long-leg cylinder cast. The waistband is connected to the cylinder cast with a hip hinge. The two polycentric knee hinges are installed next, and the heel cup and two attached ankle hinges are applied last.

BIBLIOGRAPHY

Adair, I.V.: The use of plaster casts in the treatment of fractures of the femoral shaft. Injury, *7*:194, 1976.

Anderson, R.: An ambulatory method of treating fractures of the shaft of femur. Surg. Gynecol. Obstet., *62*:865, 1936.

Arnold, W.D., Lyden, J.P., and Minkoff, J.: Treatment of intracapsular fractures of the femoral neck. J. Bone Joint Surg. [Am.], *56*:254, 1974.

Askin, S.R., and Bryan, R.S.: Femoral neck fractures in young adults. Clin. Orthop., *114*:259, 1976.

Atkinson, R.E., Kinnett, J.G., and Arnold, W.D.: Simultaneous fractures of both femoral

necks: Review of the literature and report of two cases. Clin. Orthop., *152*:284, 1980.
Bernstein, S.M.: Fractures of the femoral shaft and associated ipsilateral fractures of the hip. Orthop. Clin. North Am., *5*:799, 1974.
Branch, H.E.: March fractures of the femur. J. Bone Joint Surg., *26*:387, 1944.
Brittain, H.A.: Ischio-femoral arthrodesis. J. Bone Joint Surg. [Br.], *30*:642, 1948.
Burk, D.L., Jr., et al.: Pelvic and acetabular fractures: Examination by angled CT-scanning. Radiology, *153*:548, 1984.
Canale, S.T., and Manugian, A.H.: Irreducible traumatic dislocations of the hip. J. Bone Joint Surg. [Am.], *61*:7, 1979.
Chakraborti, S., and Miller, I.M.: Dislocation of the hip associated with fracture of the femoral head. Injury, *7*:134, 1975.
Chandler, F.A.: Hip-fusion operation. J. Bone Joint Surg., *15*:947, 1933.
Connolly, J.: Management of fractures associated with arterial injuries. Am. J. Surg., *120*:331, 1970.
Connolly, J.F., Whittaker, D., and Williams, E.: Femoral and tibial fractures combined with injuries to the femoral or popliteal artery. J. Bone Joint Surg. [Am.], *53*:56, 1971.
Dahl, E.: Mortality and life expectancy after hip fractures. Acta Orthop. Scand., *51*:163, 1980.
DeLee, J.C., Clanton, T.O., and Rockwood, C.A.: Closed treatment of subtrochanteric fractures of the femur in a modified cast brace. J. Bone Joint Surg. [Am.], *63*:773, 1981.
Denker, H.: Shaft fractures of femur: A comparative study of the results of various methods of treatment in 1003 cases. Acta Chir. Scand., *130*:173, 1965.
Doherty, J.H., and Lyden, J.P.: Intertrochanteric fractures of the hip treated with the hip compression screw. Clin. Orthop., *141*:184, 1979.
Dowd, G.S.E., and Johnson, R.: Successful conservative treatment of a fracture-dislocation of the femoral head. J. Bone Joint Surg. [Am.], *61*:1244, 1979.
Ernst, J.: Stress fracture of the neck of the femur. J. Trauma, *4*:71, 1964.
Fraser, R.D., Hunter G.A., and Waddell, J.P.: Ipsilateral fracture of the femur and tibia. J. Bone Joint Surg. [Br.], *60*:510, 1978.
Ghormley, R.K.: Use of the anterior superior spine and crest of ilium in surgery of the hip joint. J. Bone Joint Surg., *13*:784, 1931.
Gunterberg, B., Goldie, I., and Slatis, P.: Fixation of pelvic fractures and dislocations. Acta Orthop. Scand., *49*:278, 1978.
Henderson, M.S.: Combined intra-articular and extra-articular arthrodesis for tuberculosis of the hip joint. J. Bone Joint Surg., *15*:51, 1933.
Henderson, O.L., Morrissy, R.T., Gerdes, M.H., and McCarthy, R.E.: Early casting of femoral shaft fractures in children. J. Pediatr. Orthop., *4*:16, 1984.
Henson, J.S.: Treatment of intracapsular fracture of the hip with primary pedicle bone graft from greater Trochanter. Clin. Orthop., *76*:100, 1971.
Hirasawa, Y., Oda, R., and Nakatani, K.: Sciatic nerve paralysis in posterior dislocation of the hip. Clin. Orthop., *126*:172, 1977.
Ingman, A.M., Paterson, D.C., and Sutherland, A.D.: A comparison between innominate osteotomy and hip spica in the treatment of Legg-Perthes' disease, Clin. Orthop., *163*:141, 1982.
Irani, R.N., Nicholson, J.T., and Chung, S.M.: Long-term results in the treatment of femoral-shaft fractures in young children by immediate spica immobilization. J. Bone Joint Surg. [Am.], *58*:945, 1976.
Judet, R., Judet, J., and Letournel, E.: Fractures of the acetabulum: Classification and surgical approaches for open reduction. J. Bone Joint Surg. [Am.], *46*:1615, 1964.
Katznelson, A.M.: Traumatic anterior dislocation of the hip. J. Bone Joint Surg. [Br.], *44*:129, 1962.
Kewenter, Y.: A case of isolated fracture of the lesser trochanter. Acta Orthop. Scand., *2*:160, 1931.
Kirkaldy-Willis, W.H., and Mbuthia, A.S.: Abduction arthrodesis of the hip. J. Bone Joint Surg. [Br.], *34*:433, 1952.
Kostuik, J.P., and Harrington, I.J.: Treatment of infected ununited femoral shaft fractures. Clin. Orthop., *108*:90, 1975.
Kyle, R.F., Gustilo, R.B., and Premer, R.F.: Analysis of six hundred and twenty-two intertrochanteric hip fractures. J. Bone Joint Surg. [Am.], *61*:216, 1979.
Looser, K.G., and Crombie, H.D., Jr.: Pelvic fractures: An anatomic guide to severity of injury. Am. J. Surg., *132*:638, 1976.
McCarthy, R.E.: A method for early spica cast application in treatment of pediatric femoral shaft fractures. J. Pediatr. Orthop., *6*:89, 1986.
Mears, D.C., and Fu, F.: External fixation in pelvic fractures. Orthop. Clin. North Am., *11*:465, 1980.
Meggitt, B.F., and Vaughan-Lane, T.: Hip hinge thigh brace for early mobilization of proximal femoral shaft fractures. Prosthet. Orthot. Int., *4*:150, 1980.
Merlino, A.F., and Nixon, J.E.: Isolated fractures of the greater trochanter. Int. Surg., *52*:117, 1969.

Meyer, M.H., Telfer, N., and Moore, T.M.: Determination of the vascularity of the femoral head with technetium-99M-sulfur-colloid. Diagnostic and prognostic significance. J. Bone Joint Surg. [Am.], *59:*658, 1977.
Montgomery, S., and Mooney, V.: Femur fractures: Treatment with roller traction and early ambulation. Clin. Orthop., *156:*196, 1981.
Muller, J., Bachmann, B., and Berg, H.: Malgaigne fracture of the pelvis: Treatment with percutaneous pin fixation. J. Bone Joint Surg. [Am.], *60:*992, 1978.
Naam, N.H., et al.: Major pelvic fractures. Arch. Surg., *118:*610, 1983.
Nerubay, J.: Traumatic anterior dislocation of the hip joint with vascular damage. Clin. Orthop., *116:*129, 1976.
Pankovich, A.M., and Tarabishy, I.E.: Ender nailing of intertrochanteric and subtrochanteric fractures of the femur. J. Bone Joint Surg. [Am.], *62:*635, 1980.
Peltier, L.F.: Complications associated with fractures of the pelvis. J. Bone Joint Surg. [Am.], *47:*1060, 1965.
Polesky, R.E., and Polesky, F.A.: Intrapelvic dislocation of the femoral head following anterior dislocation of the hip. J. Bone Joint Surg. [Am.], *54:*1097, 1972.
Roeder, L.F., and DeLee, J.C.: Femoral head fractures associated with posterior hip dislocation. Clin. Orthop., *147:*121, 1980.
Roper, B.A., and Provan, J.L.: Late thrombosis of femoral artery complicating fracture of the femur. J. Bone Joint Surg. [Br.], *47:*510, 1965.
Seinsheimer, F.: Subtrochanteric fractures of the femur. J. Bone Joint Surg. [Am.], *60:*300, 1978.
Shirkhoda, B., Brashear, H.R., and Staab, E.V.: Computed tomography of metabular fractures. Radiology, *134:*683, 1980.
Slatis, P., and Karaharju, E.D.: External fixation of unstable pelvic fractures: Experiences in 22 patients treated with a trapezoid compression frame. Clin. Orthop., *151:*73, 1980.
Stewart, H.D.: The hip cast-brace for hip prosthesis instability. Ann. R. Coll. Surg. Engl., *65:*404, 1983.
Templeton, T.S., and Saunders, E.A.: A review of fractures in the proximal femur treated with the Zickel nail. Clin. Orthop., *141:*213, 1979.
Tile, M.: Pelvic fractures: Operative versus nonoperative treatment. Orthop. Clin. North Am., *11:*423, 1980.
Upadhyay, S.S., Moulton, A., and Burwell, R.G.: Biological factors predisposing to traumatic posterior dislocation of the hip. A selection process in the mechanism of injury. J. Bone Joint Surg. [Br.], *67:*232, 1985.
Watson-Jones, R.: Arthrodesis of the osteoarthritic hip. JAMA, *110:*278, 1938.
Weil, G.S., Kuehner, H.G., and Henry, J.P.: The treatment of 278 consecutive fractures of the femur. Surg. Gynecol. Obstet., *62:*435, 1936.
Williams, J.F., Gottesman, M.J., and Mallory, T.H.: Dislocation after total hip arthroplasty. Treatment with an above-knee hip spica cast. Clin. Orthop., *171:*53, 1982.
Worland, R.L., and Keim, H.A.: Displaced fractures of the major pelvis: A method of management. Clin. Orthop., *112:*215, 1975.
Zickel, R.E.: An intramedullary fixation device for the proximal part of the femur. J. Bone Joint Surg. [Am.], *58:*866, 1976.

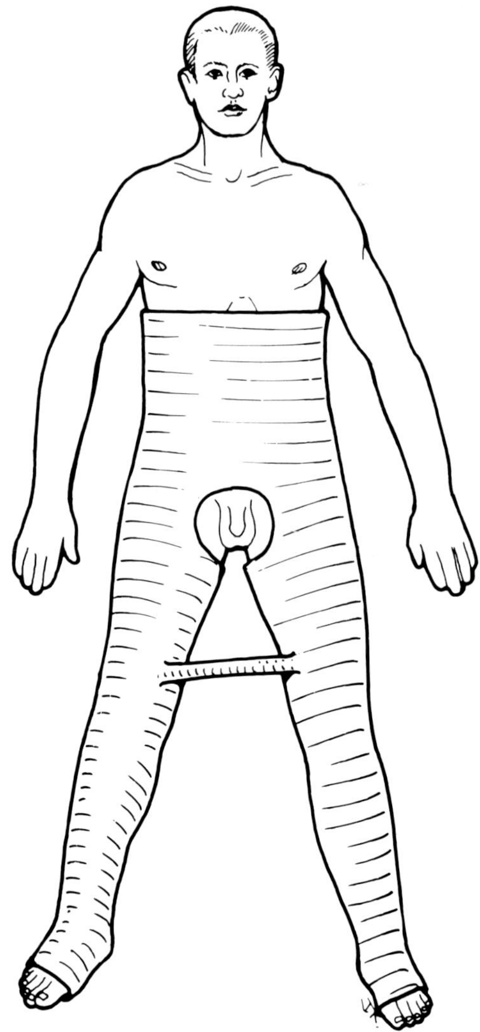

Fig. 10–1. Anterior view of a double hip spica cast.

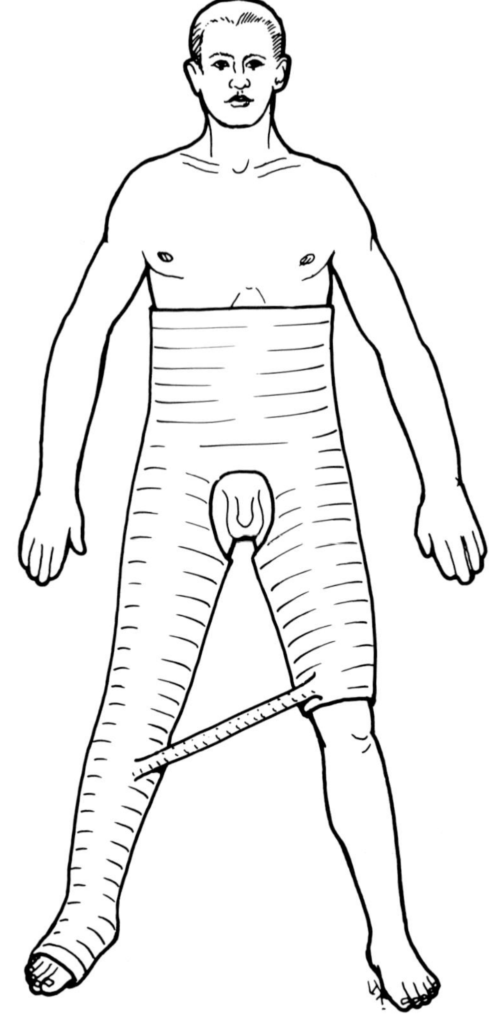

Fig. 10–2. Anterior view of a one and one-half hip spica cast.

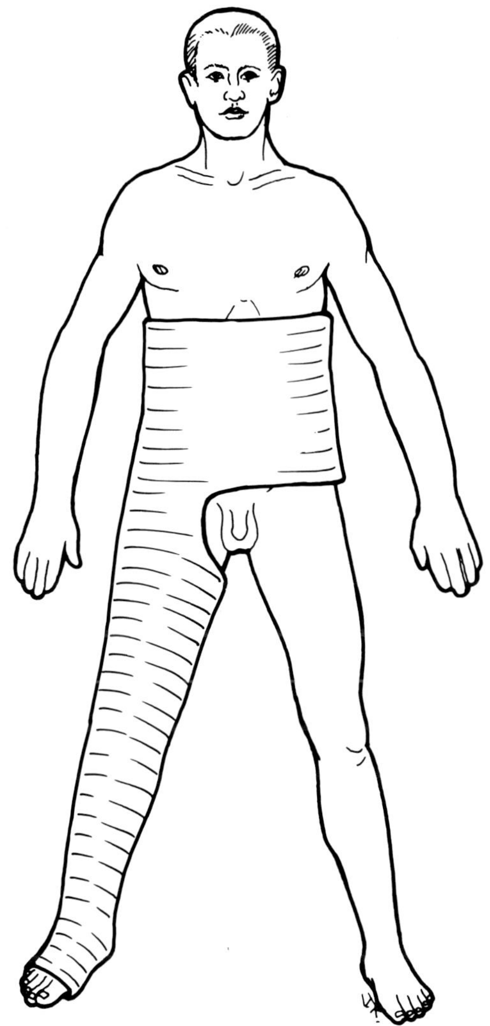

Fig. 10–3. Anterior view of a single hip spica cast.

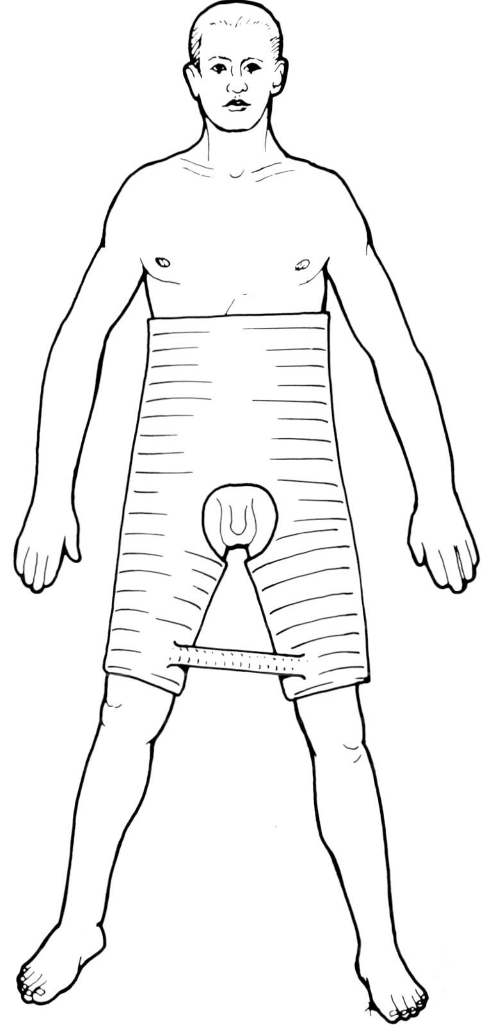

Fig. 10–4. Anterior view of a double pantaloon hip spica cast.

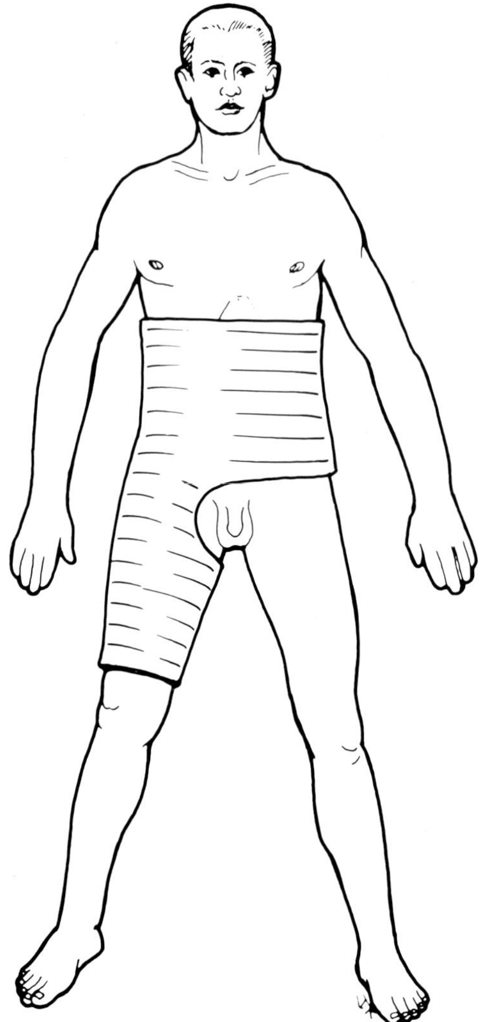

Fig. 10–5. Anterior view of a single pantaloon hip spica cast.

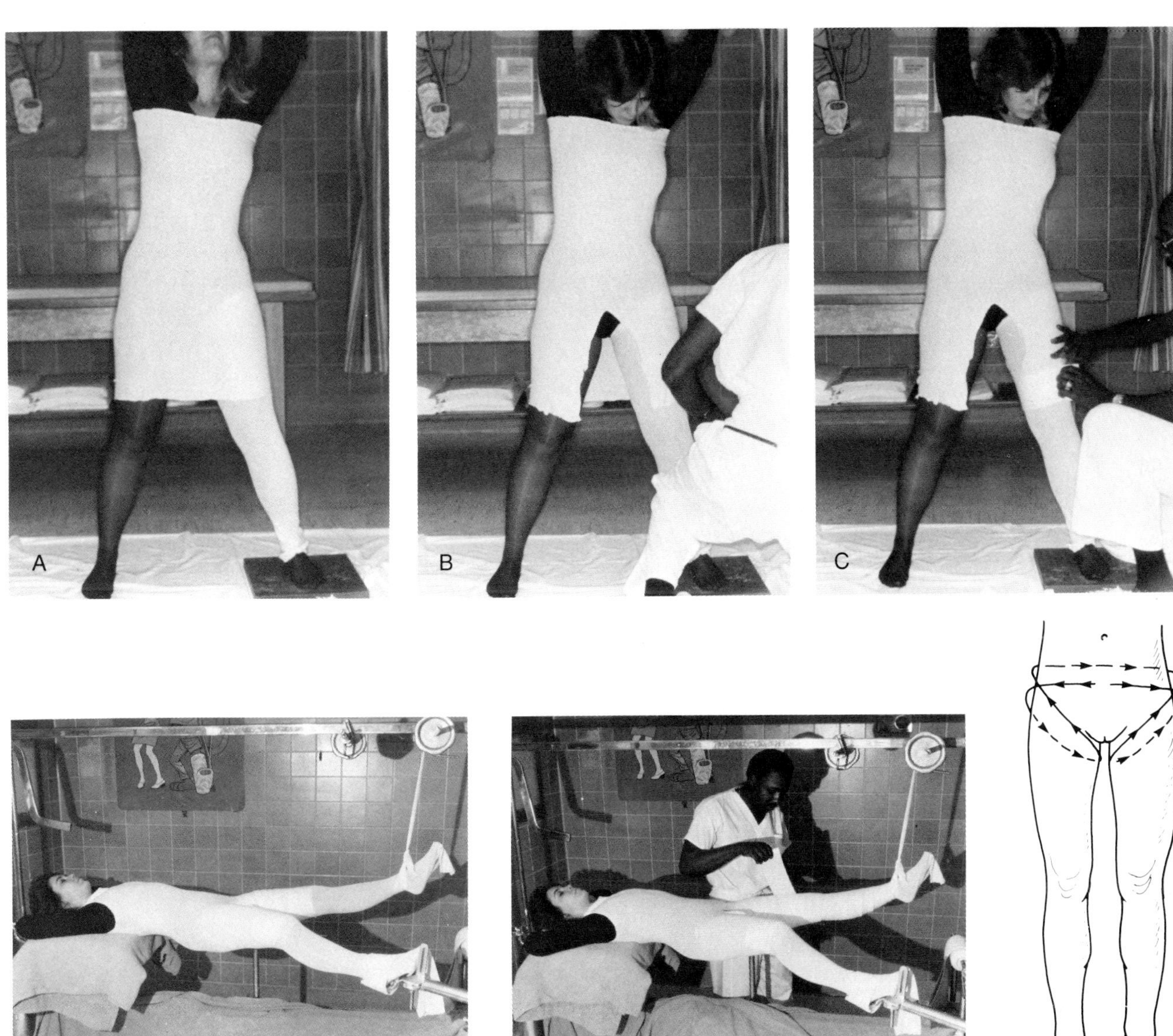

Fig. 10–6. The making of a fiberglass double hip spica cast. *A*, Application of the body and leg stockinets. *B*, The distal end of the body stockinet is split longitudinally between the thighs. *C*, To cover the upper thigh region, the leg stockinets can be rolled up to cover the cut ends of the body stockinet. An alternate method (shown here) is to roll the leg stockinet to the base of the thigh and then lap the two free ends of the split body stockinet over the leg stockinet and hold them in place with a few turns of 4″ Webril bandage. *D*, An alternative method for applying a body stockinet is to cut out two armholes from one end of the body stockinet, working the stockinet on like a T-shirt. After the patient's body and both legs are covered with stockinet, the patient is placed on a fracture table with the upper back supported by the upper end of the fracture table, the sacrococcygeal region by a small padded seat, and the feet by a foot rest and a cloth sling. *E*, 4″ Webril bandage is being applied to the leg. *F*, The junction between the body and the thighs is covered with 4″ Webril bandages, which are applied in an overlapping figure-8 fashion.

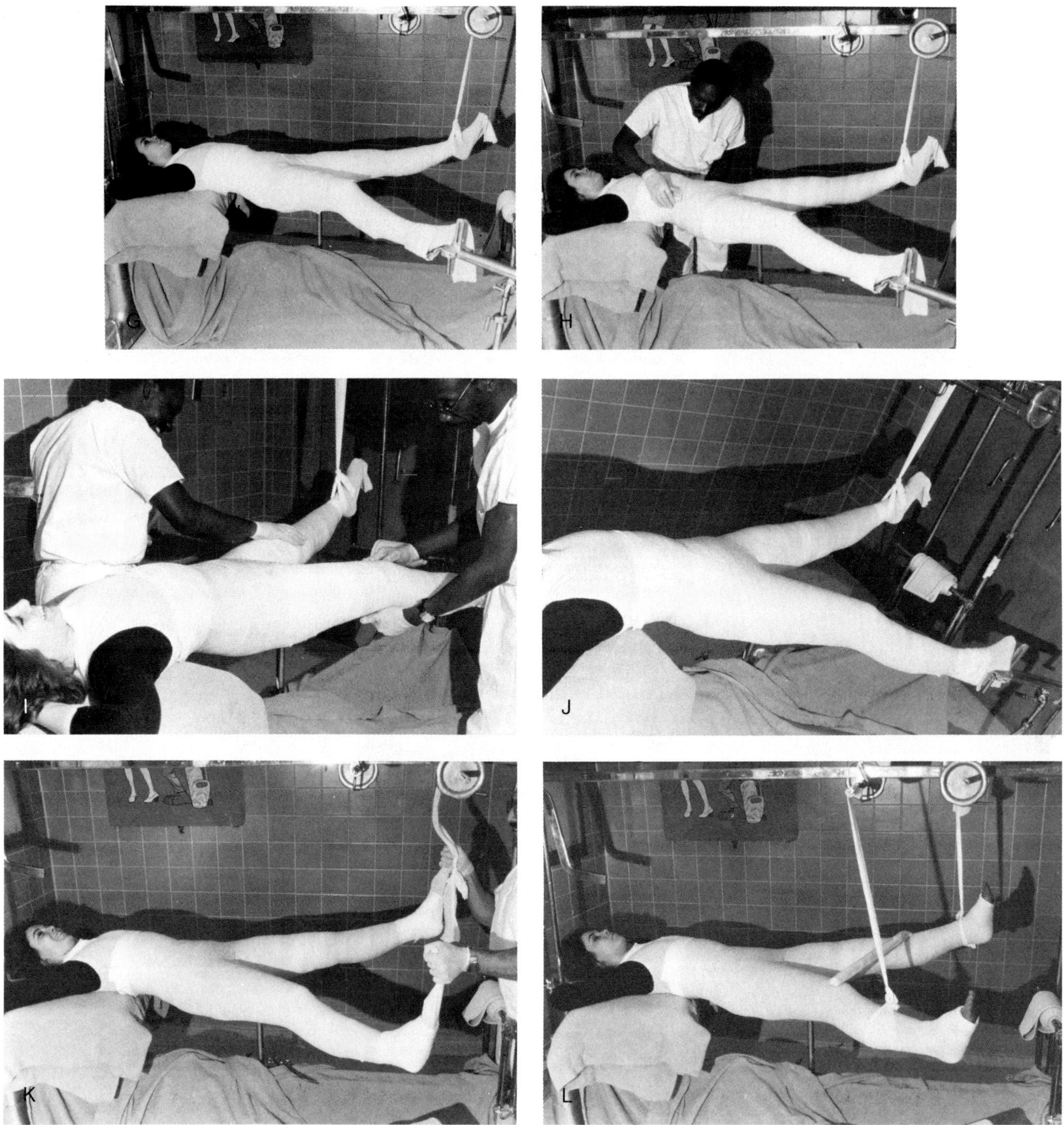

Fig. 10–6 (cont.). *G*, The body has been covered with 6″ Webril bandages, and the legs with 4″ Webril bandages. *H,I,J*, 5″ fiberglass bandages are applied to the body and legs from about 3″ below the nipple line to the ankle. *K*, Ankles and feet are covered with 4″ Webril. *L*, Ankles and feet have been covered with 4″ fiberglass bandages, and an 18″ wooden bar has been laid across the legs of the cast.

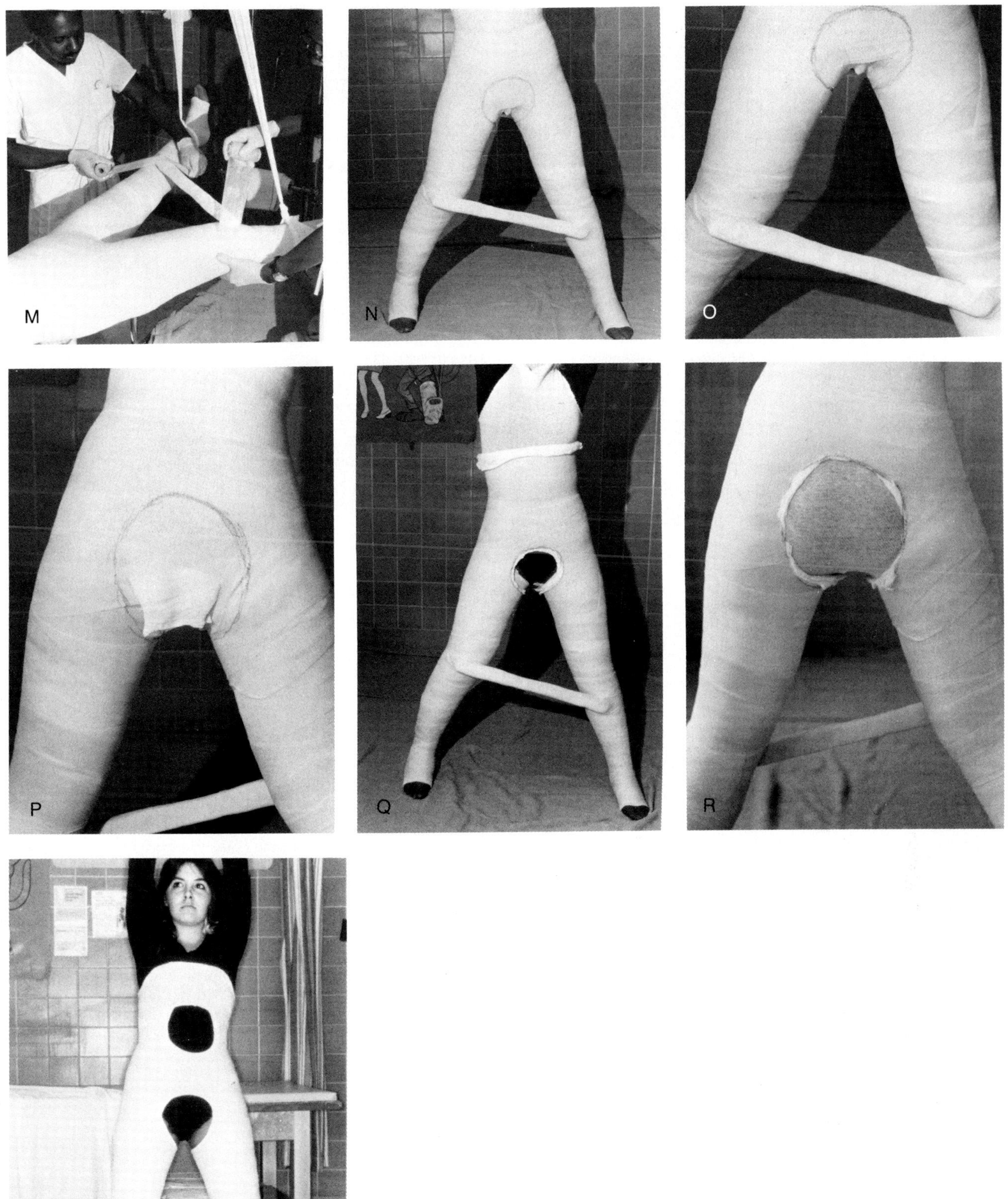

Fig. 10–6 (cont.). *M,N,* The wooden bar is attached to the legs of the cast by means of 2 rolls of 4″ fiberglass bandage. *O,P,* The anterior and posterior perineal openings of the cast have been marked on the cast with a wax pencil. *Q,R,* The anterior and posterior perineal openings have been made. *S,* A hole 6″ to 8″ in diameter has been cut out of the epigastric portion of the cast to minimize the chance of development of cast syndrome or other gastrointestinal disturbances.

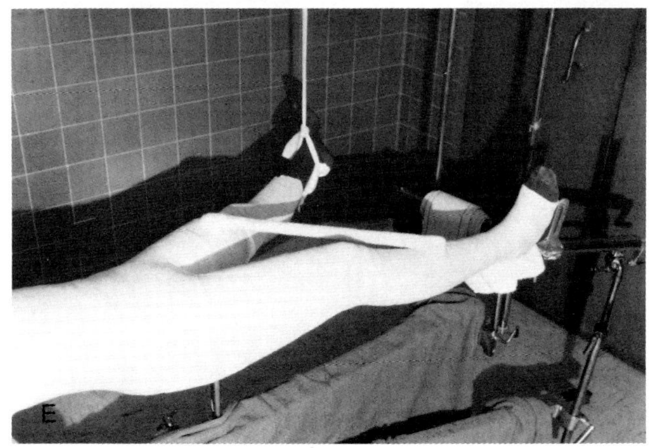

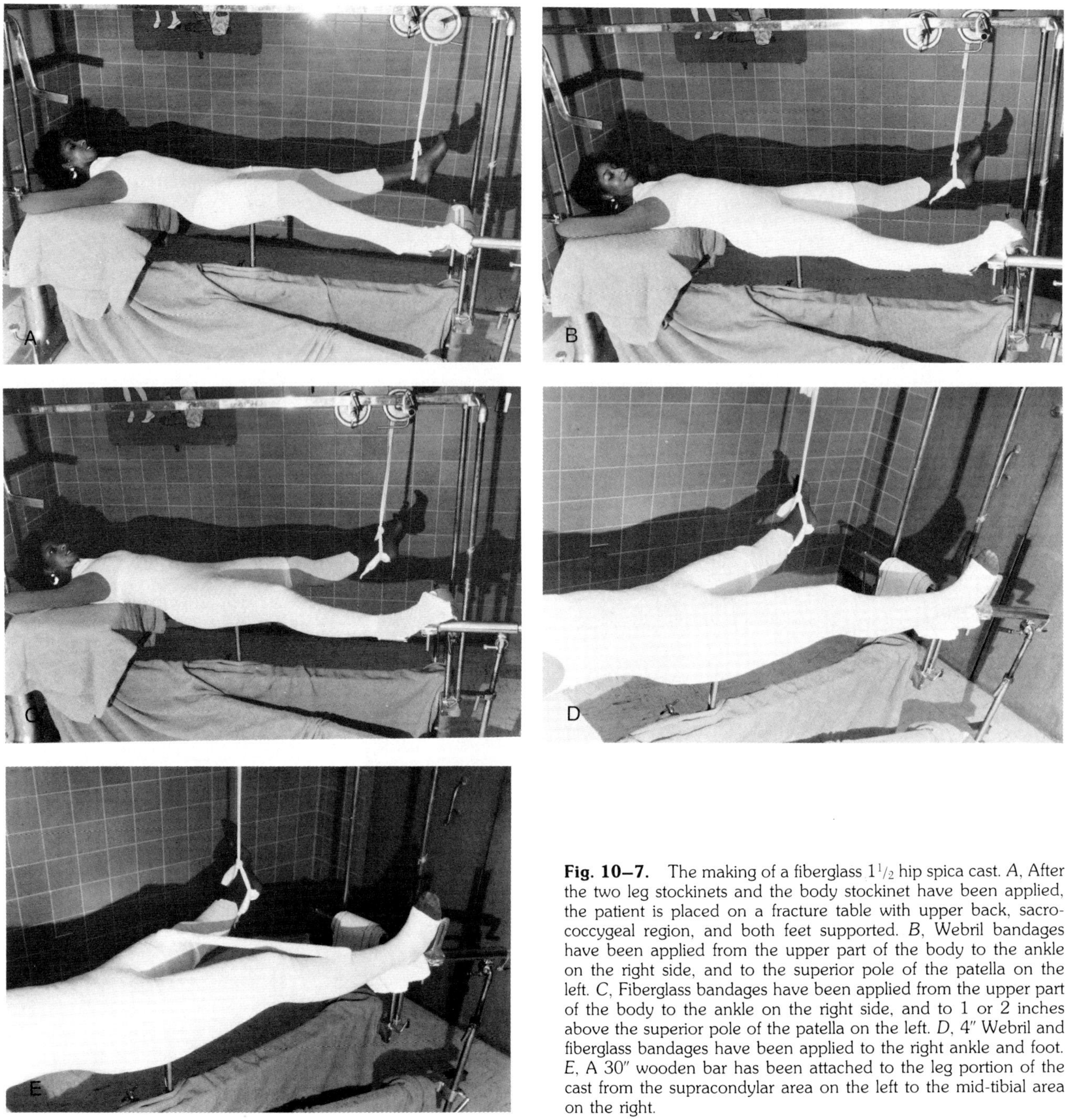

Fig. 10–7. The making of a fiberglass $1\frac{1}{2}$ hip spica cast. *A*, After the two leg stockinets and the body stockinet have been applied, the patient is placed on a fracture table with upper back, sacrococcygeal region, and both feet supported. *B*, Webril bandages have been applied from the upper part of the body to the ankle on the right side, and to the superior pole of the patella on the left. *C*, Fiberglass bandages have been applied from the upper part of the body to the ankle on the right side, and to 1 or 2 inches above the superior pole of the patella on the left. *D*, 4″ Webril and fiberglass bandages have been applied to the right ankle and foot. *E*, A 30″ wooden bar has been attached to the leg portion of the cast from the supracondylar area on the left to the mid-tibial area on the right.

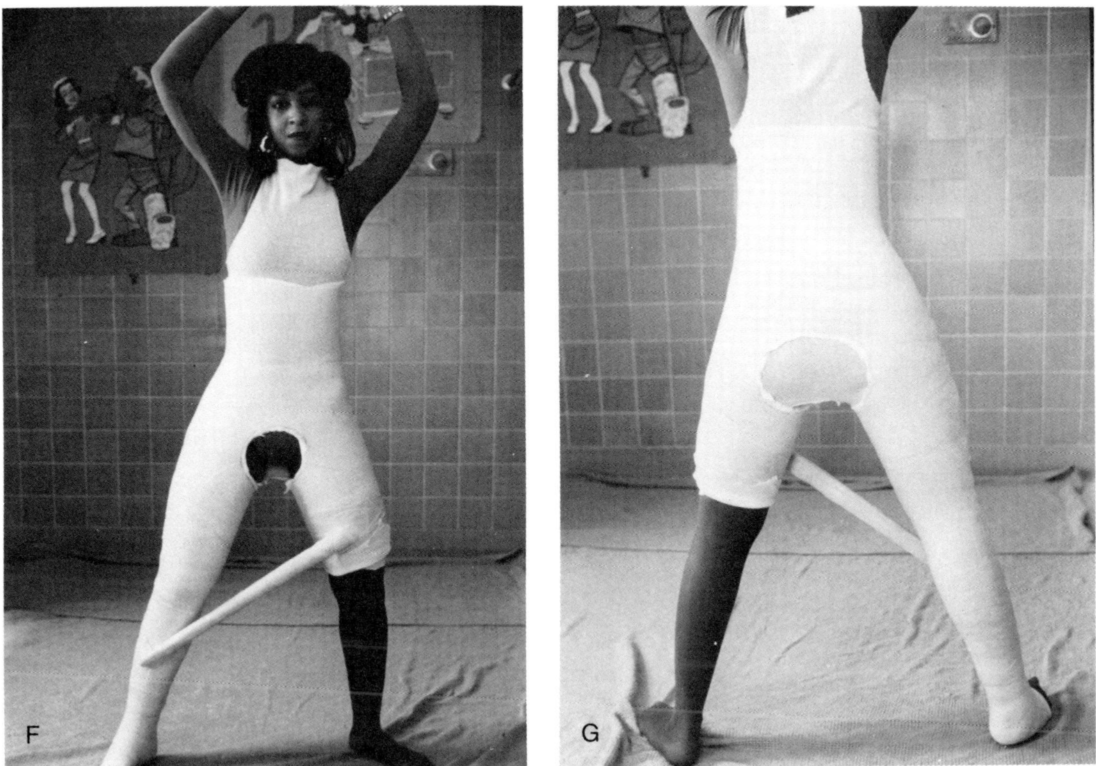

Fig. 10–7 (cont.). *F,G,* Anterior and posterior views of the cast after the perineal area has been trimmed.

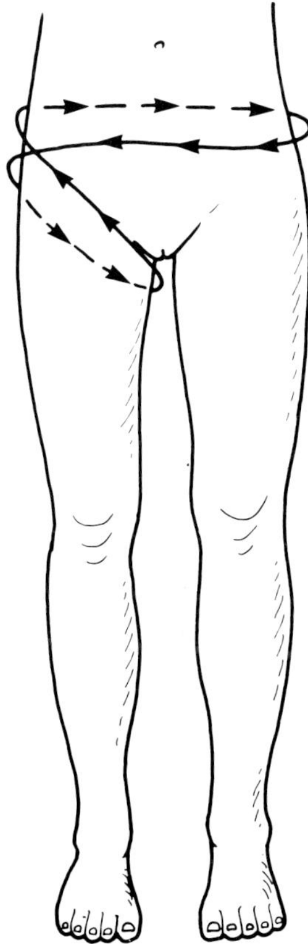

Fig. 10–8. In a single hip spica cast, an asymmetrical figure-8 is usually used to wrap the junction between the legs and the body on the involved side. Two rolls of 4" Webril bandage are used.

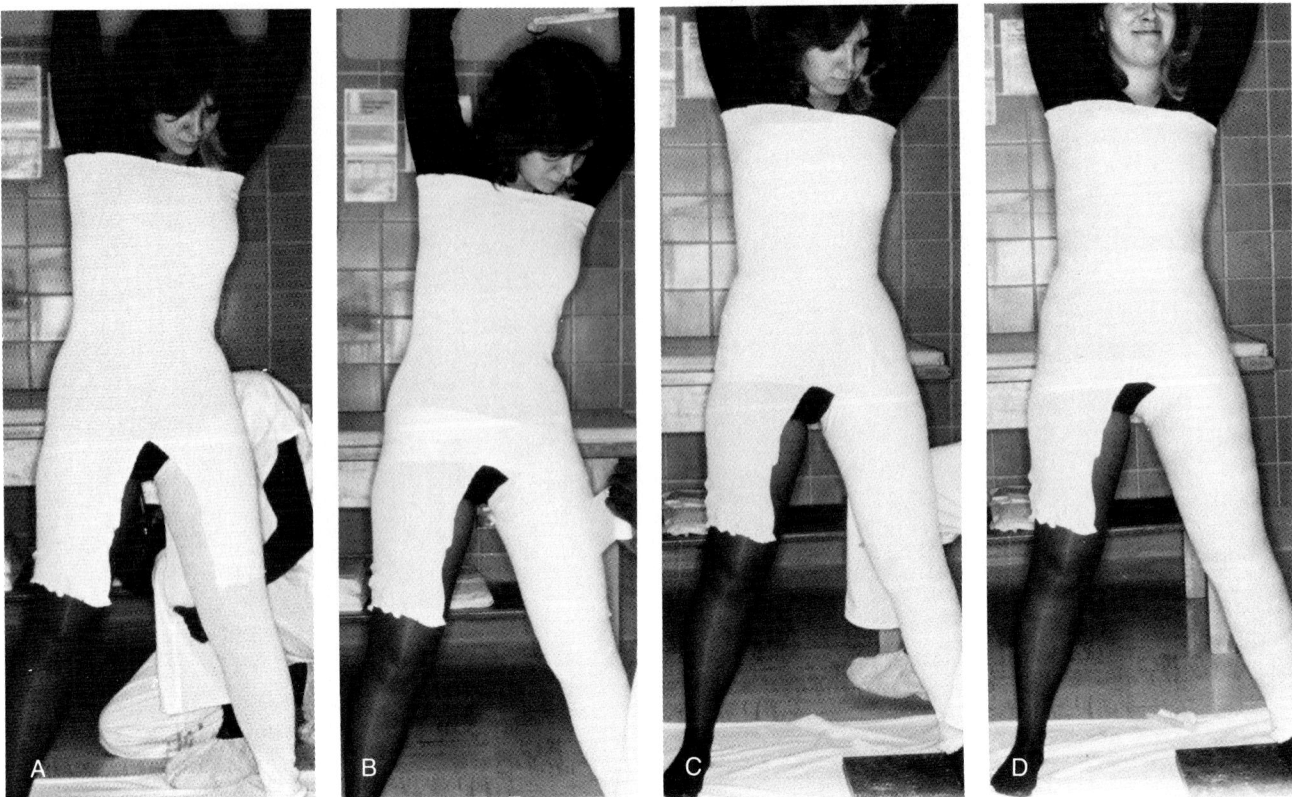

Fig. 10–9. The making of a fiberglass single hip spica cast. *A*, Body stockinet and leg stockinet have been applied. *B*, The junction between leg and body is covered with 4″ Webril wrapped in an asymmetrical fashion. *C*, Webril bandages have been applied to the body and leg. *D*, Fiberglass bandages have been applied to the body and leg. All the cast needs now is application of Webril and fiberglass bandages to the left ankle and foot.

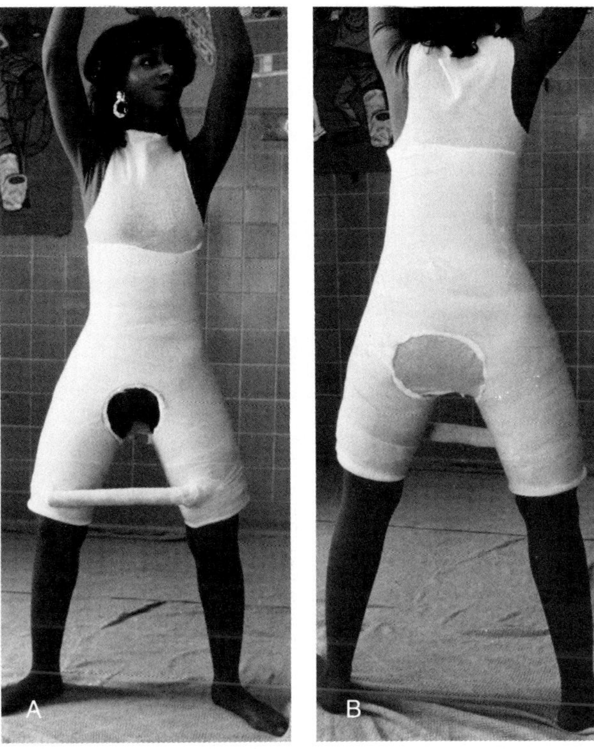

Fig. 10–10. Anterior (*A*) and posterior (*B*) views of a fiberglass double pantaloon hip spica cast without an opening over the epigastrium.

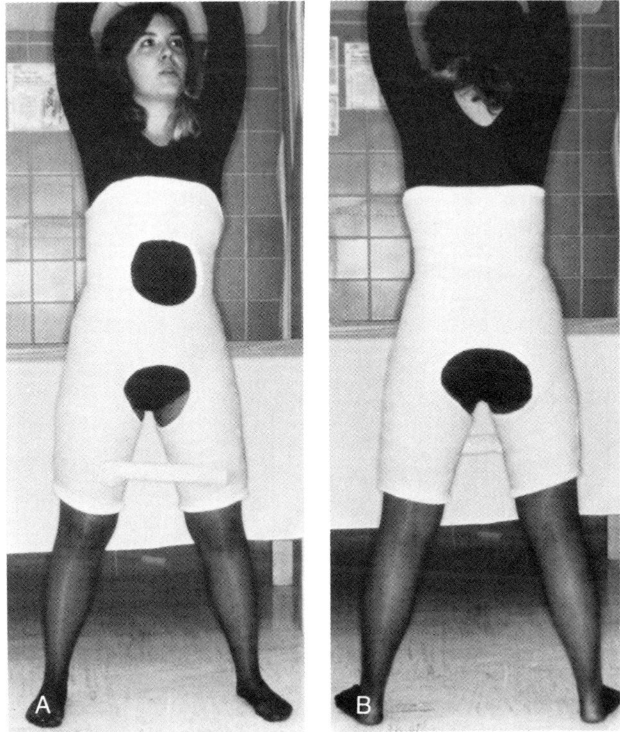

Fig. 10–11. Anterior (*A*) and posterior (*B*) views of a fiberglass double pantaloon hip spica cast with a round opening over the epigastrium.

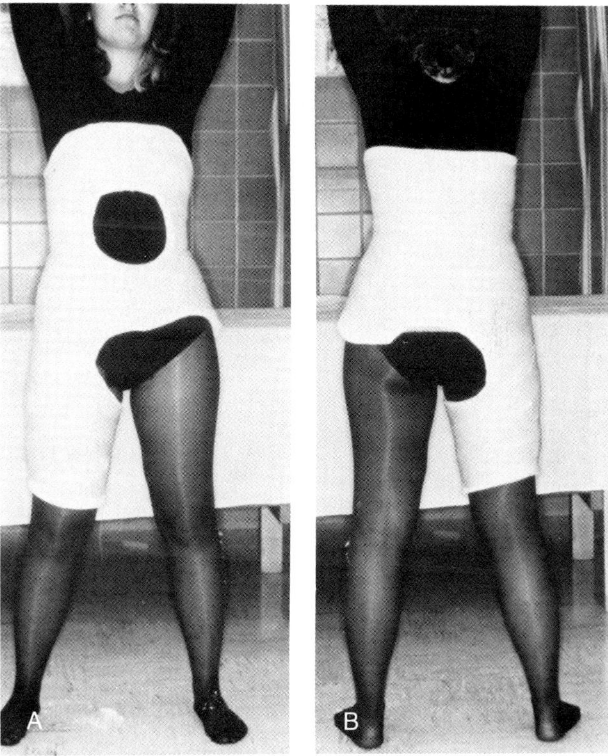

Fig. 10–12. Anterior (*A*) and posterior (*B*) views of a single pantaloon hip spica cast with an 8-inch hole over the epigastric region.

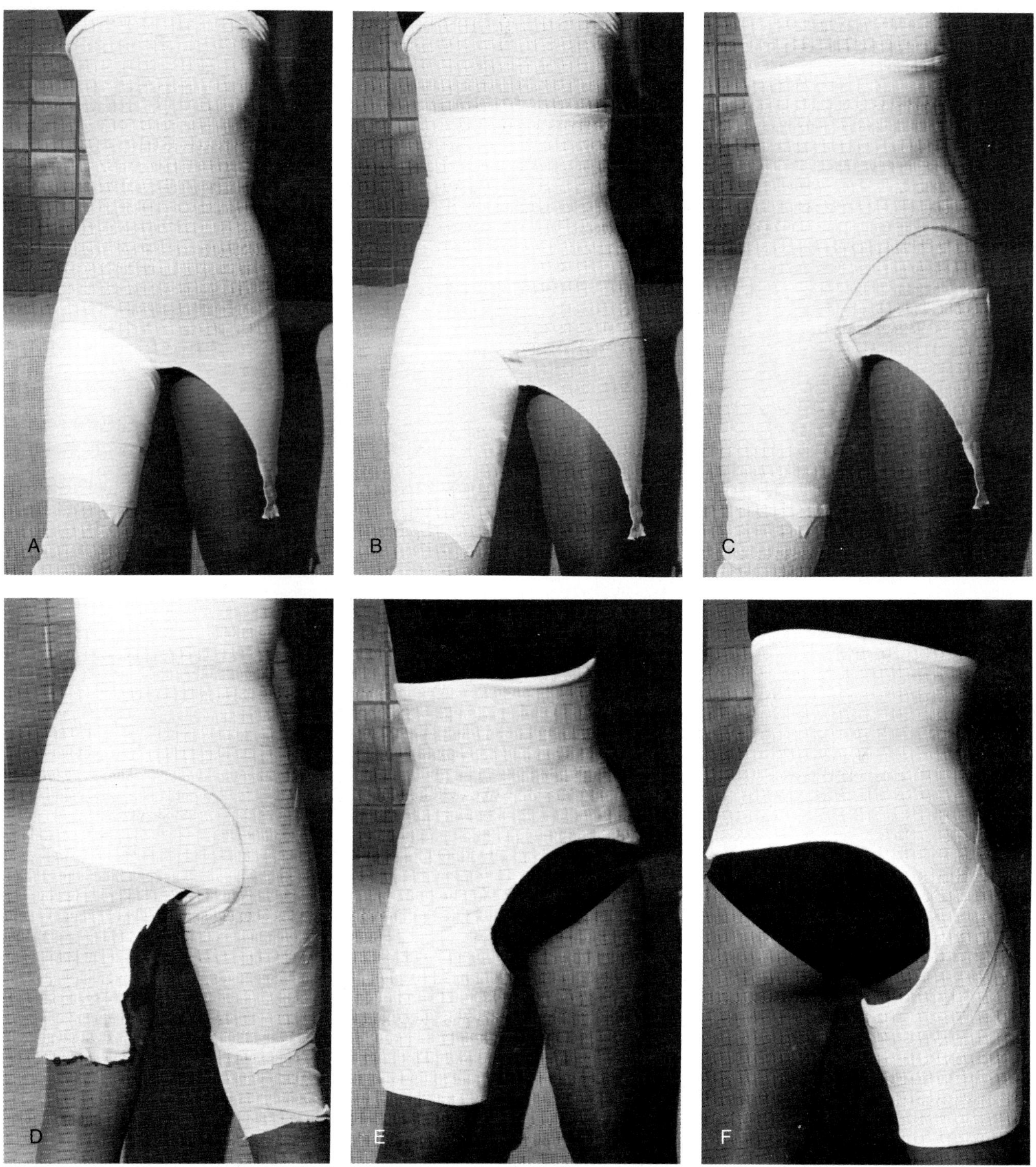

Fig. 10–13. The making of a fiberglass single pantaloon hip spica cast. *A*, A 10″ body stockinet has been applied to the body, and a short 4″ leg stockinet and some 4″ Webril bandages have been applied to the right thigh. *B*, 6″ Webril bandages have been applied to the body. *C,D*, After the 5″ fiberglass bandages have been applied to the body and the right thigh, a wax pencil is used to mark the cast materials that have to be removed from the left hip and gluteal region. *E,F*, Anterior and posterior views of the finished cast.

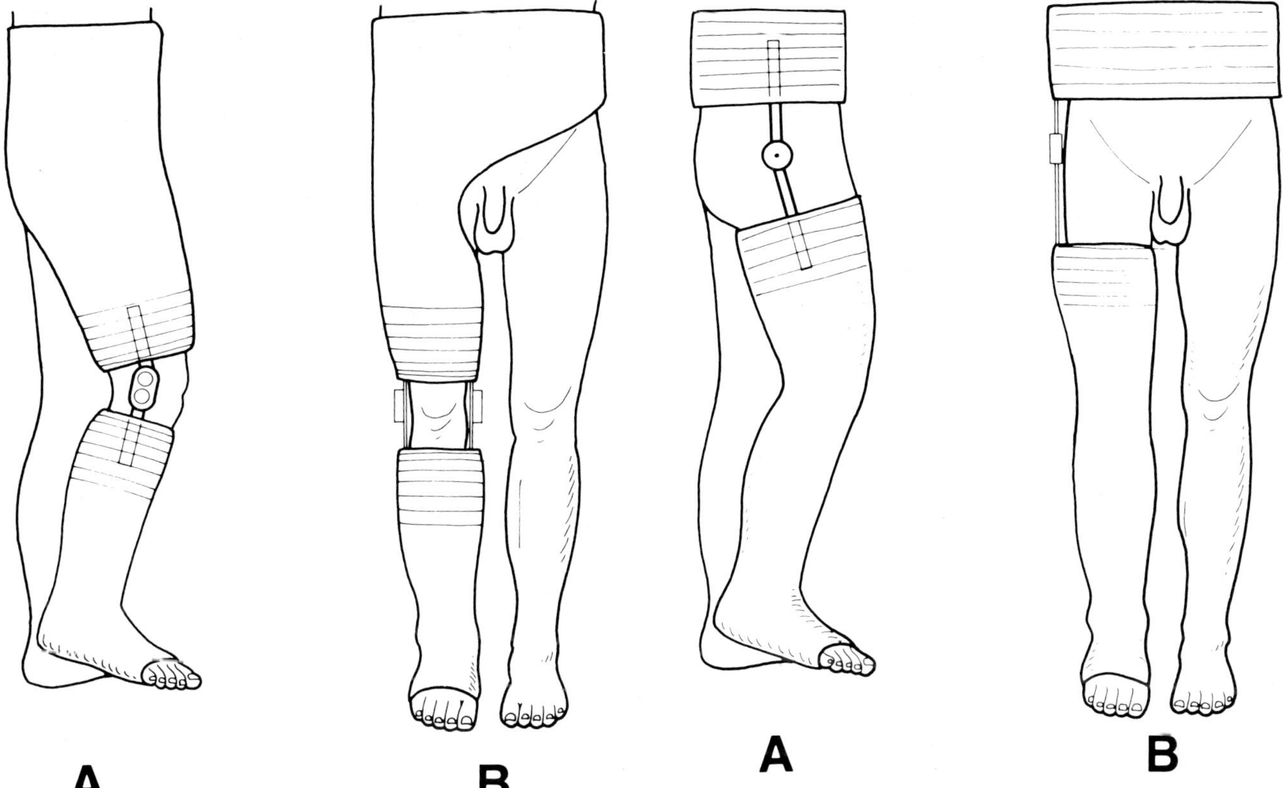

Fig. 10–14. Lateral (*A*) and anterior (*B*) views of a single hip spica cast with two polycentric knee hinges.

Fig. 10–15. Lateral (*A*) and anterior (*B*) views of a single hip spica cast with a hip hinge.

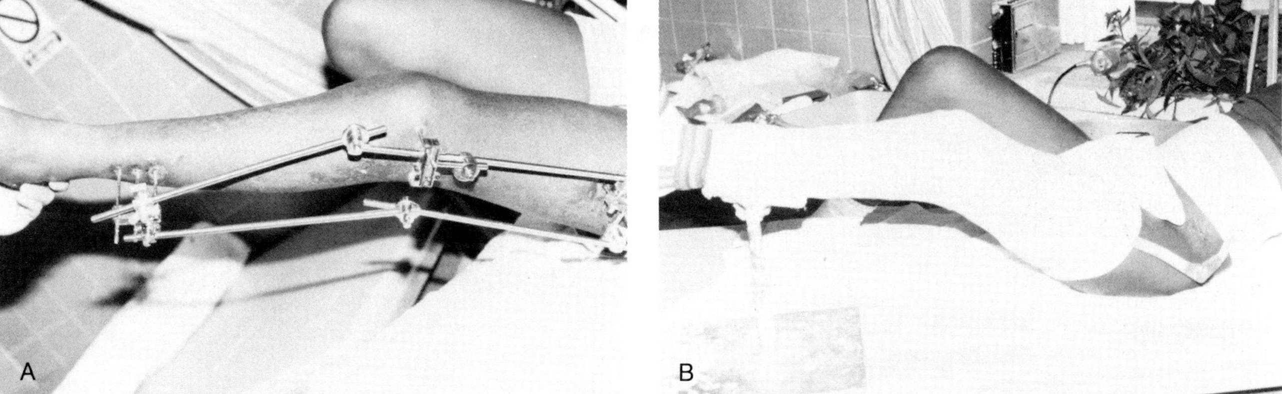

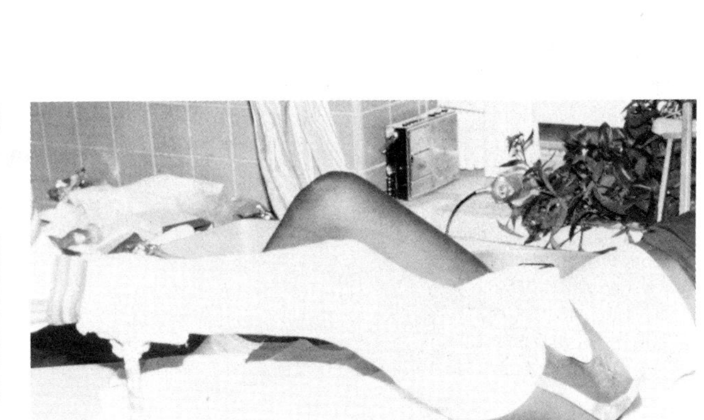

Fig. 10–16. This 15-year-old boy had an osteogenic sarcoma resected from his left distal femur, and the bony gap was bridged with a tibial, a fibular, and two bicortical iliac grafts plus an 18-inch compression plate. Hoffmann apparatus was subsequently used to provide external support (*A*). The Hoffmann apparatus was subsequently replaced by a long-leg cast and a waistband with a hip hinge (*B*).

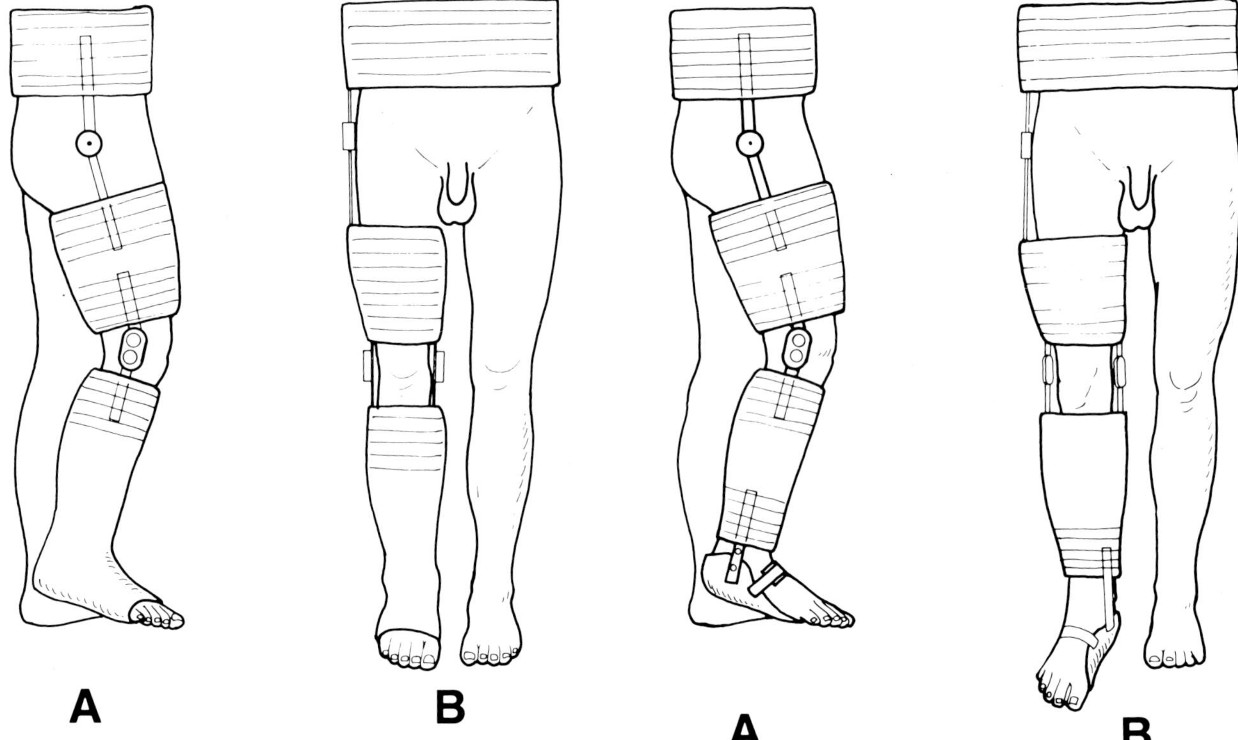

Fig. 10–17. Lateral (*A*) and anterior (*B*) views of a single hip spica cast with a hip hinge and two polycentric knee hinges.

Fig. 10–18. Lateral (*A*) and anterior (*B*) views of a single hip spica cast with a hip hinge, two knee hinges, two ankle hinges, and a heel cup.

CHAPTER 11. BODY CASTS

The various body casts include the standard body cast, the halo cast, the clavicular cast, the Risser cast, and the Minerva cast. These body casts enclose the major portion of the body, and their primary use is in treating disorders of the spine. Many orthopedic surgeons are not familiar with the methods for application of these body casts because they do not often use them.

STANDARD BODY CAST

Indications

A standard body cast (Fig. 11-1) is most commonly used in immobilizing the lumbar spine following a lower lumbar or lumbosacral fusion. It can also be used for treating fractures and dislocations and other disorders of the lower thoracic and lumbar spine.

Cast Materials Needed

Plaster Standard Body Cast

1 10″ or 12″ stockinet

4 rolls of 6″ Webril bandage

5 rolls of 6″ plaster bandage

2 boxes of 5″ × 30″ plaster splints (10 splints per box)

2 felt pads for the anterior iliac crests

Fiberglass Standard Body Cast

1 10″ or 12″ stockinet

4 rolls of 6″ Webril bandage

5 rolls of 5″ fiberglass bandage

2 felt pads for the anterior iliac crests

Patient's Position

A standard body cast can be applied with the patient recumbent on a fracture table, or in a standing or sitting position with both hands tightly holding on to an overhead horizontal bar.

Technique for Applying a Plaster Standard Body Cast

A long piece of 10″ or 12″ stockinet with armholes is worn by the patient like a T-shirt from the neck to the lower leg (Fig. 11-2A). Four rolls of 6″ Webril bandage are wrapped around the body from the upper axillary region to the level of the greater trochanters (Fig. 11-2B,C). After felt pads have been applied to the anterior iliac crests, 2 rolls of 6″ plaster bandage are used to cover the Webril bandages (Fig. 11-2D,E). The 2 boxes of 5″ × 30″ plaster splints are applied over the plaster bandages in either a horizontal or vertical manner, overlapping each other by about $^1/_2$ inch (Fig. 11-2F). Two rolls of 6″ plaster bandage are used to cover the splints, and the cast is carefully molded to fit the contours of the body, especially the iliac crest regions (Fig. 11-2G,H,I).

The upper and lower margins of the cast are then marked on the cast. The lower trimming line starts from the pubic symphysis and arches slightly upward and then slightly downward above the flexion crease of the hip joint to the greater trochanters. The line continues across the lower buttock region in a slightly curved fashion to the sacrococcygeal junction, where it meets the opposite trimming line. To avoid pressure on the sacrococcygeal region, a small half-moon-shaped piece of plaster should be cut out. The upper trimming line starts from the upper sternum, going laterally and slightly downward to the lower portion of the axilla and then proceeding in a medial and slightly upward direction to the lateral border of the scapula, where it levels off to meet the opposite trimming line (Fig. 11-2J,K).

The redundant cast materials are removed (Fig. 11-2L,M). The upper and lower stockinet ends are folded over the carefully trimmed cast ends and are fixed to the adjacent cast surfaces with a roll of 6″ plaster bandage (Fig. 11-2N,O,P). If the cast has been properly applied, the patient should be able to sit comfortably with hips flexed to at least 90° (Fig. 11-2Q,R).

Technique for Applying a Fiberglass Standard Body Cast

The stockinet, Webril bandages, and felt pads are applied as for a plaster standard body cast (Fig. 11-3A,B). Next, 4 rolls of 5″ fiberglass bandage are wrapped evenly around the Webril bandages (Fig. 11-3C,D). After the proximal and distal ends of the cast have been trimmed (Fig. 11-3E–I), the stockinet ends are folded over them and a roll of 5″ fiberglass bandage is used to fix the stockinet ends to the adjacent portions of the cast (Fig. 11-3J,K,L). A properly applied body cast should allow at least 90° of hip flexion (Fig. 11-3M,N).

In order to allow exercise, wound care, and bathing, a standard body cast can be bivalved. Velcro straps or webbings with buckles can be attached to the two halves of the cast so that it can be reapplied to the body (Fig. 11-4A–F). For an obese patient, a standard body cast should be suspended with two shoulder straps (Fig. 11-5).

HALO CAST

Indications

A halo cast (Fig. 11-6) is usually used to treat fractures and dislocation of the cervical spine or to replace a Minerva cast, which is much harder to apply and less comfortable to wear because of the many layers of cast materials around the head and neck, which impede dissipation of heat and moisture and can produce skin irritation and pressure sores. The drawbacks of a halo cast include the possibility of loosening of the pins through the outer table of the skull and infection of the pin tracts (Fig. 11-7).

Cast Materials Needed

Plaster Halo Cast

1 10″ or 12″ stockinet

6 rolls of 6″ Webril bandage

8 rolls of 6″ plaster bandage

3 rolls of 4″ plaster bandage

2 boxes of 5″ × 30″ plaster splints

5 felt pads for the shoulders, lower sacrum, and anterior iliac crests

Fiberglass Halo Cast

1 10″ or 12″ stockinet

6 rolls of 6″ Webril bandage

7 rolls of 5″ fiberglass bandage

3 rolls of 4″ fiberglass bandage

5 felt pads for the shoulders, lower sacrum, and anterior iliac crests

Patient's Position

A halo cast can be applied with the patient either in a recumbent position on a fracture table or in a sitting or standing position. Head traction can be provided either by a head halter or by a halo ring.

Technique for Applying a Plaster Halo Cast

A 10″ or 12″ stockinet with 2 armholes is applied to the body like a sleeveless T-shirt, and the patient is placed on a fracture table with cephalopelvic traction (Fig. 11-8A,B). Four rolls of 6″ Webril bandage are applied to the body from the armpits to the level of the greater trochanters. Four long strips of 6″ Webril (obtained from 2 rolls of 6″ Webril bandage) are applied to the tops of the shoulders, the free ends going downward to cover the chest and scapular regions (Fig. 11-8C,D).

After felt pads have been applied to the shoulders, the lower sacrum, and the anterior iliac crests, 2 rolls of 6″ plaster bandage are applied to the body. Another 2 rolls of 6″ plaster bandage are used to cover the shoulders and the upper chest and scapular regions in a figure-8 manner (Fig. 11-8E,F). Two 5″ × 30″ plaster splints are applied from the top of both shoulders, their free ends going to the chest and scapular regions. The remaining plaster splints are applied to the body in a transverse and circular manner, overlapping each other by about $^1/_2$ (Fig. 11-8G,H,I). Two rolls of 6″ plaster bandage are used to cover both shoulders and the upper chest and scapular regions in a figure-8 manner, and another 2 rolls are wrapped around the rest of the body (Fig. 11-8J). The upright bars of the halo apparatus are fixed to the cast with 2 rolls of 6″ plaster bandage (Fig. 11-8K,L). Then the cast ends and the shoulder openings are trimmed and all the free stockinet ends are fixed to the adjacent cast surfaces with 3 rolls of 4″ plaster bandage to finish the cast (Fig. 11-8M).

Technique for Applying a Fiberglass Halo Cast

The stockinet, Webril bandages, and felt pads are applied as for a plaster halo cast. Next, 3 rolls of 5″ fiberglass bandage are applied to the body from the upper axillary region to the level of the greater trochanters. Two more rolls of 5″ fiberglass bandage are used to cover the shoulders, upper chest, and scapular regions of the cast in a figure-8 fashion. The lower end of the cast is trimmed like that of the plaster halo cast, and the distal stockinet end is folded up and fixed to the adjacent cast surface with a roll of 4″ fiberglass bandage. The neck and shoulder openings are then trimmed, plastic adhesive is applied to the cast surfaces around the openings, and the stockinet ends are pulled over the cut edges of the openings and allowed to stick to the nearby cast surfaces. Two rolls of 4″ fiberglass bandage are used to cover and fix these stockinet ends. The upright bars of the halo apparatus are fixed to the upper portion of the cast with 2 rolls of 5″ fiberglass bandage.

CLAVICULAR CAST

Indications

A clavicular cast (Fig. 11-9) is basically a modified shoulder spica cast and is usually used to treat fracture of the middle third of the clavicle. It exerts constant upward and backward pressure on the anterior shoulder region to keep the clavicular fracture in alignment.

Cast Materials Needed

Plaster Clavicular Cast

1 10″ or 12″ stockinet

1 3″ stockinet

6 rolls of 6″ Webril bandage

2 rolls of 4″ Webril bandage

4 rolls of 6″ plaster bandage

6 rolls of 4″ plaster bandage

2 boxes of 5″ × 30″ plaster splints (10 splints per box)

Fiberglass Clavicular Cast

1 10″ or 12″ stockinet

1 3″ stockinet

6 rolls of 6″ Webril bandage

2 rolls of 4″ Webril bandage

5 rolls of 5″ fiberglass bandage

5 rolls of 4″ fiberglass bandage

Patient's Position

A clavicular cast is applied with the patient in either a sitting or a standing position.

Technique for Applying a Plaster Clavicular Cast

A 10″ or 12″ stockinet with 2 armholes is applied to the body, and a 3″ stockinet is applied to 1 arm. The proximal end of the 3″ stockinet is split longitudinally in the armpit area, and the cut ends are allowed to overlap the adjacent body stockinet. One or 2 turns of 4″ Webril bandage are used to hold the overlapped stockinet ends together (Fig. 11-10). Four strips 6″ Webril bandage are applied over the fractured clavicle from the lower pectoral region across the top of the shoulder to the lower scapular region (Fig. 11-11). Two rolls of 6″ Webril bandage are applied to the upper thoracic region in a figure-8 manner, and another 3 rolls of 6″ Webril bandage are wrapped around the lower part of the body to the level of the greater trochanters (Fig. 11-12). Two rolls of 4″ Webril bandage are used to cover the upper arm and the adjacent shoulder region (Fig. 11-13).

Two rolls of 6″ plaster bandage are used to cover the body part of the cast, and 2 rolls of 4″ plaster bandage are used to cover the arm and adjacent shoulder portion of the cast (Fig. 11-14). A 5″ × 30″ plaster splint is applied to the top of each shoulder; the free ends of the splints cross each other in the middle of the upper chest and back (Fig. 11-15). A third 5″ × 30″ plaster splint is applied from the top of the shoulder along the lateral aspect of the arm to the supracondylar level (Fig. 11-16), and the remaining 17 splints are applied to the lower part of the body down to the level of the greater trochanters. After the distal end of the arm portion of the cast has been trimmed, the stockinet is folded over the cast end and 2 rolls of 4″ plaster bandage are used to cover the arm and adjacent shoulder portion of the cast. A roll of 6″ plaster bandage is applied to the upper half of the body part of the cast in a figure-8 manner (Fig. 11-17).

The neck and shoulder openings are trimmed carefully to allow full neck and shoulder motion, and the stockinet ends are folded over the edges of these 2 cast openings and temporarily fixed to the cast with thumbtacks (Fig. 11-18, 11-19). Two rolls of 4″ plaster bandage are applied in a figure-8 fashion to the upper half of the cast to cover all the stockinet ends bordering the neck and shoulder openings. The distal portion of the cast is trimmed, and the distal end of the body stockinet is folded over the cast before a roll of 6″ plaster bandage is applied to finish the lower half of the cast (Figs. 11-20, 11-21).

Technique for Applying a Fiberglass Clavicular Cast

The stockinet and Webril bandages are applied as for a plaster clavicular cast. The upper arm and adjacent shoulder region are covered with 2 rolls of 4″ fiberglass bandage. The distal end of the arm stockinet is folded up over the cast end. Next, 2 rolls of 5″ fiberglass bandage are wrapped around the upper half of the body portion of the cast in a figure-8 fashion, and another 2 rolls of 5″ fiberglass bandage are applied in a circular manner to the lower half of the body portion of the cast. The distal end of the body stockinet is turned up over the distal cast end and fixed to the adjacent cast surface with a roll of 5″ fiberglass bandage.

The neck and shoulder openings are trimmed to allow full neck and shoulder motion. The cast surfaces around these 2 openings are painted with plastic adhesive, and the corresponding stockinet ends are pulled tightly over the edges of the 2 openings and allowed to stick to the adjacent cast surfaces. Three rolls of 4″ fiberglass bandage are used to cover the turned down arm, neck, and shoulder stockinet ends in a multiple figure-8 manner (Fig. 11-22) to complete the cast.

RISSER CAST

Indications

A Risser cast (Figs. 11-23, 11-24) is usually used to provide correction for scoliosis and to maintain correction after spinal fusion.

Cast Material Needed

Plaster Risser Cast

1 10″ or 12″ stockinet

3 rolls of 4″ Webril bandage

6 rolls of 6″ Webril bandage

5 rolls of 6″ plaster bandage

6 rolls of 4″ plaster bandage

2 boxes of 5″ × 30″ plaster splints (10 splints per box)

2 felt pads for the anterior superior iliac spines

Fiberglass Risser Cast

1 10″ or 12″ stockinet

3 rolls of 4″ Webril bandage

6 rolls of 6″ Webril bandage

5 rolls of 5″ fiberglass bandage

6 rolls of 4″ fiberglass bandage

2 felt pads for the anterior superior iliac spines

Patient's Position

The patient is usually placed in a supine position on a fracture table, with a head halter for applying head traction and two straps criss-crossed over the iliac crests for applying pelvic traction.

Because of the difficulty of illustrating the technique with the patient on a fracture table, the steps involved in the application of a Risser cast are shown here with the patient in a sitting position.

Technique for Applying a Plaster Risser Cast

A 10″ or 12″ body stockinet with 2 armholes is used. The stockinet should extend from the mid-thigh level to the top of the head (Fig. 11-25). Three rolls of 4″ Webril bandage are wrapped around the neck, chin, angles of the mandible, and postauricular and occipital areas to a level about 1 inch above the superior nuchal line (Fig. 11-26). Eight strips of 6″ Webril obtained from 2 rolls of 6″ Webril bandage are applied from the tops of both shoulders to cover the anterior and posterior aspects of the upper part of the body. Another 4 rolls of 6″ Webril bandage are applied to the body from the axillary level to the level of the greater trochanters, and felt pads are placed over the anterior superior iliac spines (Figs. 11-27, 11-28).

One roll of 6″ plaster bandage is applied from the level of the greater trochanters to the axillary region (Fig. 11-29). Another roll of 6″ plaster bandage is used to cover the upper part of the body and both shoulders in a figure-8 manner (Fig. 11-30). Two rolls of 4″ plaster bandage are applied to the neck, chin, both angles of the mandible, and the postauricular and occipital regions of the skull (Fig. 11-31).

Two 5″ × 30″ plaster splints are applied diagonally across the upper thoracic and scapular regions and across both shoulders (Fig. 11-32). Another plaster splint is wrapped around the neck, mandible, and occipital region of the skull (Fig. 11-33). Two more plaster splints are applied, from the superior nuchal line straight down the posterior aspect of the spinal column to the lower thoracic level and across the upper chest (Fig. 11-34). The remaining 15 5″ × 30″ plaster splints are applied to the lower body portion of the cast in a circular and slightly overlapping manner, and then all the plaster splints around the body are covered with 2 rolls of 6″ plaster bandage (Fig. 11-35). Two rolls of 4″ plaster bandage are applied to the neck, chin, mandibular angles, and postauricular and occipital regions (Fig. 11-36).

The margins of the proximal and distal ends and the shoulder openings of the cast are carefully marked on the cast with a wax pencil (Fig. 11-37). After the proximal end of the cast and the 2 shoulder openings have been trimmed, the stockinet ends are folded over the edges of these 3 openings and temporarily fixed to the adjacent cast surface with thumbtacks (Fig. 11-38). The distal end of the cast is trimmed laterally from the pubic symphysis in a slightly arched manner to allow hip flexion to the greater trochanters. The trimming line then crosses the lower buttock region to the sacrococcygeal junction to meet the opposite trimming line. The distal end of the body stockinet can now be turned up over the trimmed cast end (Fig. 11-39). One roll of 6″ plaster bandage is used to cover the distal stockinet end (Fig. 11-40), and 2 rolls of 4″ plaster bandage are used to cover the stockinet ends at the neck and shoulder openings (Fig. 11-41). The completed Risser cast is shown in Fig. 11-42.

Technique for Applying a Fiberglass Risser Cast

The stockinet, Webril bandages, and felt pads are applied as for a plaster Risser cast. Then, 3 rolls of 5″ fiberglass bandage are applied to the body from the level of the greater trochanters to the axillary level. The upper part of the body, both shoulders, and the base of the neck are covered with 2 rolls of 5″ fiberglass bandage, which should be applied in a figure-8 fashion. The neck, chin, and postauricular and occipital regions are wrapped with 2 rolls of 4″ fiberglass bandage.

The lower end of the cast is trimmed, and the distal stockinet end is folded up over the distal cast end and fixed to the adjacent cast surface with a roll of 4″ fiberglass bandage. Next, the 2 shoulder openings are trimmed, and the cast surfaces near the shoulder openings are painted with plastic adhesive. The stockinet ends are pulled over the edges of the shoulder openings to stick to the adjacent cast surfaces. Two rolls of 4″ fiberglass bandage are used to fix the stockinet ends to the cast surfaces next to the shoulder openings.

Finally, the upper end of the cast is trimmed slightly below the chin, across the lower part of the mandibular angles to the external occipital protuberance, where a small half-moon shaped piece should be removed to prevent pressure sore. The adjacent cast surface is painted with plastic adhesive, and the proximal stockinet end is turned down over the cast end to stick to the cast surface. A roll of 4″ fiberglass bandage is used to cover the proximal stockinet end around the neck to finish the cast.

MINERVA CAST

Indications

A Minerva cast (Fig. 11-43) is usually used for the treatment of fractures and dislocations of the cervical spine and for immobilization of the cervical spine following a spinal fusion.

Cast Materials Needed

Plaster Minerva Cast

1 10″ or 12″ stockinet

6 rolls of 6″ Webril bandage

3 rolls of 4″ Webril bandage

1 roll of 3″ Webril bandage

5 rolls of 6″ plaster bandage

7 rolls of 4″ plaster bandage

2 rolls of 3″ plaster bandage

2 boxes of 5″ × 30″ plaster splints (10 per box)

4 felt pads for the forehead, chin, and anterior superior iliac spines

Fiberglass Minerva Cast

1 10″ or 12″ stockinet

6 rolls of 6″ Webril bandage

3 rolls of 4″ Webril bandage

1 roll of 3″ Webril bandage

5 rolls of 5″ fiberglass bandage

6 rolls of 4″ fiberglass bandage

2 rolls of 3″ fiberglass bandage

4 felt pads for the forehead, chin, and anterior superior iliac spines

Patient's Position

A Minerva cast can be applied with the patient either in a supine position on a fracture table (Fig. 11-44) or in a sitting position. We routinely apply head halter traction, and lateral views of the cervical spine are usually taken to confirm the presence of satisfactory reduction of cervical fracture or dislocation prior to application of the cast.

Technique for Applying a Plaster Minerva Cast

With the patient in a sitting position under head halter traction, a 10″ or 12″ body stockinet is applied from the mid-thigh level to the top of the head (Fig. 11-45). A pair of plaster scissors is used to cut out the stockinet over the face to expose the eyes, nose, cheeks, and lips (Fig. 11-46). Four rolls of 6″ Webril bandage are applied to the body from the upper axillary level to the level of the greater trochanters (Fig. 11-47). Two rolls of 6″ Webril bandage are cut into 8 strips, and 4 strips are applied to each shoulder from the top of the shoulder obliquely downward to cover the upper part of the body (Fig. 11-48). Three rolls of 4″ Webril bandage are wrapped around the neck, chin, angles of the mandible, and postauricular and occipital regions, and 3″ Webril bandage is wrapped around the forehead, ears, and the temporal, upper occipital, and posterior parietal regions of the skull (Fig. 11-49).

After felt pads have been applied to the forehead, chin, and anterior superior iliac spines (Fig. 11-50), 2 rolls of 4″ plaster bandage are wrapped around the neck, chin, mandible, and postauricular and occipital portions of the skull, and a roll of 3″ plaster bandage is used to cover the headband from the frontal area across the temporal area to the upper occipital and posterior parietal regions. In addition, 1 roll of

6″ plaster bandage is applied to the shoulders and the upper part of the body in a figure-8 manner, and a 2nd roll of 6″ plaster bandage is used to cover the lower part of the body down to the level of the greater trochanters (Fig. 11-51).

One 5″ × 30″ plaster splint is applied from the tops of each shoulder obliquely across the upper chest and back (Fig. 11-52). One plaster splint is applied from the chin down the anterior surface of the neck to the upper abdominal region (Fig. 11-53), another splint is folded longitudinally and applied to the headband in a circumferential manner (Fig. 11-54), and 2 splints are applied from the mid-level of the headband to the mid-back region (Fig. 11-55). The remaining 14 plaster splints are applied to the lower part of the body in a circular and slightly overlapping manner (Fig. 11-56). The plaster splints around the head and neck are covered with 3 rolls of 4″ plaster bandage, and the plaster splints over the body are covered with 2 rolls of 6″ plaster bandage (Fig. 11-57).

The final margins of the headband and face and shoulder openings are marked on the cast with a wax pencil (Fig. 11-58). Excess plaster is then removed from the shoulder openings with a cast saw (Fig. 11-59). Similarly, excess plaster is removed from the headband (Fig. 11-60) and from around the face (Fig. 11-61). The distal end of the cast is trimmed from the pubic symphysis to the greater trochanters in a slightly arched manner to allow good hip flexion; the trimming from the greater trochanters to the sacrococcygeal junction should go across the lower portion of the buttock. A small half-moon shaped piece of plaster should be cut out of the cast over the lower sacral region to prevent development of pressure sores (Fig. 11-62).

Several cuts are made in the stockinet ends at the shoulder openings, and the cut ends are folded tightly over the edges of the shoulder openings and fixed to the adjacent cast surfaces with thumbtacks (Fig. 11-63). The distal stockinet end, the proximal stockinet end, and the stockinet at the margins of the face opening can be folded over the edges of the cast and fixed to the adjacent cast surfaces with thumbtacks. Care should be taken to make sure that the chin is not compressed by the cast and that the head and neck portion of the cast does not touch the ears. The head halter can be removed at this point (Fig. 11-64).

When the stockinet ends have been fixed to the headband and the face opening with 1 roll of 3″ plaster bandage, to the shoulder openings with 2 rolls of 4″ plaster bandage, and to the distal cast end with 1 roll of 6″ plaster bandage, the Minerva cast is finally finished (Fig. 11-65).

Technique for Applying a Fiberglass Minerva Cast

The stockinet, Webril bandages, and felt pads are applied as for a plaster Minerva cast. At this point, 3 rolls of 5″ fiberglass bandage are applied to the body from the level of the axillae to the level of the greater trochanters. Two more rolls of 5″ fiberglass bandage are used to cover the shoulders and the upper parts of the chest and back in a figure-8 fashion. Two rolls of 4″ fiberglass bandage are applied to the neck, chin, angles of the mandible, and postauricular and occipital regions, and 1 roll of 3″ fiberglass bandage is wrapped around the headband to cover the frontal, temporal, upper occipital, and posterior parietal regions of the skull in a circumferential manner.

The lower end of the cast is trimmed from the pubic symphysis to the two greater trochanters in a slightly arched manner to allow good hip flexion; the posterior trimming from the greater trochanters to the sacrococcygeal junction should include removal of a small half-moon-shaped piece of fiberglass cast material from the lower sacral area. The distal stockinet is folded up over the distal cast end, and a roll of 4″ fiberglass bandage is used to fix the stockinet end to the adjacent cast surface.

Next, the shoulder openings are carefully trimmed to allow full shoulder motion. The cast surfaces near the shoulder openings are painted with plastic adhesive. The stockinet ends at the shoulders are split superiorly and inferiorly, pulled tightly over the cast edges of the shoulder openings, and allowed to stick to the adjacent cast surfaces. Two rolls of 4″ fiberglass bandage are wrapped around the shoulder region in a figure-8 manner to fix the stockinet ends.

The margins of the head portion of the cast are trimmed in such a way that the chin is free of cast impingement and the ears are completely free of cast edge irritation. The headband and the margins of the cast at the face opening are painted with plastic adhesive, and the remaining loose stockinet is folded over the trimmed edges of the headband and the face opening and allowed to stick to the adjacent cast surfaces. A roll of 3″ fiberglass bandage is used to cover the headband, and the stockinet ends bordering the face opening are covered with another roll of 4″ fiberglass bandage to finish the cast.

BIBLIOGRAPHY

Adkins, E.W.O.: Lumbo-sacral arthrodesis after laminectomy. J. Bone Joint Surg. [Br.], *37:*208, 1955.

Anderson, L.D., and D'Alonzo, R.T.: Fractures of the odontoid process of the axis. J. Bone Joint Surg. [Am.], *56:*1663, 1974.

Anderson, S., and Bradford, D.S.: Lo-profile halo. Clin. Orthop., *103:*72, 1974.

Apuzzo, M.L., et al.: Acute fractures of the odontoid process. An analysis of 45 cases. J. Neurosurg., *48:*85, 1978.

Bailey, R.W., and Badgley, C.E.: Stabilization of the cervical spine by anterior fusion. J. Bone Joint Surg. [Am.], *42:*565, 1960.

Bohlman, H.H.: Acute fractures and dislocations of the cervical spine. An analysis of three hundred hospitalized patients and review of the literature. J. Bone Joint Surg. [Am.], *61:*1119, 1979.

Bradford, D.S., Akbarnia, B.A., Winter, R.B., and Seljoskog, E.L.: Surgical stabilization of fracture and fracture dislocations of thoracic spine. Spine, *2:*185, 1977.

Byrnes, D.P., Russo, G.L., Ducker, T.B., and Cowley, R.A.: Sacrum fractures and neurological damage. J. Neurosurg., *47:*459, 1977.

Cleveland, M., Bosworth, D.M., Fielding, J.W., and Smyrnis, P.: Fusion of the spine for tuberculosis in children. A long-range follow-up study. J. Bone Joint Surg. [Am.], *40:*91, 1958.

Convery, F.R., Minteer, M.A., Smith, R.W., and Emerson, S.M.: Fracture-dislocations of the dorsal-lumber spine: Acute operative stabilization by Harrington instrumentation. Spine, *3:*160, 1978.

Coria, F., et al.: Occipitoatlantal instability and vertebrobasilar ischemia: Case report. Neurology, *32:*303, 1982.

Danzig, L.A., Resnick, D., and Akeson, W.H.: The treatment of cervical spine metastasis from the prostate with a halo cast. Spine, *5:*395, 1980.

Davies, W.E., Morris, J.H., and Hill, V.: An analysis of conservative (non-surgical) management of thoracolumbar fractures and fracture-dislocations with neural damage. J. Bone Joint Surg. [Am.], *62:*1324, 1980.

Dickson, J.H., Harrington, P.R., and Windell, D.E.: Results of reduction and stabilization of the severely fractured thoracic and lumbar spine. J. Bone Joint Surg. [Am.], *60:*799, 1974.

Dubousset, J.: Torticollis in children caused by congenital anomalies of the atlas. J. Bone Joint Surg. [Am.], *68:*178, 1986.

Ferlic, D.C., Clayton, M.L., Leidholt, J.D., and Gamble, W.E.: Surgical treatment of the symptomatic unstable cervical spine in rheumatoid arthritis. J. Bone Joint Surg. [Am.], *57:*349, 1975.

Garrett, A.L., Perry, J., and Nickel, V.L.: Stabilization of the collapsing spine. J. Bone Joint Surg. [Am.], *43*:474, 1961.
Goldstein, L.A.: Surgical management of scoliosis. J. Bone Joint Surg. [Am.], *48*:167, 1966.
Henry, M.O., and Geist, E.S.: Spinal fusion by simplified technique. J. Bone Joint Surg., *15*:622, 1933.
Hibbs, R.A., and Risser, J.C.: Treatment of vertebral tuberculosis by the spinal fusion operation. A report of 286 cases. J. Bone Joint Surg., *10*:805, 1928.
Holdsworth, F.: Fractures, dislocations and fracture-dislocations of the spine. J. Bone Joint Surg. [Am.], *52*:1534, 1970.
Jacobs, R.R., Asher, M.A., and Snider, R.K.: Thoracolumbar spine injuries: A comparative study of recumbent and operative treatment in 100 patients. Spine, *5*:463, 1980.
James, J.I.P.: Infantile idiopathic scoliosis. Clin. Orthop., *77*:57, 1971.
Kaufer, H., and Hayes, J.T.: Lumbar fracture-dislocation. A study of 21 cases. J. Bone Joint Surg. [Am.], *48*:712, 1966.
Koop, S.E., Winter, R.B., and Lonstein, J.E.: The surgical treatment of instability of the upper part of the cervical spine in children and adolescents. J. Bone Joint Surg. [Am.], *63*:403, 1984.
Kostuik, J.P.: Indications for the use of the halo immobilization. Clin. Orthop., *154*:46, 1981.
Lewis, J., and McKibbin, B.: The treatment of unstable fracture-dislocations of the thoraco-lumbar spine accompanied by paraplegia. J. Bone Joint Surg. [Br.], *56*:603, 1974.
Maiman, D.J., and Larson, S.J.: Management of odontoid fractures. Neurosurgery, *14*:471, 1982.
Mir, S.R., Cole, J.R., Lardone, J., and Levine, D.B.: Early ambulation following spinal fusion and Harrington instrumentation in idiopathic scoliosis. Clin. Orthop., *110*:54, 1975.
Moe, J.H., and Gustilo, R.B.: Treatment of scoliosis. Results in 196 patients treated by cast correction and fusion. J. Bone Joint Surg. [Am.], *46*:293, 1964.
Murray, G.C., and Persellin, R.H.: Cervical fracture complicating ankylosing spondylitis: A report of eight cases and review of the literature. Am. J. Med., *70*:1033, 1981.
Nickel, V.L., Perry, J., Garrett, A., and Heppenstall, M.: The halo: A spinal skeletal traction fixation device. J. Bone Joint Surg. [Am.], *50*:1400, 1968.
Nishihara, N., et al.: Surgical treatment of cervical spondylotic myelopathy complicating athetoid cerebral palsy. J. Bone Joint Surg. [Br.], *66*:504, 1984.
Norton, P.L., and Brown, T.: The immobilizing efficiency of back braces. J. Bone Joint Surg. [Am.], *39*:111, 1957.
Norton, W.L.: Fractures and dislocations of the cervical spine. J. Bone Joint Surg. [Am.], *44*:115, 1962.
Perry, J.: The halo in spinal abnormalities: Practical factors and avoidance of complications. Orthop. Clin. North Am., *3*:69, 1972.
Risser, J.C.: The application of body casts for the correction of scoliosis. American Adacemy of Orthopaedic Surgeons Instructional Course Lectures, *12*:255, 1955.
Risser, J.C.: Scoliosis, past and present. J. Bone Joint Surg. [Am.], *46*:167, 1964.
Roberts, R.S., Price, C.T., and Riddick, M.F.: Use of a bivalved polypropylene orthosis in the postoperative management of idiopathic scoliosis. Clin. Orthop., *185*:25, 1984.
Ryan, M.D., and Taylor, T.K.: Odontoid fractures. A rational approach to treatment. J. Bone Joint Surg. [Br.], *64*:416, 1982.
Schweigel, J.F.: Halo-thoracic brace. Management of odontoid fractures. Spine, *4*:192, 1979.
Thompson, R.C., Jr., and Meyer, T.J.: Posterior surgical stabilization for atlanto-axial subluxation in rheumatoid arthritis. Spine, *10*:597, 1985.
Winter, R.B., Moe, J.H., and Eilers, V.E.: Congenital scoliosis: A study of 234 patients treated and untreated. J. Bone Joint Surg. [Am.], *50*:1, 1968.
Zagra, A., Lamartina, C., and Zerbi, A.: The Risser plaster corset as the only method of correction in the surgical treatment of scoliosis. A study of 150 cases. Ital. J. Orthop. Traumatol., *11*:67, 1985.

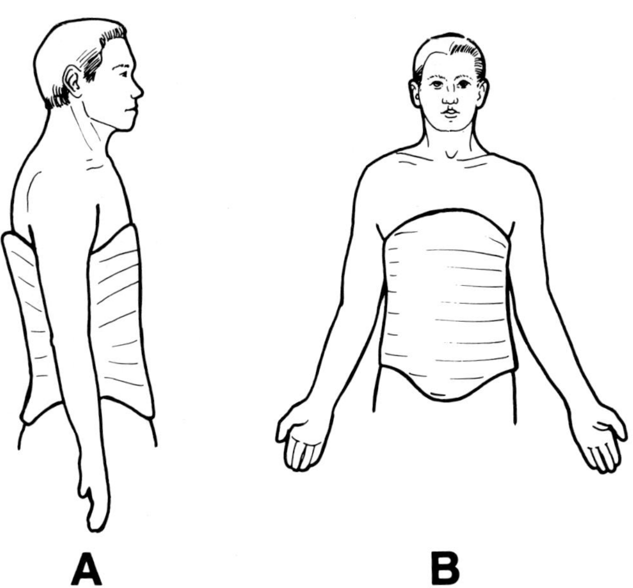

Fig. 11–1. Lateral (*A*) and anterior (*B*) views of a standard body cast.

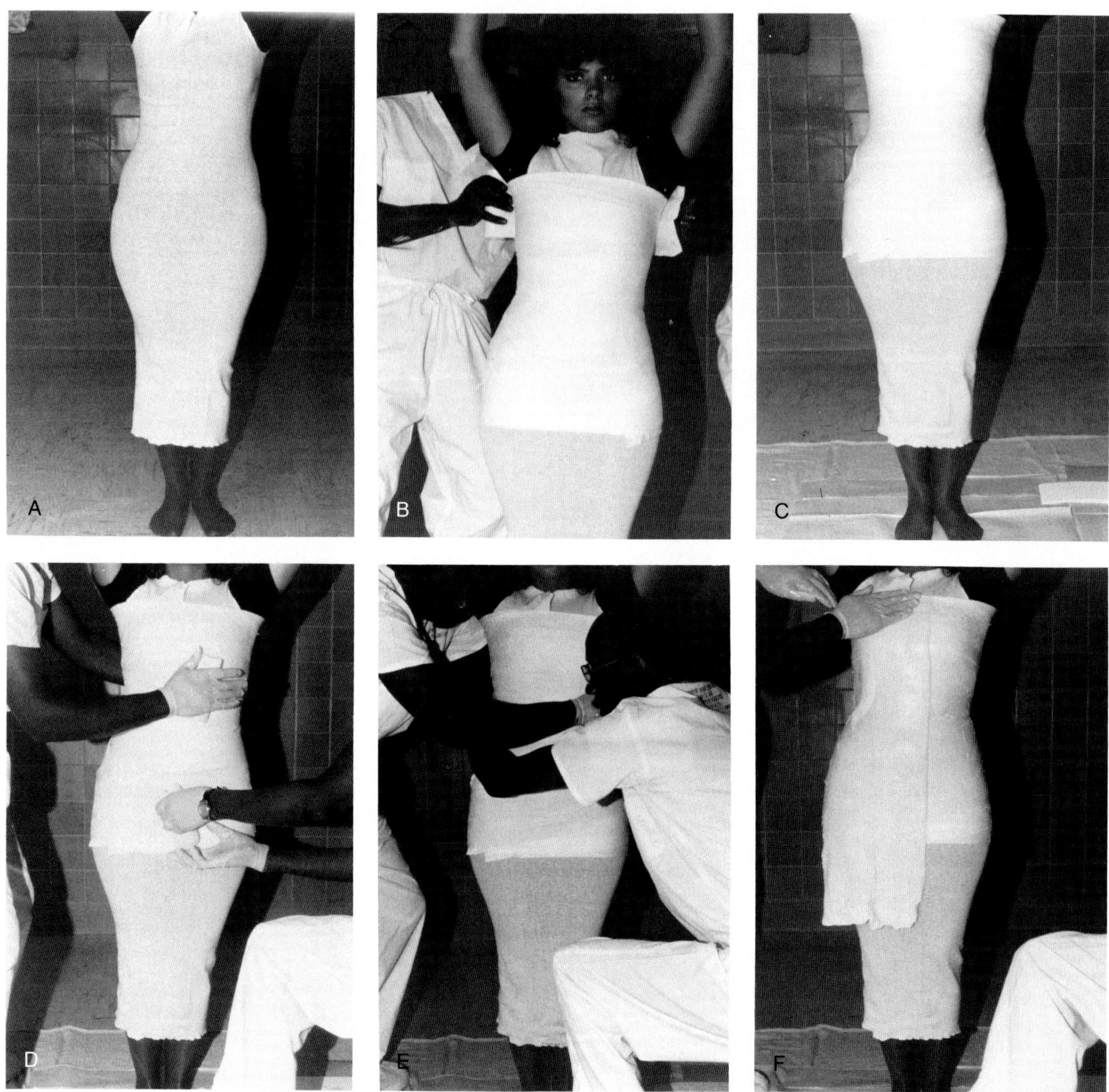

Fig. 11–2. The making of a plaster standard body cast. *A*, The patient wears a 10″ or 12″ body stockinet from the neck to the mid-calf level. *B*, *C*, The body is covered with 6″ Webril bandages from the upper axillary region to the level of the greater trochanters. *D*, *E*, The Webril bandages are covered with 6″ plaster bandages. *F*, The 5″ × 30″ plaster splints are applied to the body in a vertical manner, overlapping each other by about $^1/_2$ inch.

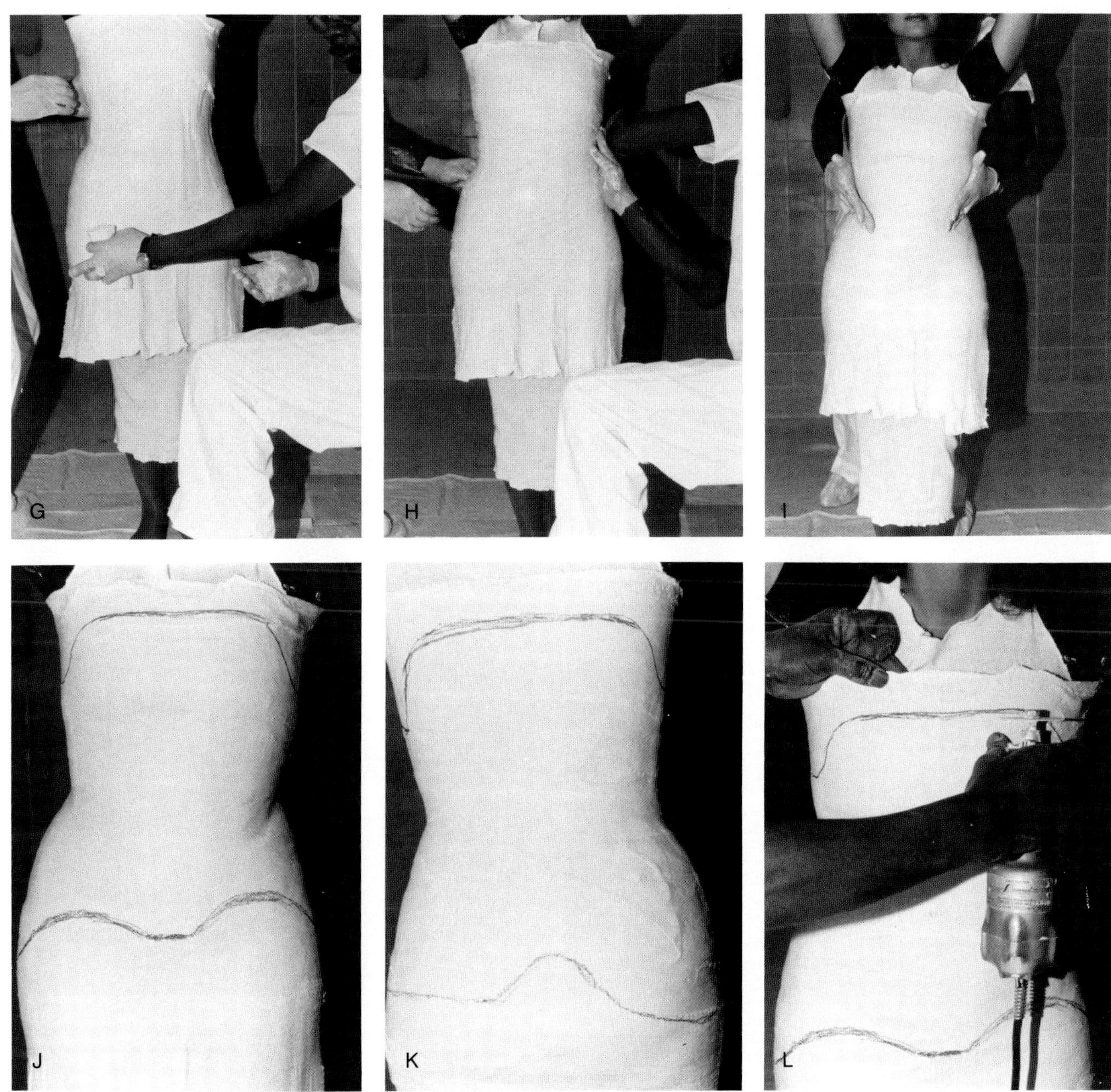

Fig. 11–2 (cont.). *G, H, I,* The plaster splints are covered with 6″ plaster bandages, and the cast is molded carefully to fit the contours of the body, particularly the iliac crest regions. *J, K,* The upper and lower margins of the cast have been marked with a wax pencil. *L,* The cast is cut with a cast saw along the wax pencil lines.

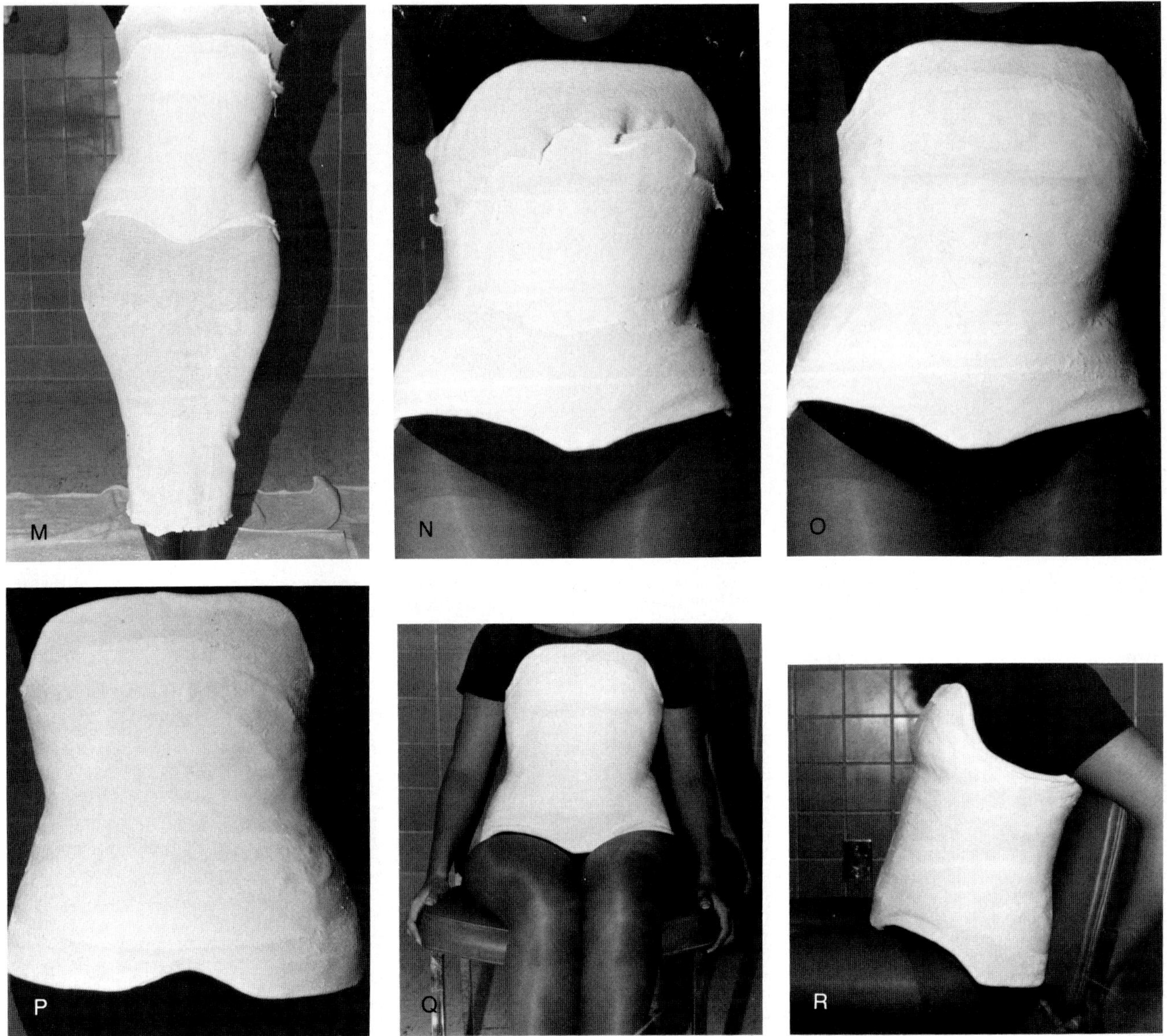

Fig. 11–2 (cont.). *M,* Redundant cast materials have been removed. *N, O, P,* After the ends of the stockinet have been folded over the upper and lower margins of the cast, a roll of 6″ plaster bandage is used to fix the stockinet ends to the adjacent cast surfaces to finish the cast. *Q, R,* Anterior and lateral views of the finished cast. The patient can sit comfortably.

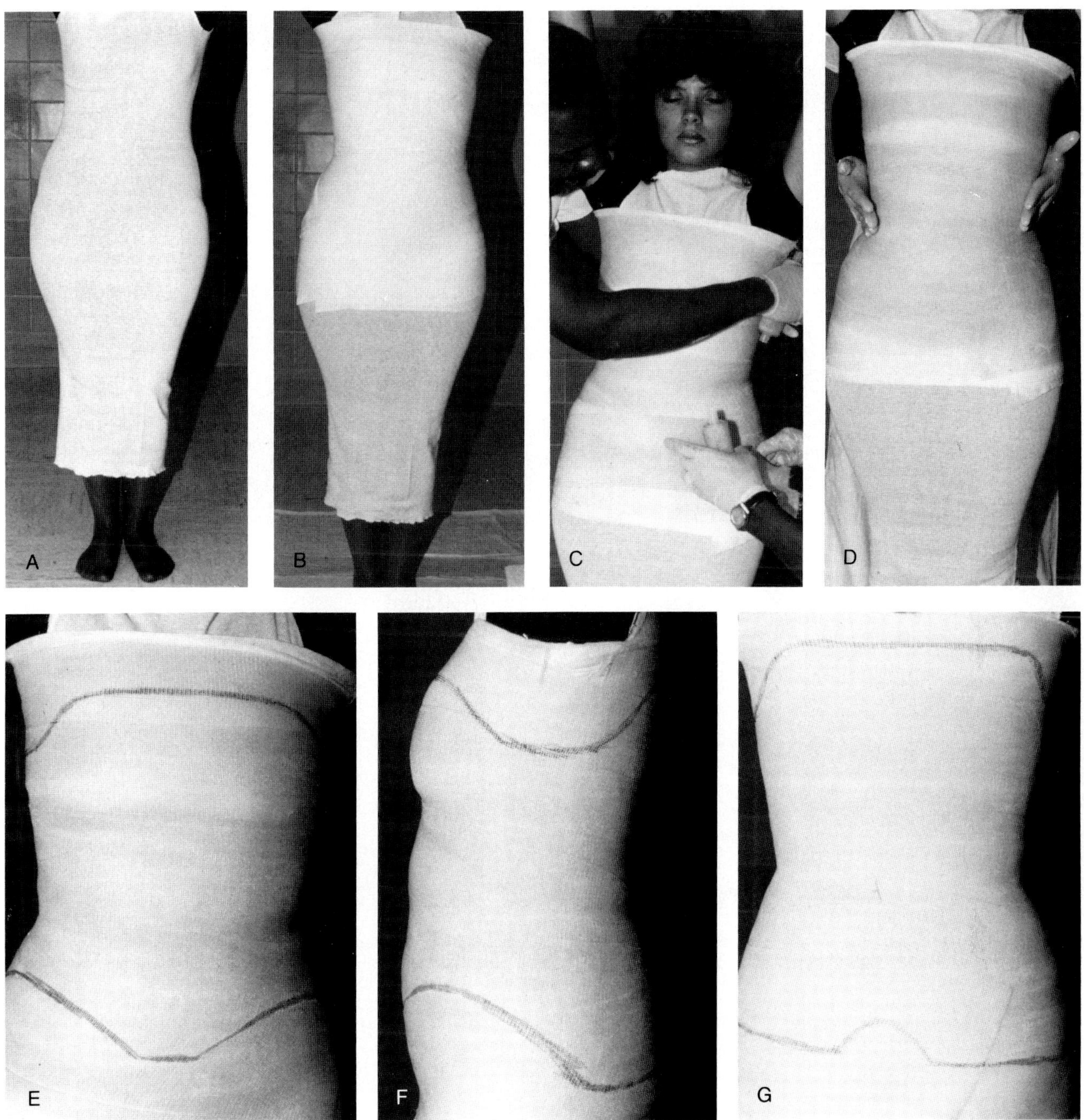

Fig. 11–3. The making of a fiberglass standard body cast. *A*, A 10″ stockinet with 2 armholes has been applied to the body. *B*, Four rolls of 6″ Webril bandage have been wrapped around the body. *C*, *D*, Four rolls of 5″ fiberglass bandage are applied to the body. *E*, *F*, *G*, The upper and lower margins of the cast have been marked with a wax pencil.

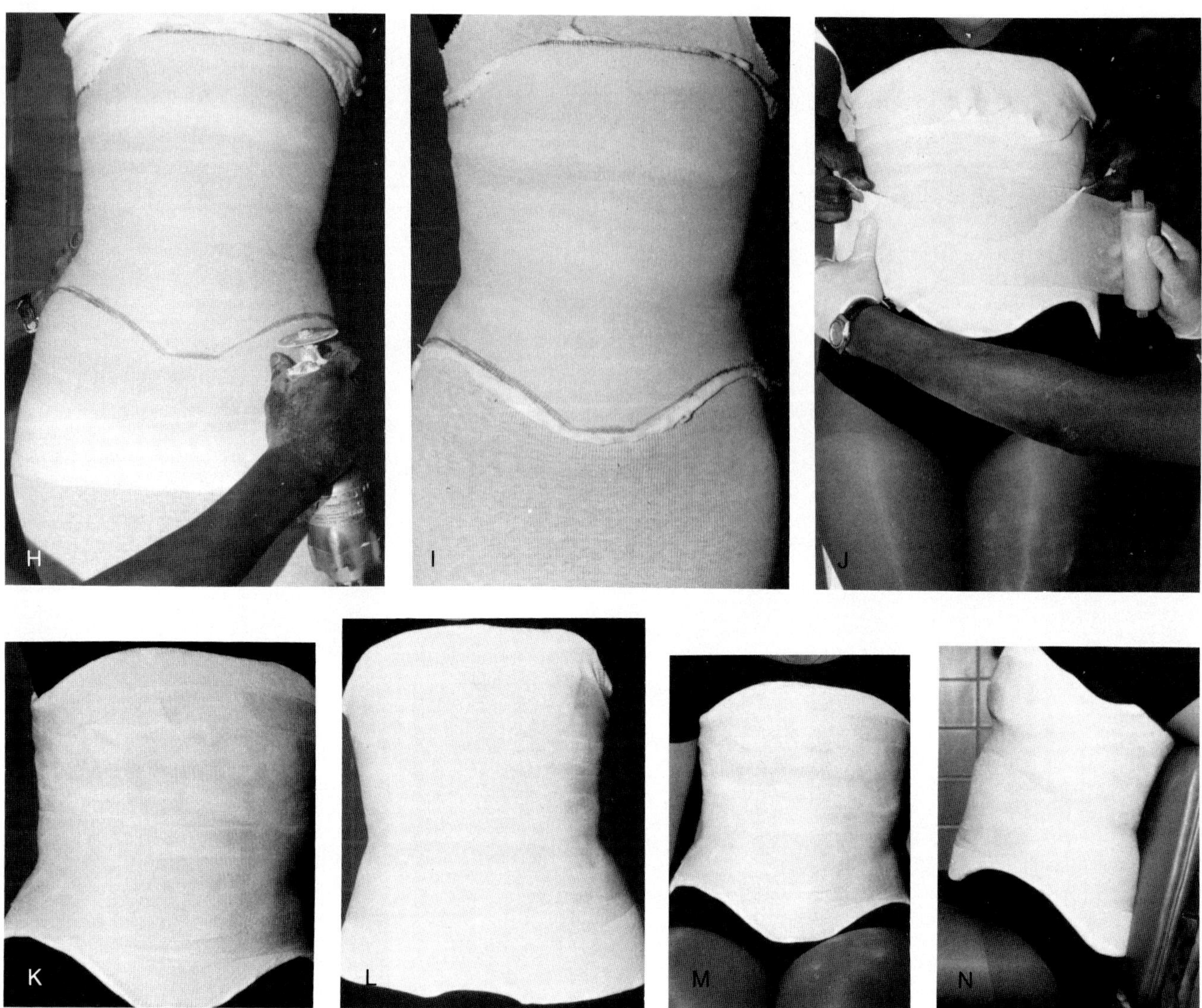

Fig. 11–3 (cont.). *H, I,* The excess cast materials are removed. *J,* The stockinet ends have been folded over the proximal and distal margins of the cast, and a roll of 5″ fiberglass bandage is applied to fix the stockinet ends of the cast. *K, L,* Anterior and posterior views of the finished cast. *M, N,* Anterior and lateral views of the cast show that the hips can be flexed easily to 90°.

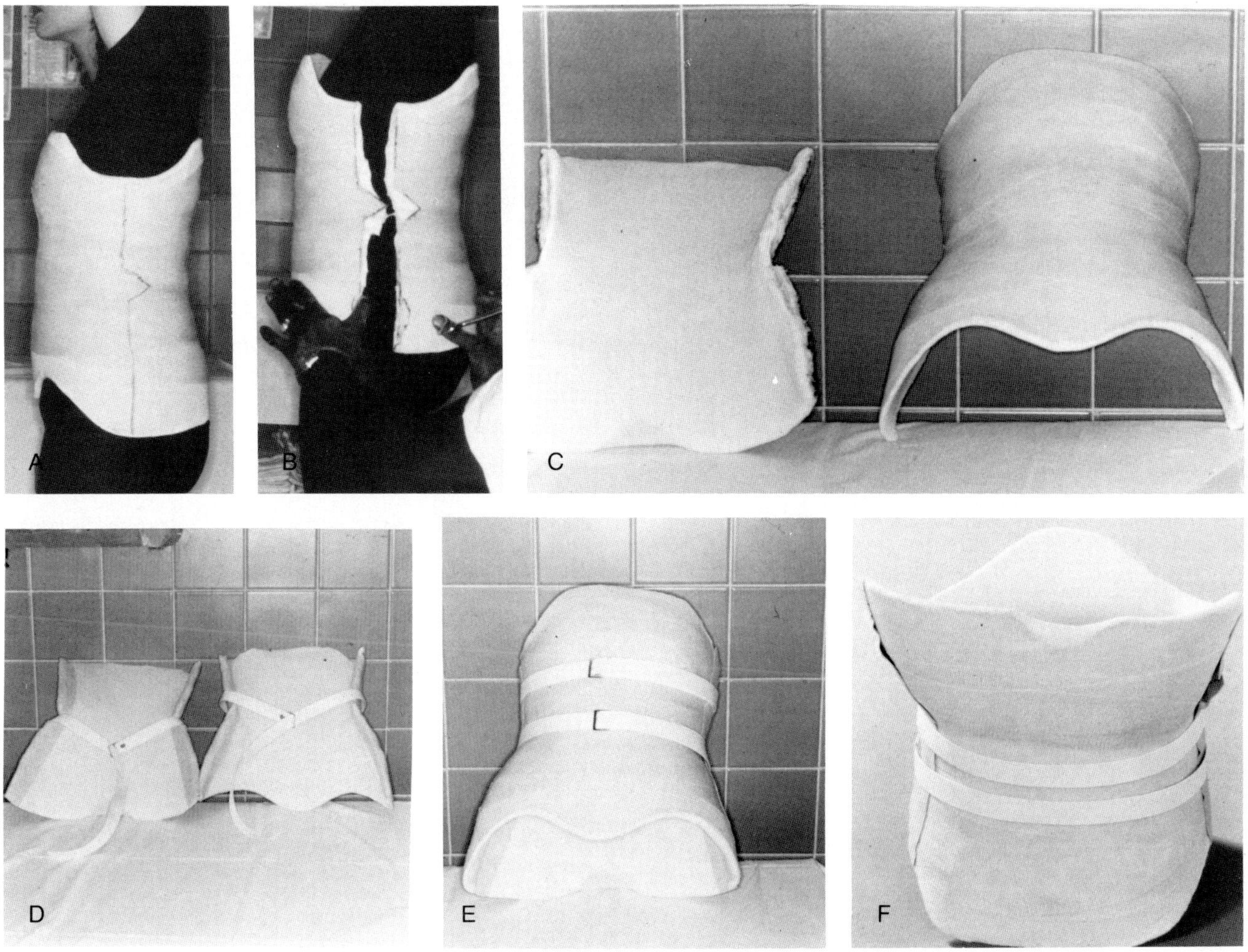

Fig. 11–4. Bivalving a standard body cast. *A,* Bivalving line with an interlocking notch on each side of the cast. *B,* Separation of the two halves of the cast. *C,* Two halves of a bivalved body cast. *D,* The margins have been lined, and two webbings and buckles have been attached to the bivalved cast. *E, F,* The two halves of the cast have been put together and are held together with webbings and buckles.

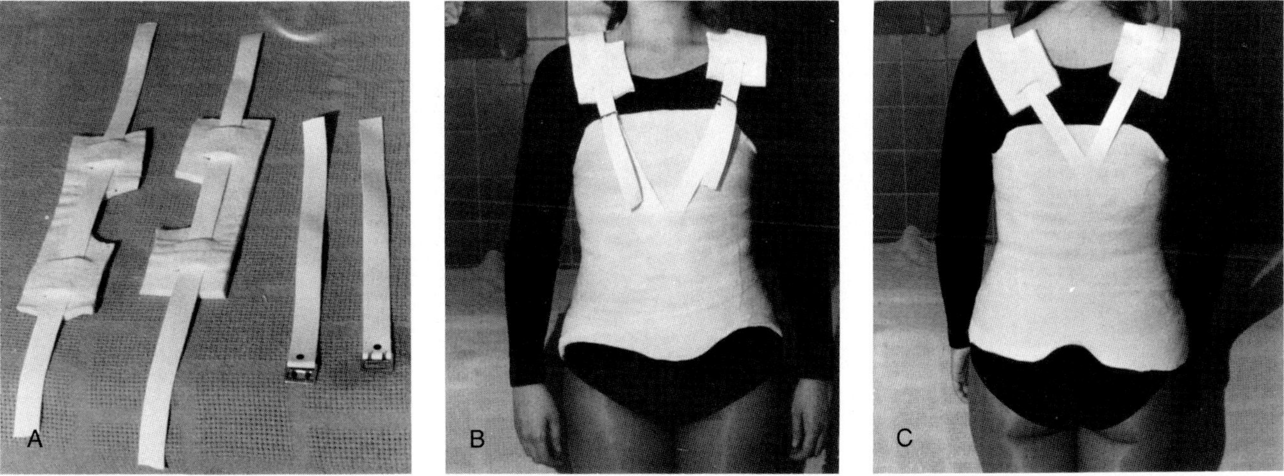

Fig. 11–5. Suspenders for a body cast. *A,* Felt shoulder pads and webbings with attached buckles. *B, C,* Anterior and posterior views of a fiberglass body cast with suspenders, which are attached to the anterior and posterior surfaces of the body cast with a roll of fiberglass bandage.

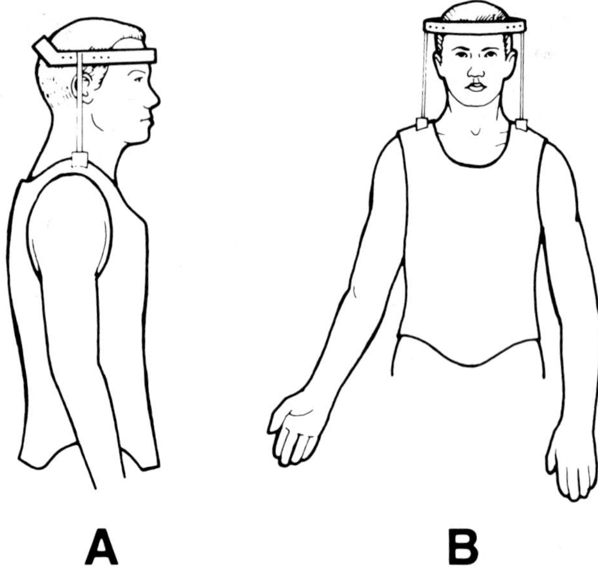

Fig. 11–6. Lateral (*A*) and anterior (*B*) views of a halo cast.

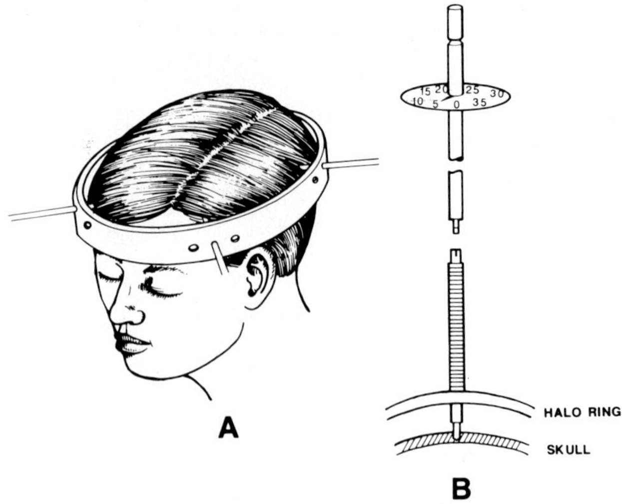

Fig. 11–7. Application of a halo ring. *A*, Oblique view of a head showing placement of the 4 halo pins. *B*, A torque wrench is used to tighten a halo pin through the outer table of the skull to about 5 pounds per square inch.

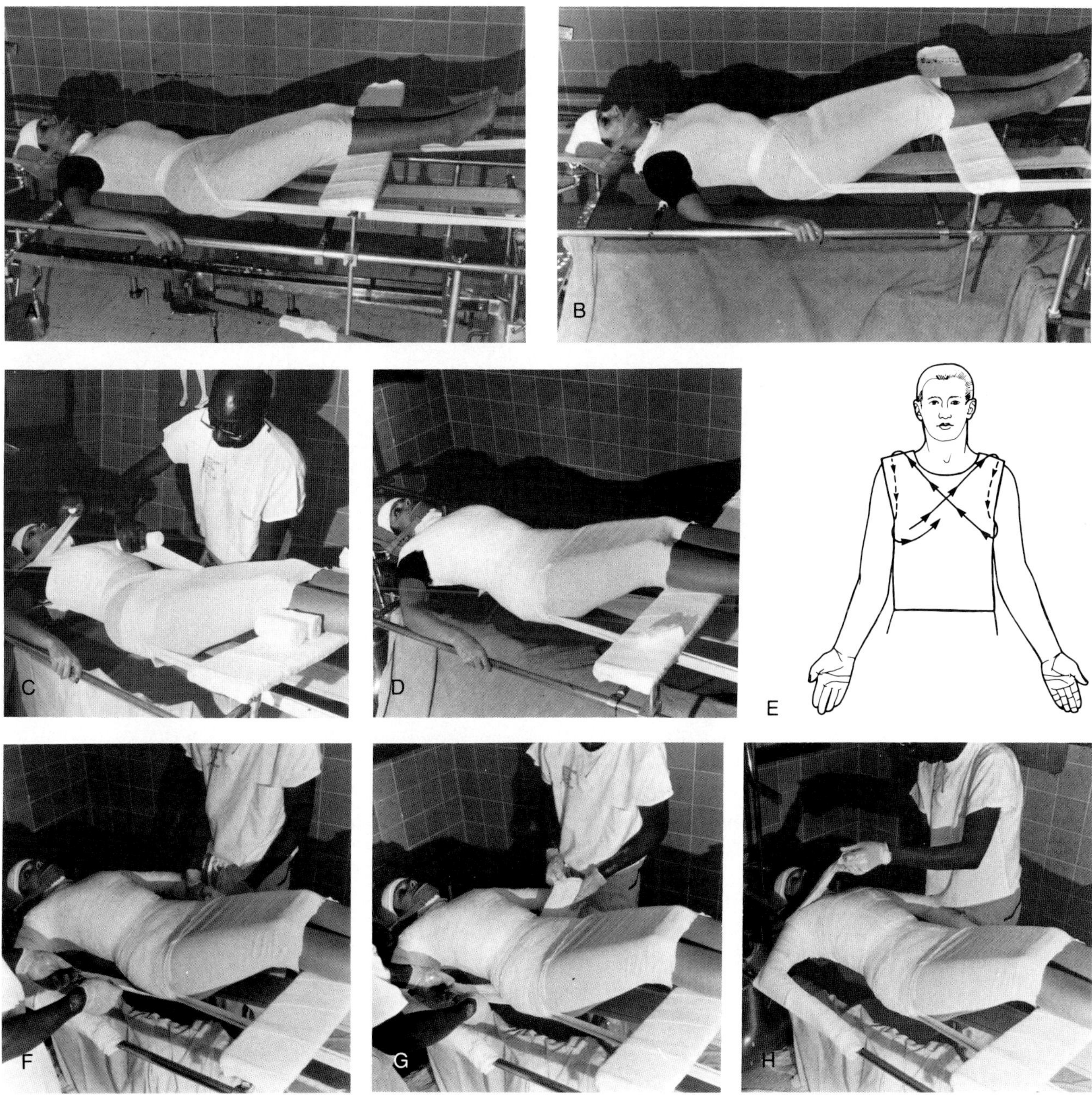

Fig. 11–8. The making of a plaster halo cast. *A,* The patient is placed on a fracture table under cephalopelvic traction. *B,* A close-up view of the same patient shows that head traction is provided by a head halter and that pelvic traction is provided by two cloth slings applied to the iliac crests in a crisscross manner. *C, D,* 6″ Webril bandages are wrapped around the body, and strips of the same Webril are applied from the tops of both shoulders to the pectoral region anteriorly and inferiorly, and the scapular region posteriorly and inferiorly. *E,* Plaster bandages are applied in a figure-8 manner to cover the shoulders and the anterior and posterior aspects of the pectoral and scapular regions. *F,* The body has been covered with 4 rolls of 6″ plaster bandage from the tops of the shoulders to the level of the greater trochanters. *G, H,* Application of 5″ × 30″ splints to the body.

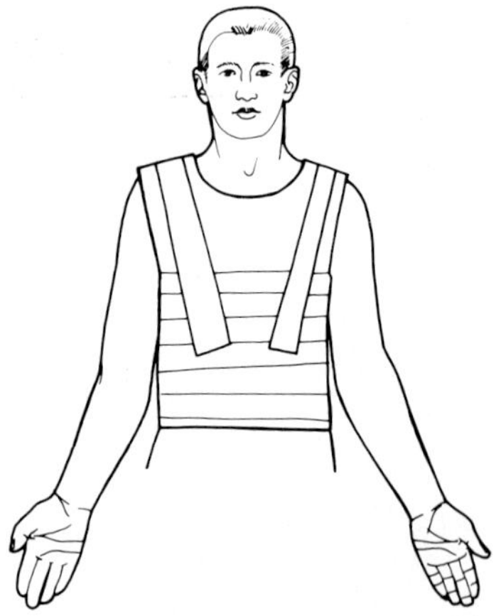

Fig. 11–8 (cont.). *I*, Application of the two boxes of the plaster splints to the body. *J*, The plaster splints are covered by plaster bandages, which are molded to fit the body contours. *K*, *L*, The upright bars of the halo apparatus are fixed to the cast with 2 rolls of 6″ plaster bandage. *M*, The upper and lower ends of the cast and the shoulder openings have been properly trimmed, and turning down and fixing the free stockinet ends will finish the cast.

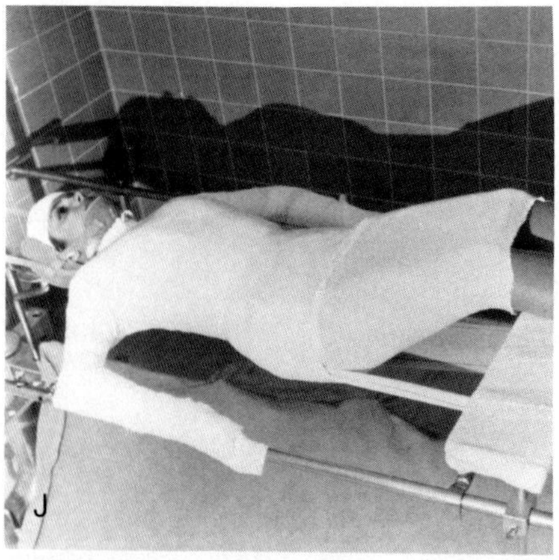

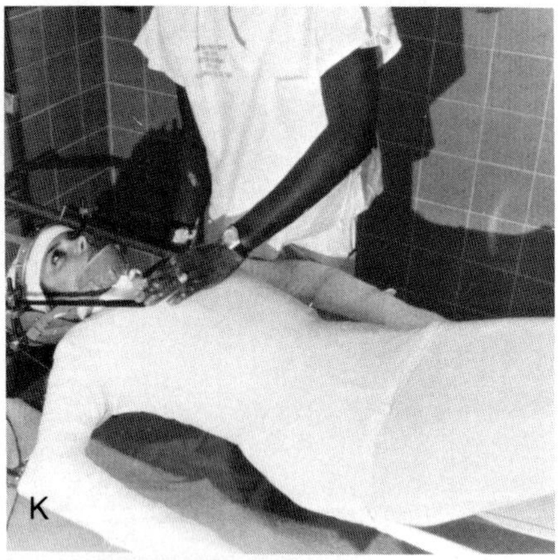

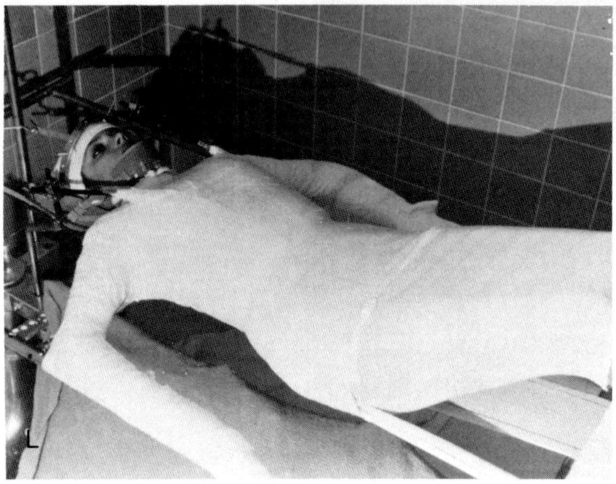

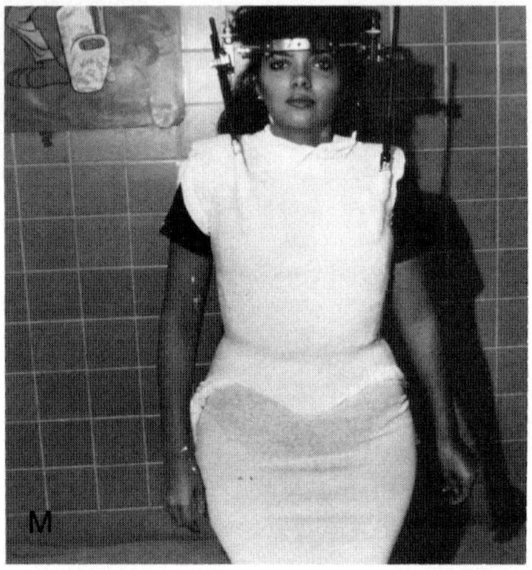

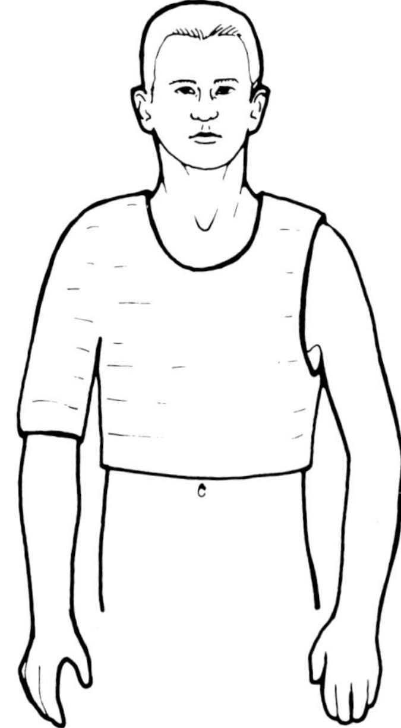

Fig. 11–9. Anterior view of a clavicular cast.

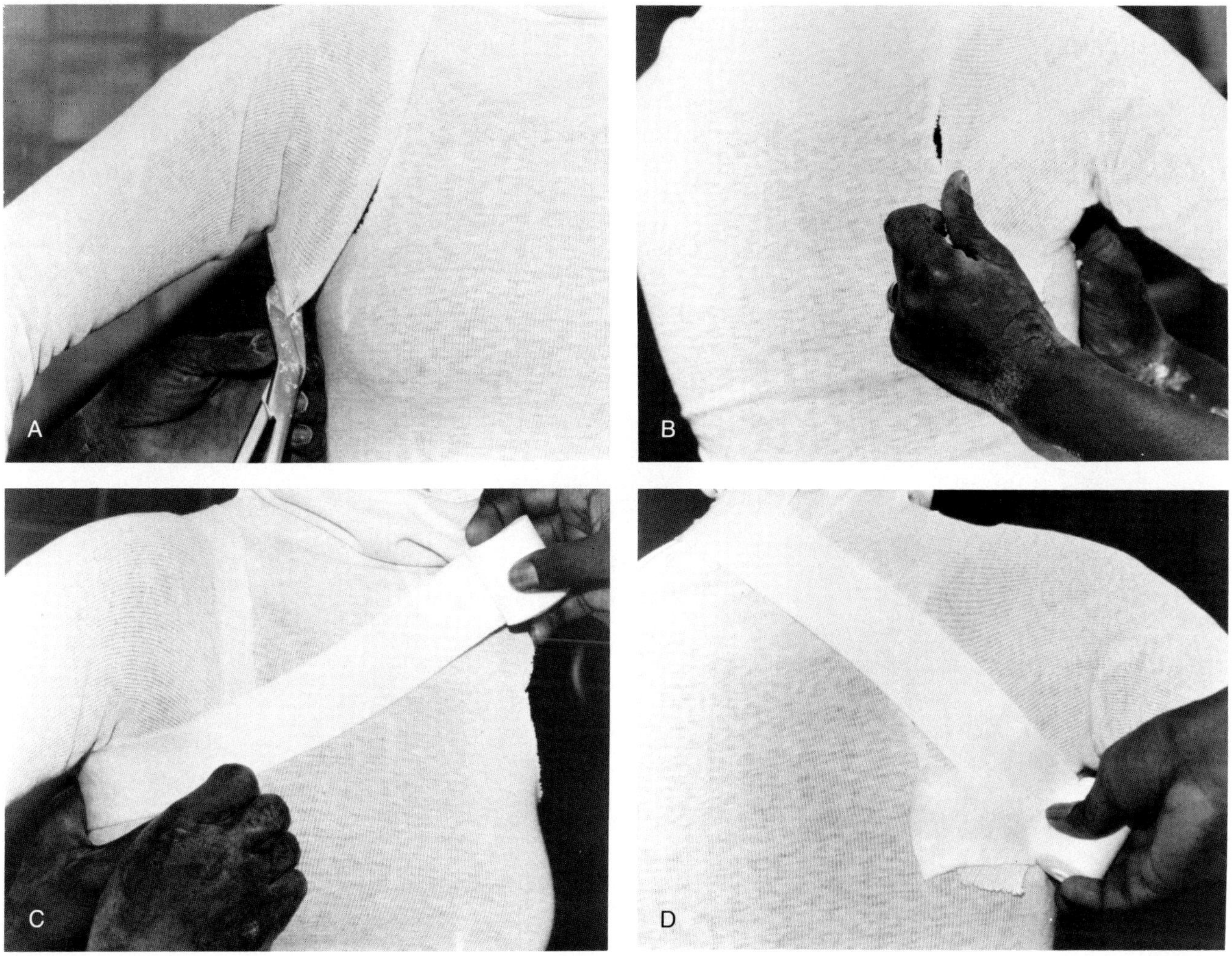

Fig. 11–10. Overlapping the body and arm stockinet ends in making a clavicular cast. *A*, Longitudinally splitting the end of the arm stockinet. *B*, Lapping the 2 cut ends of the arm stockinet over the adjacent body stockinet. *C*, *D*, Holding the overlapped stockinet ends together with 1 or 2 turns of 4″ Webril bandage.

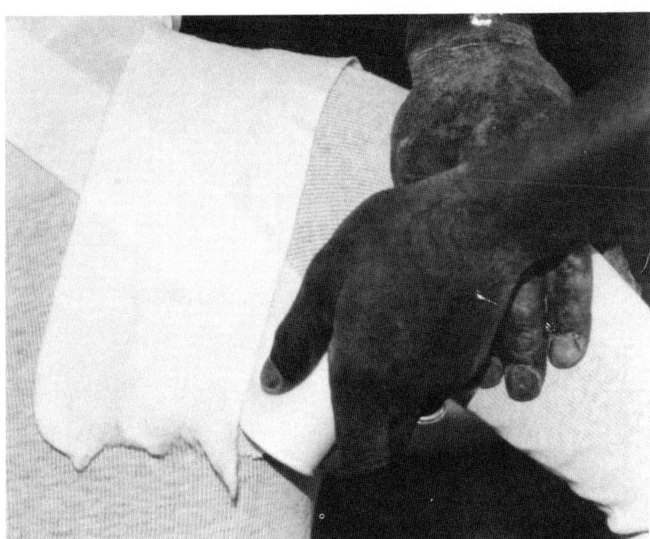

Fig. 11–11. Application of 6″ Webril strips from the lower pectoral region across the top of the shoulder to the lower scapular region.

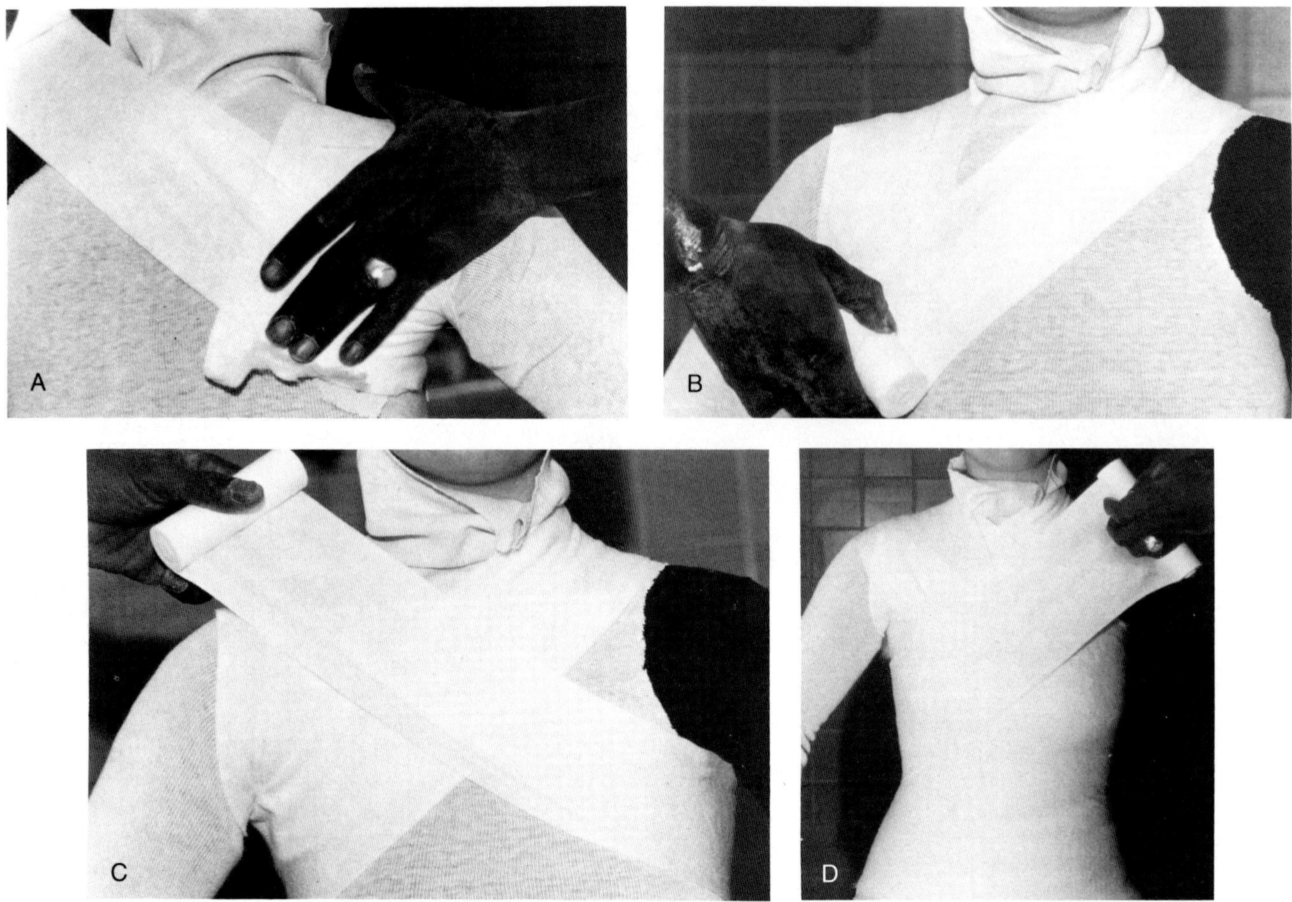

Fig. 11–12. Application of 6″ Webril bandages to the body. *A, B, C,* Webril bandages are applied to the thoracic region in a figure-8 manner. *D,* Webril bandages are applied to the lower thoracic and abdominal area in a circular and horizontal manner.

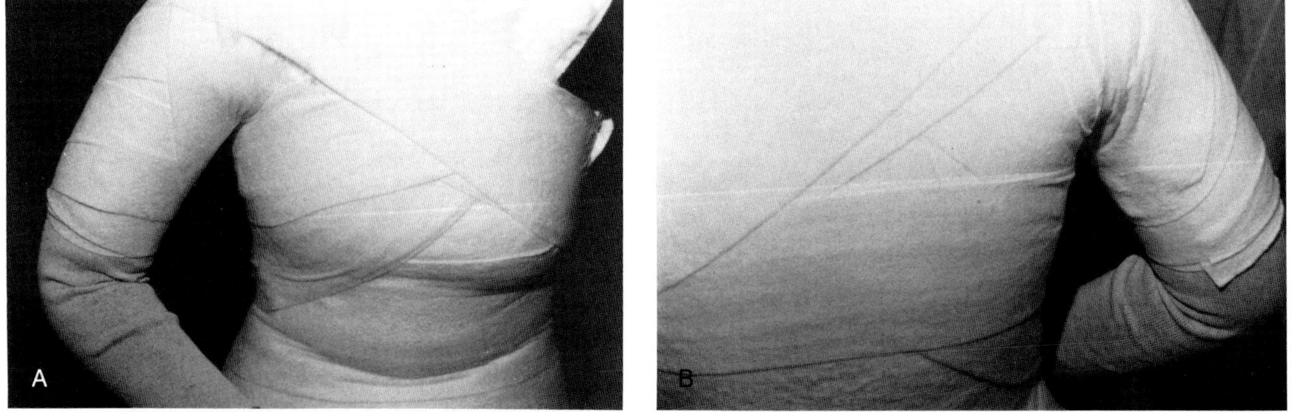

Fig. 11–13. *A, B,* Application of 4″ Webril bandages to the upper arm and adjacent shoulder region.

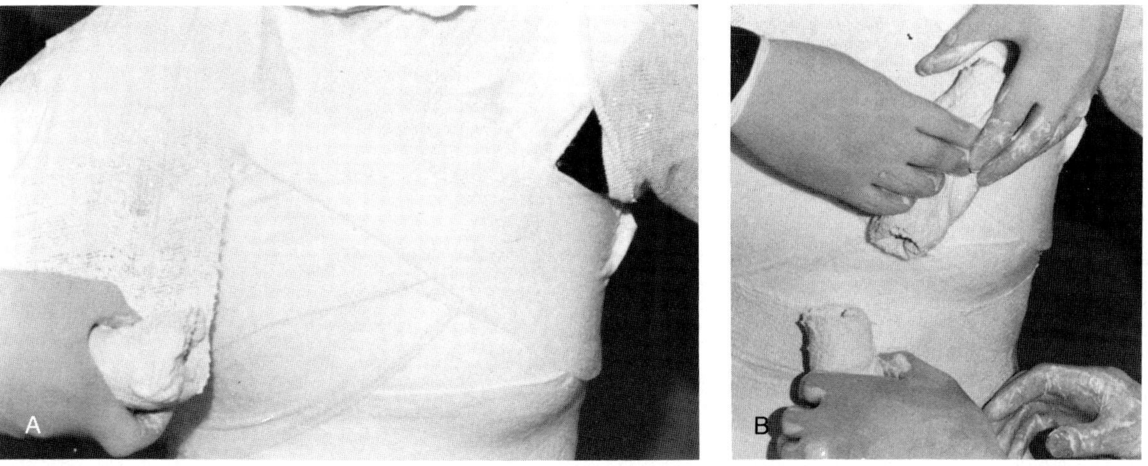

Fig. 11–14. *A, B,* Application of 2 rolls of 6″ plaster bandage to the body and 2 rolls of 4″ plaster bandage to the arm and adjacent shoulder portion of the cast.

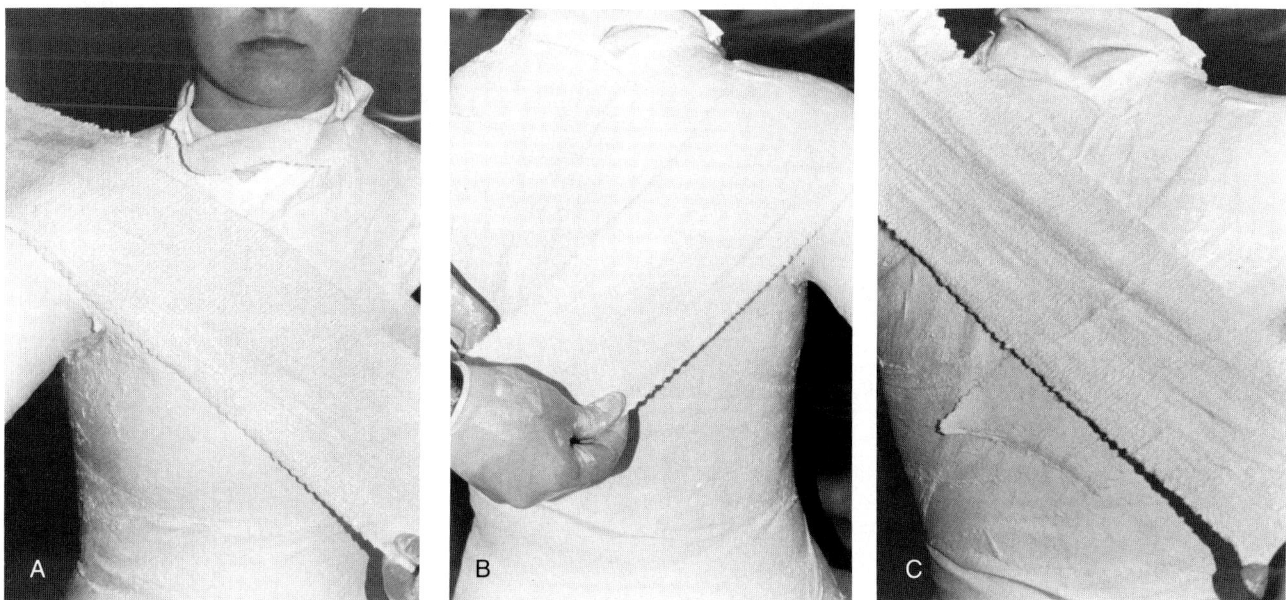

Fig. 11–15. *A, B, C,* Application of 2 5″ × 30″ plaster splints to the upper chest and back regions in a crisscross manner.

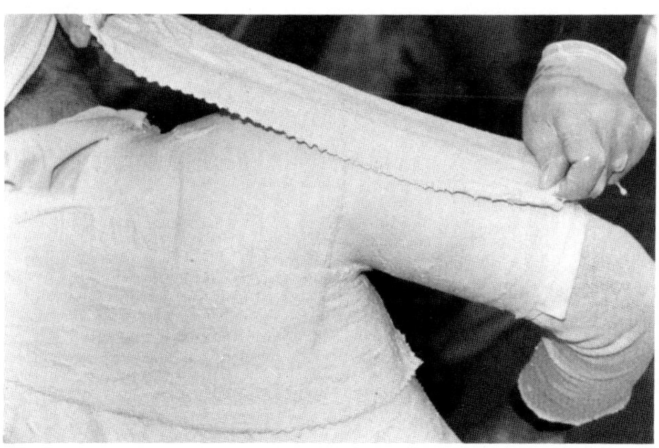

Fig. 11–16. Application of a 5″ × 30″ plaster splint from the top of the shoulder along the lateral aspect of the arm to the supracondylar level of the elbow.

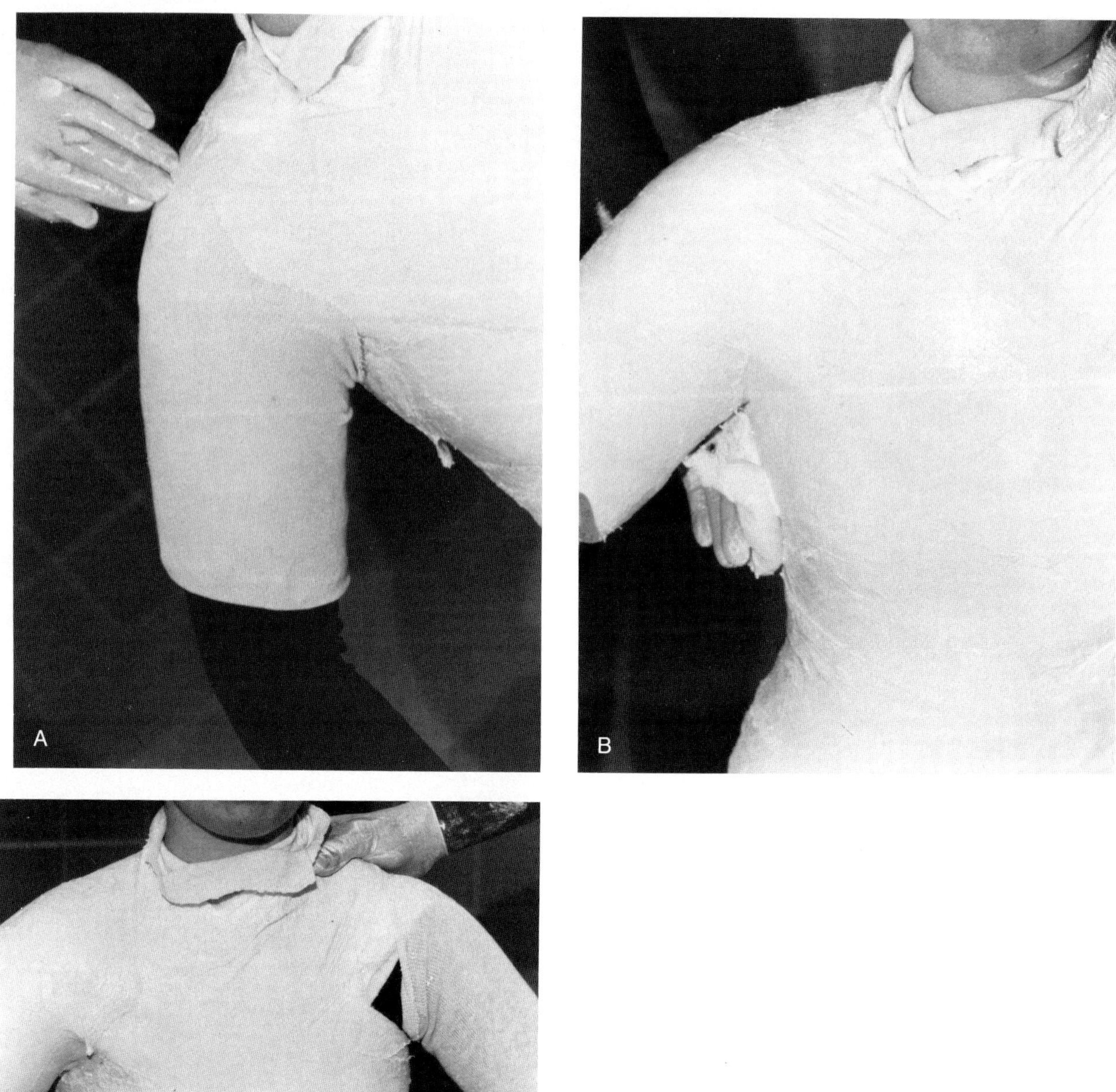

Fig. 11–17. *A, B, C,* The arm and upper portion of the body part of the cast have been covered with 4″ and 6″ plaster bandages, respectively.

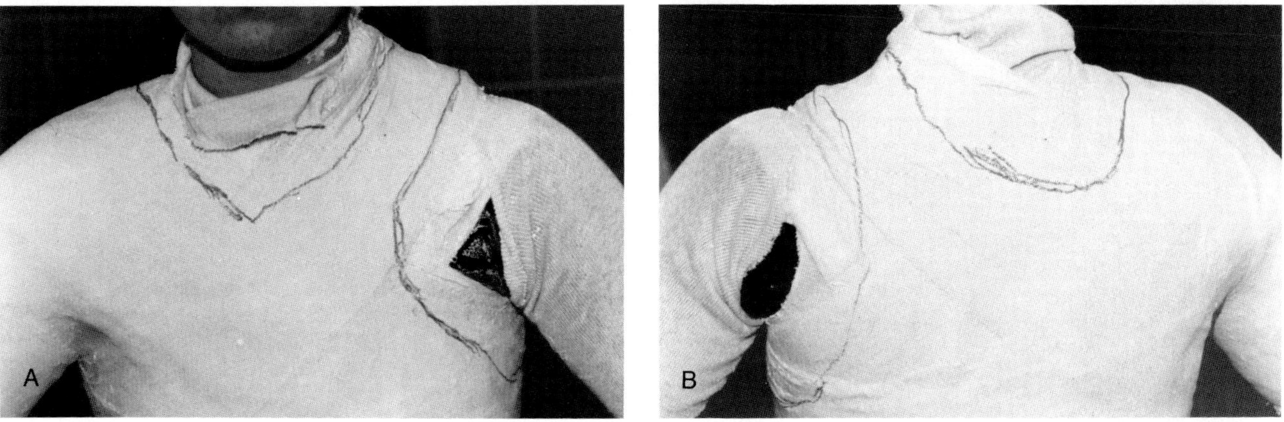

Fig. 11–18. *A, B,* The final shoulder and neck openings have been marked with a wax pencil.

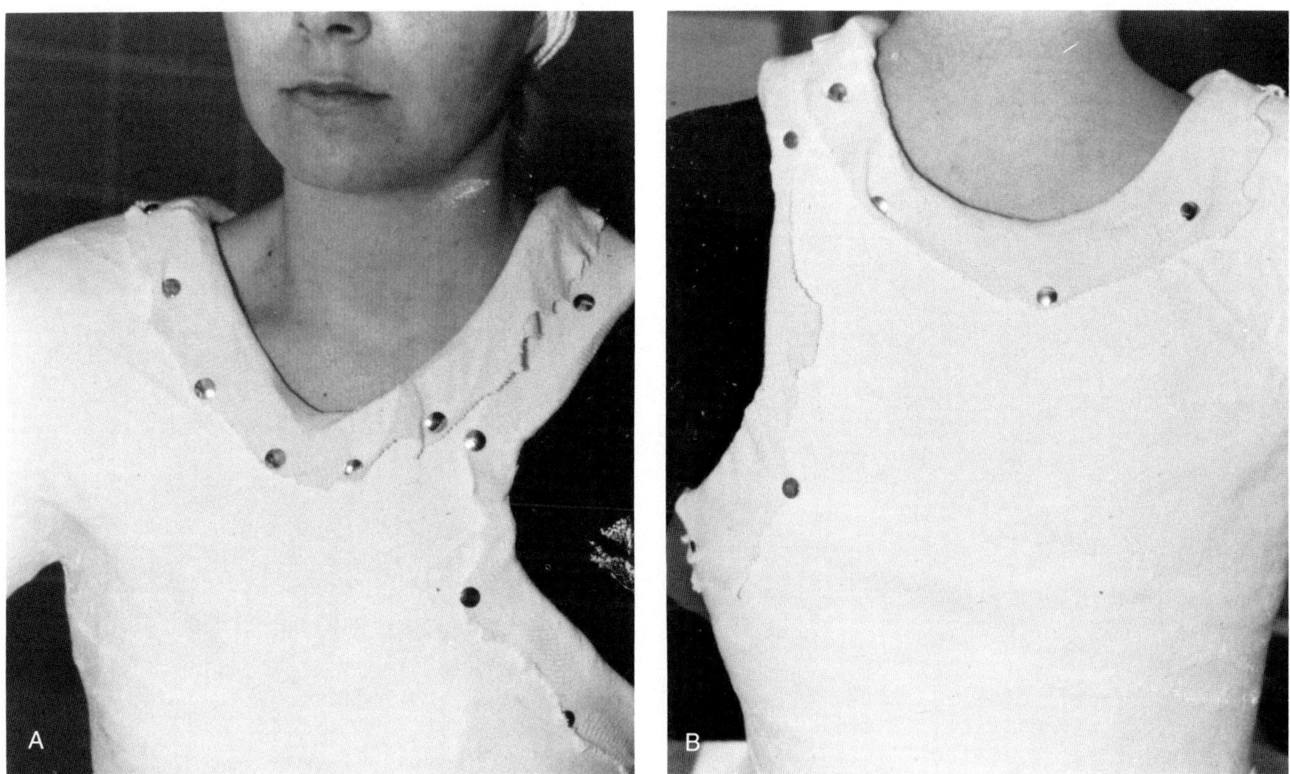

Fig. 11–19. *A, B,* The neck and shoulder openings have been trimmed, and the stockinet ends have been folded over them and temporarily fixed to the cast with thumbtacks.

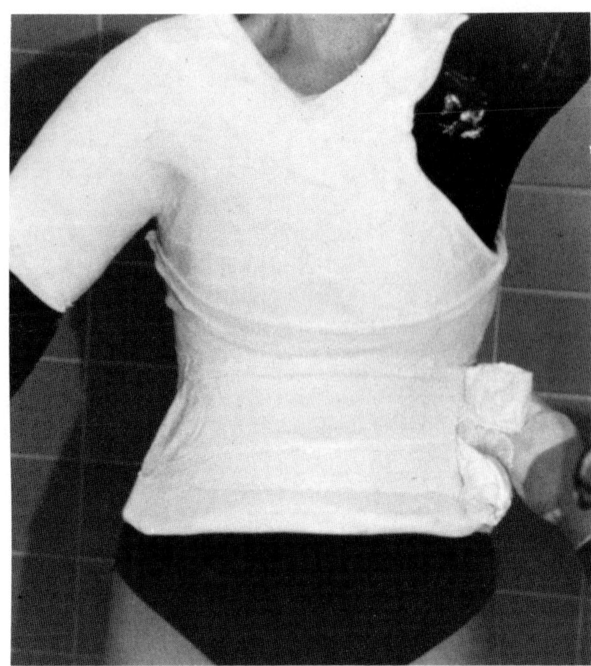

Fig. 11–20. After the distal end of the cast has been trimmed and the distal end of the body stockinet has been turned up, a roll of 6″ plaster bandage is used to finish the lower half of the body part of the cast.

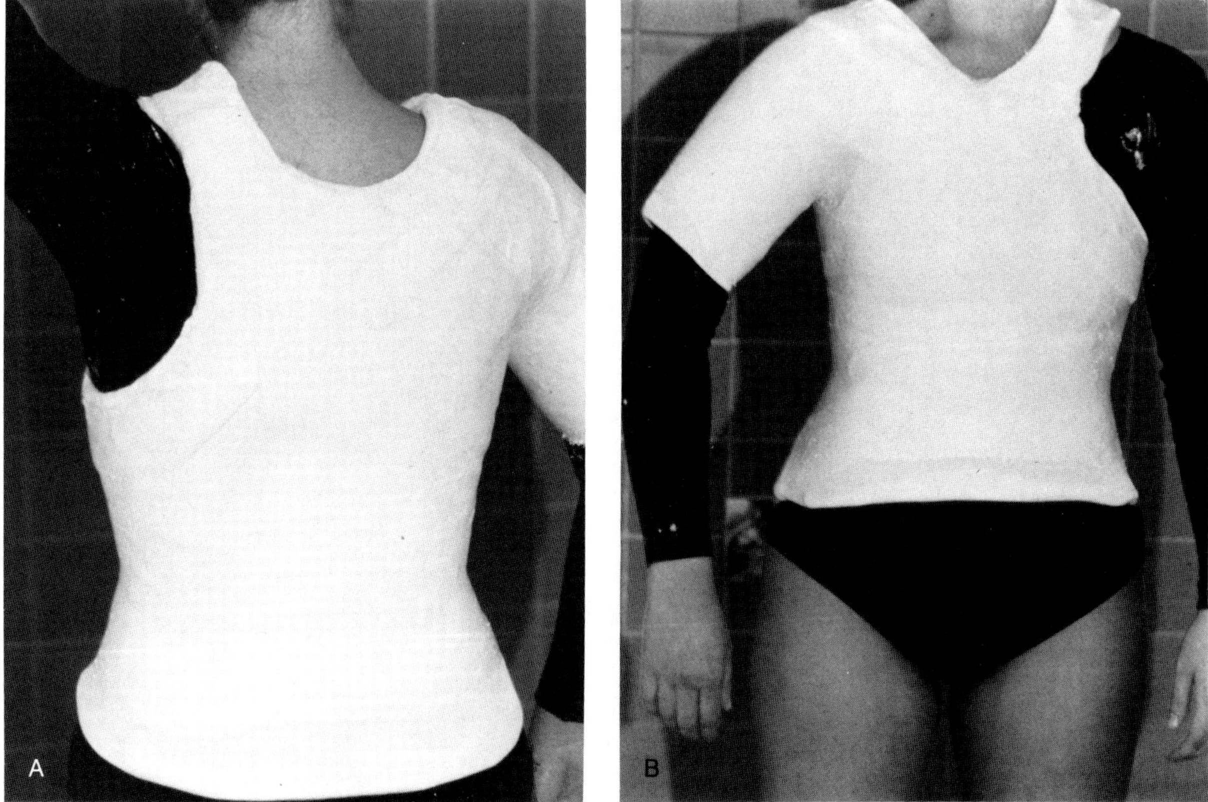

Fig. 11–21. *A, B,* Posterior and anterior views of the finished clavicular cast show that the neck and the uninvolved shoulder have full range of motion.

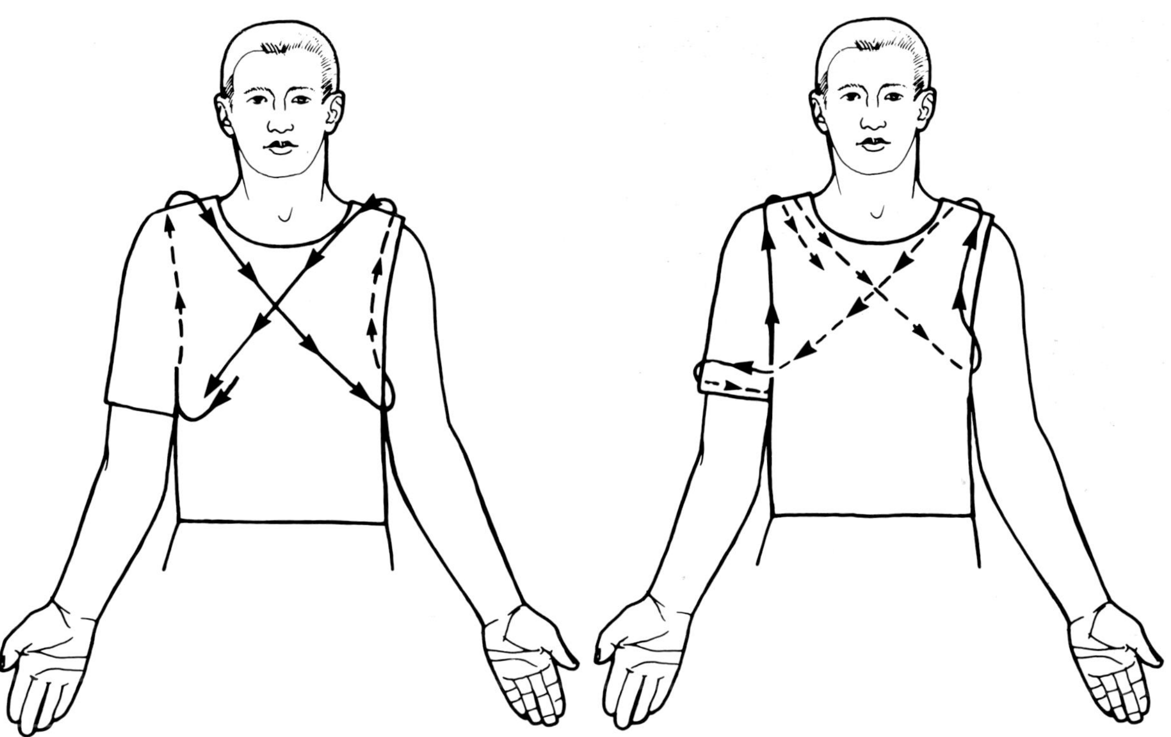

Fig. 11–22. Finishing the arm, shoulder, and neck openings by applying 4″ fiberglass bandages in a multiple figure-8 manner. The solid lines indicate the anterior surface of the cast, and the dotted lines indicate the posterior surface of the cast.

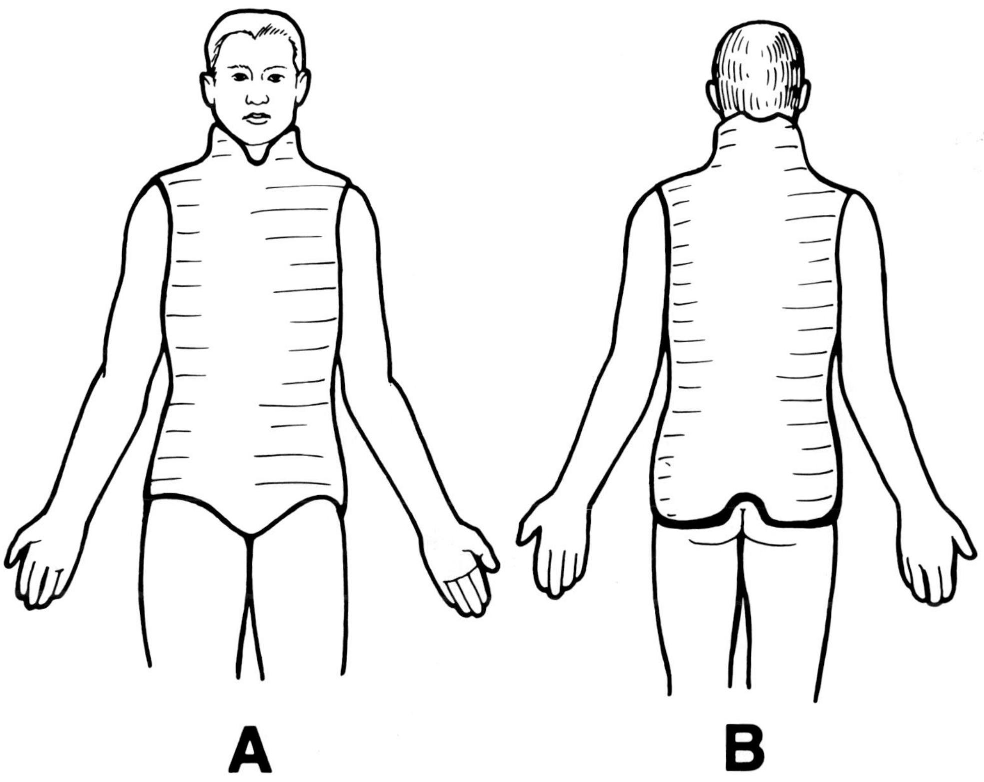

Fig. 11–23. Anterior (*A*) and posterior (*B*) views of a Risser cast.

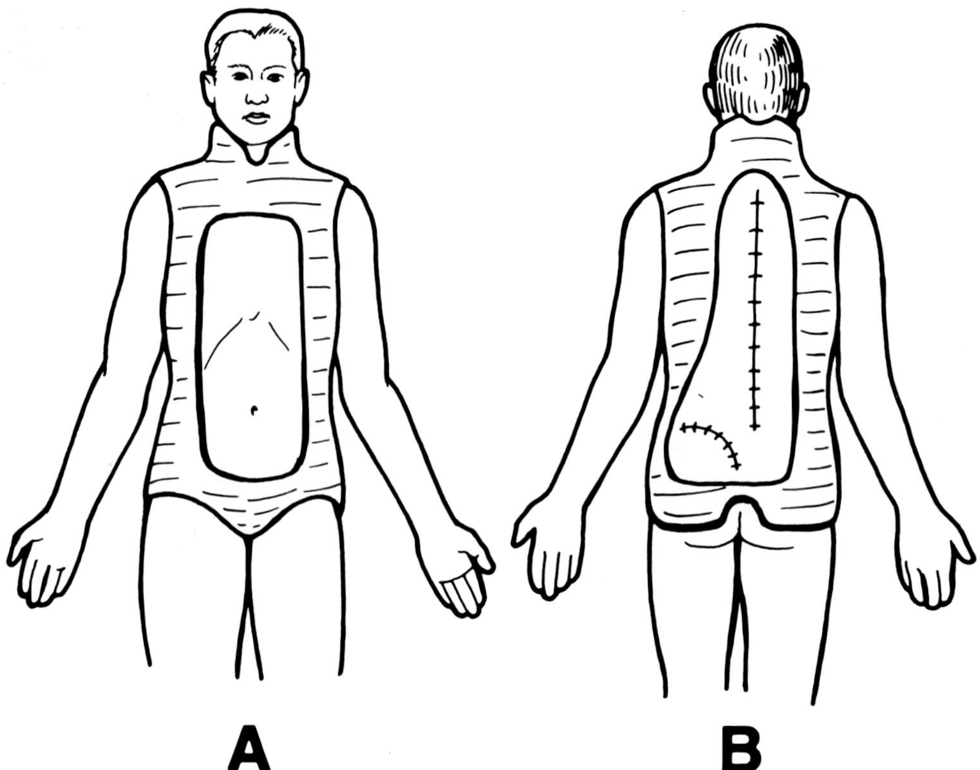

Fig. 11–24. Anterior (*A*) and posterior (*B*) views of a Risser cast with parts of the cast removed for performing spinal fusions, obtaining iliac bone grafts, and for treatment of cardiopulmonary and gastrointestinal complications.

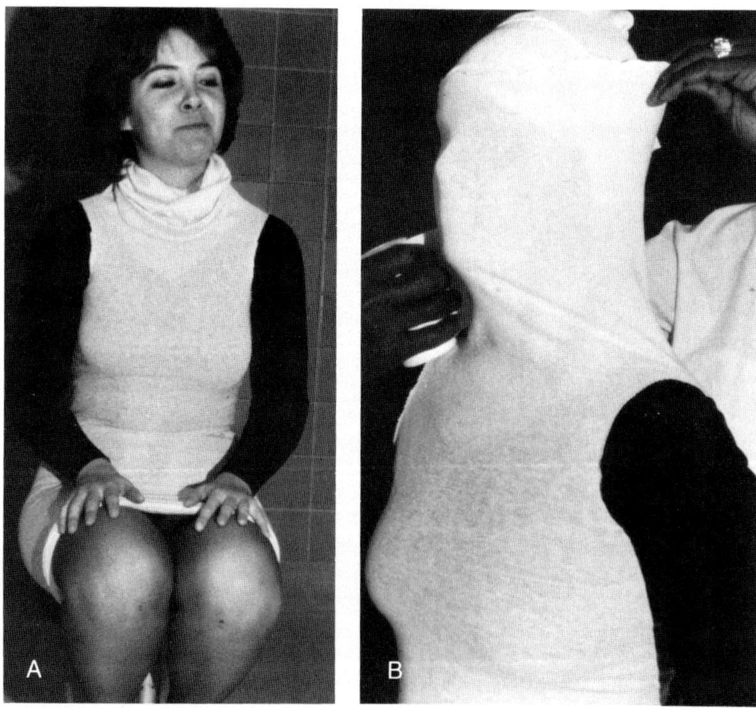

Fig. 11–25. *A, B,* Application of a body stockinet with two armholes from the mid-thigh level to the top of the head.

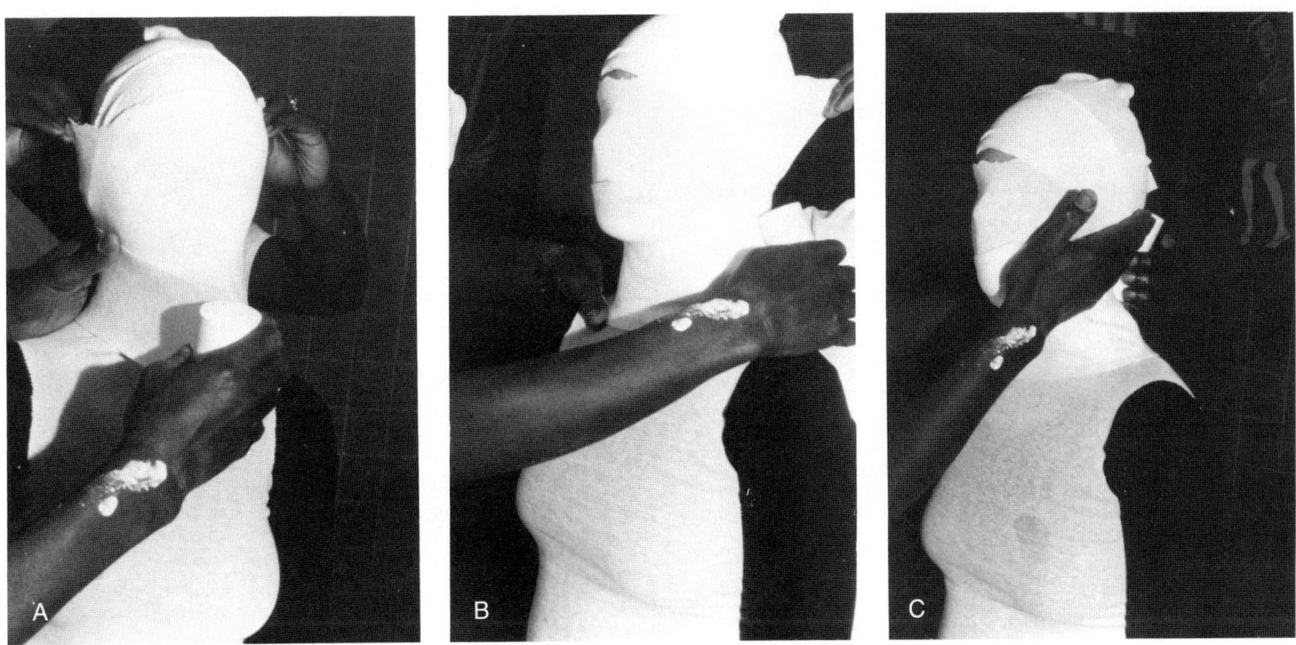

Fig. 11–26. *A, B, C,* Application of Webril bandages to the head and neck.

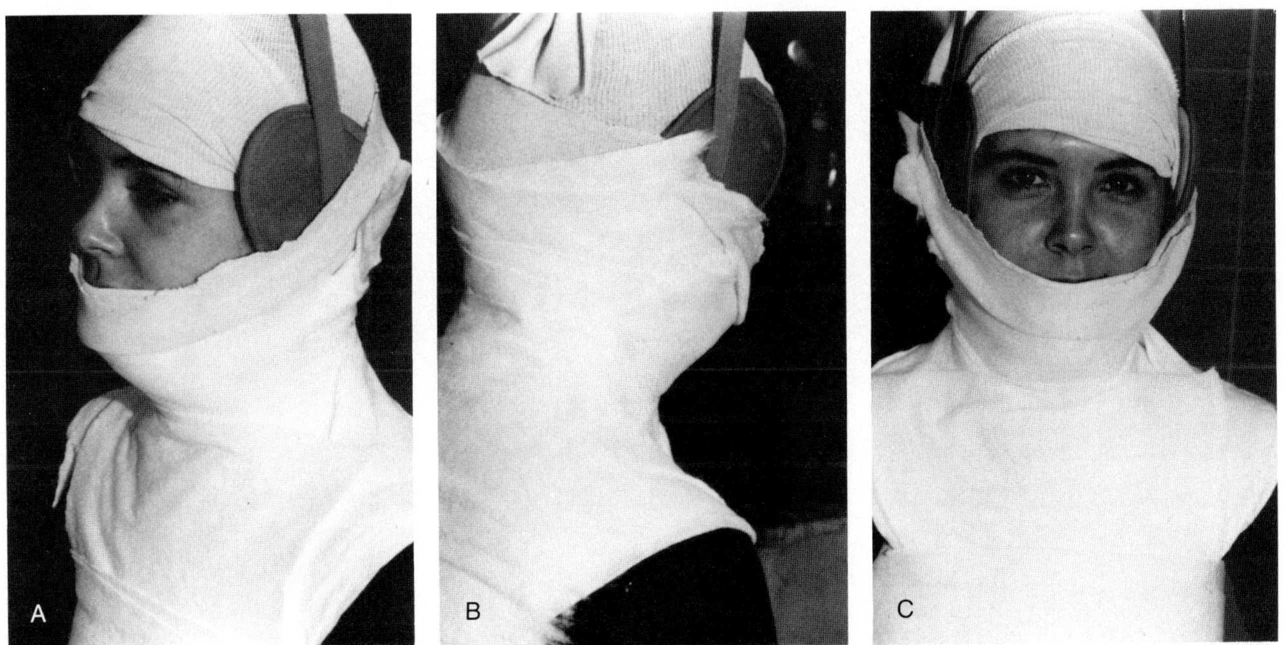

Fig. 11–27. *A, B, C,* Application of Webril bandages to the head, neck, and body.

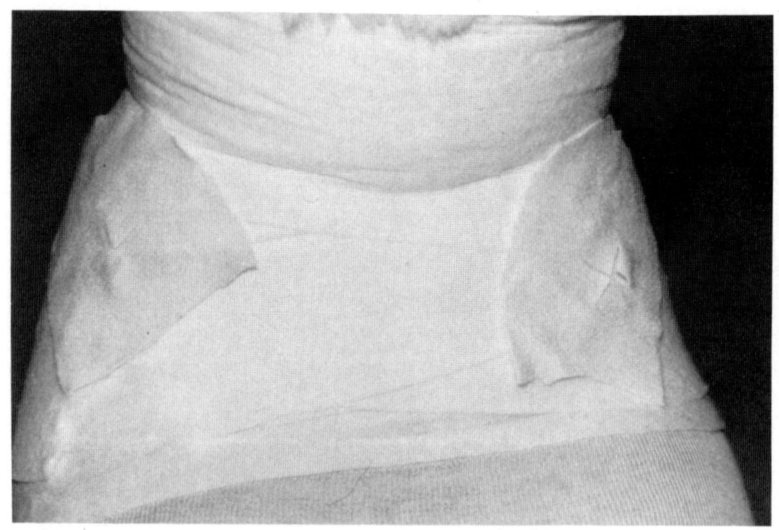

Fig. 11–28. Application of felt pads to the anterior superior iliac spines.

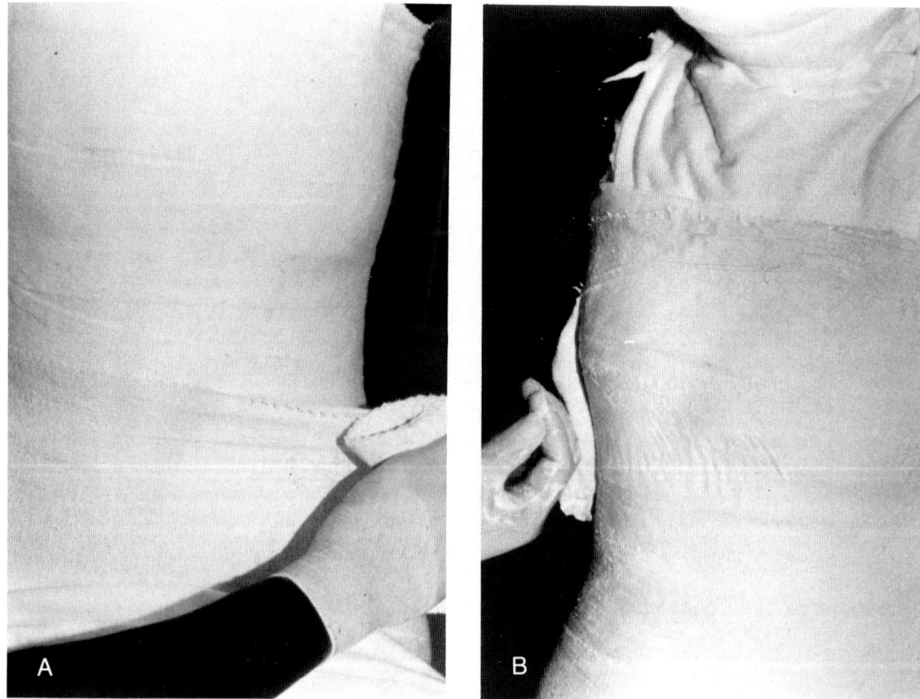

Fig. 11–29. *A, B,* Application of a roll of 6″ plaster bandage from the level of the greater trochanters to the axillary region.

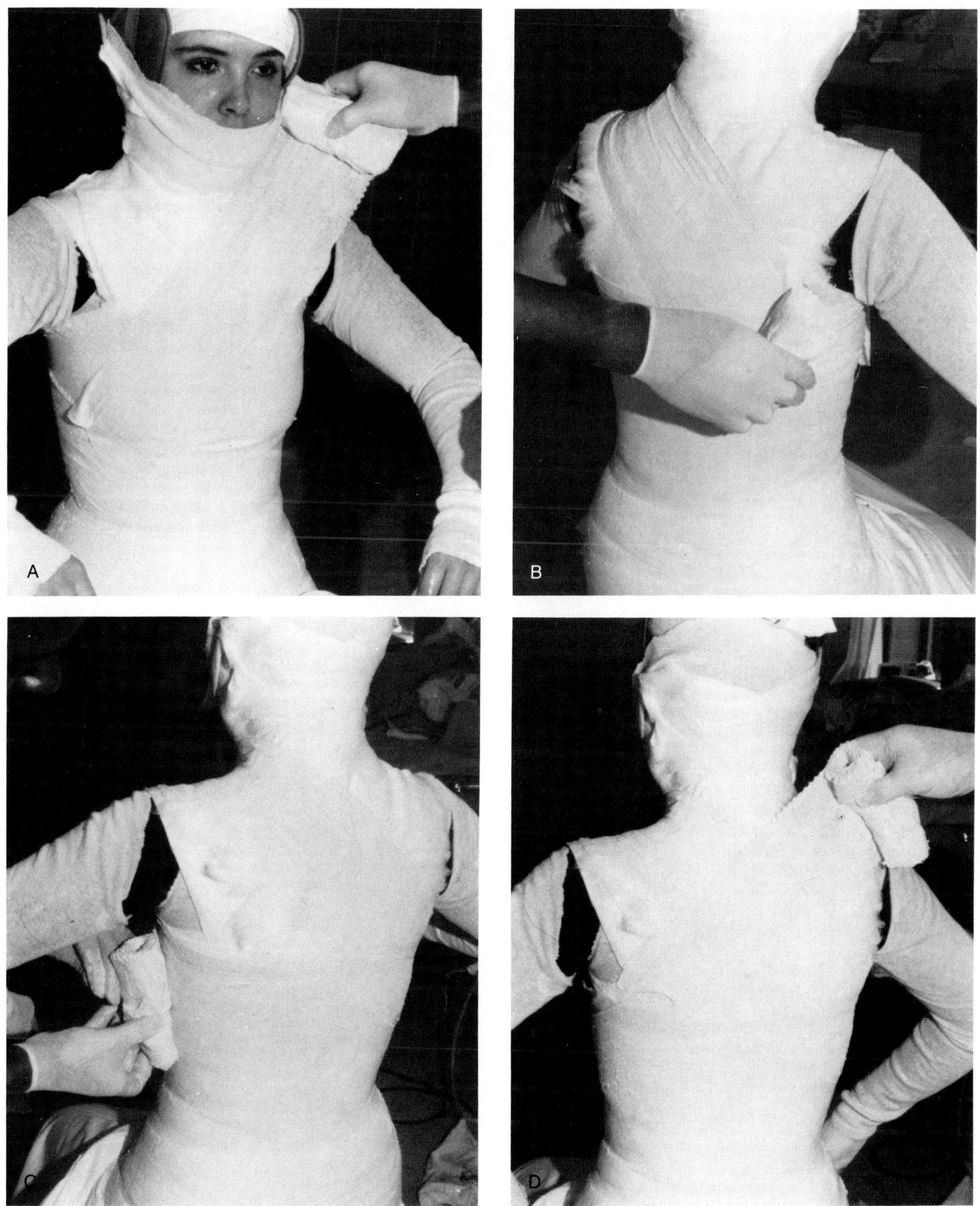

Fig. 11–30. *A–D*, Covering the upper part of the body and both shoulders with a roll of 6″ plaster bandage in a figure-8 manner.

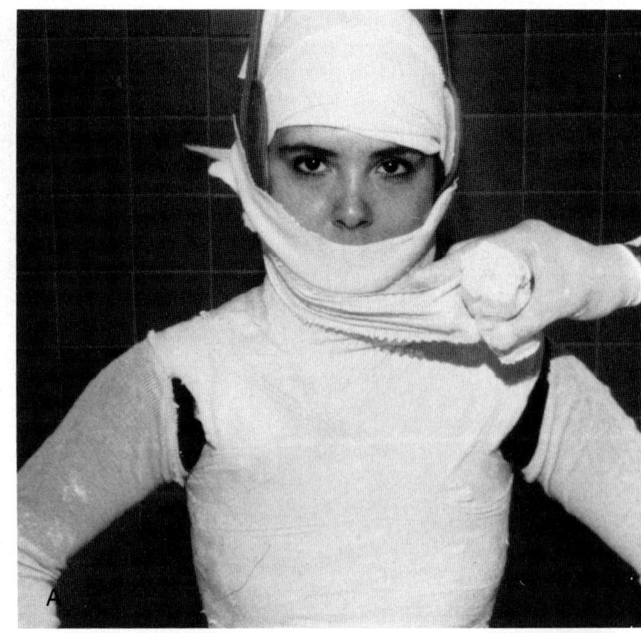

Fig. 11–31. *A, B, C,* Application of 4″ plaster bandages to the neck and the lower part of the skull.

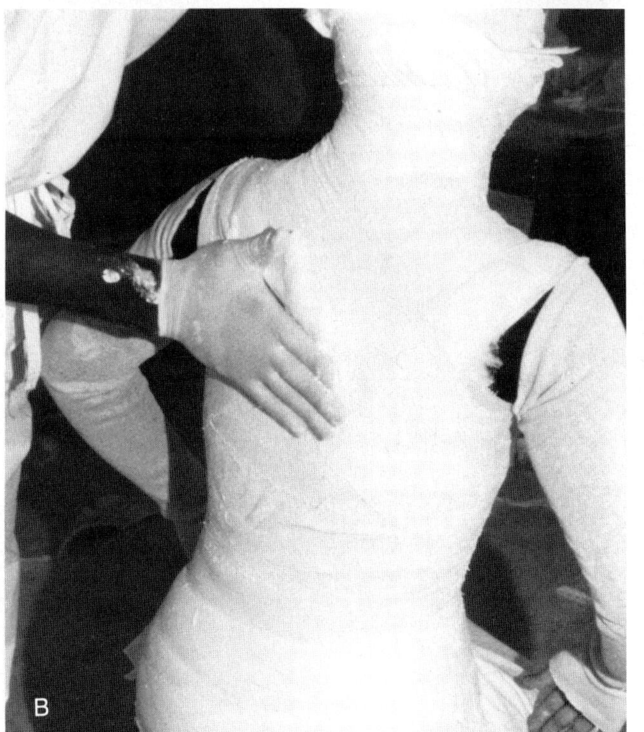

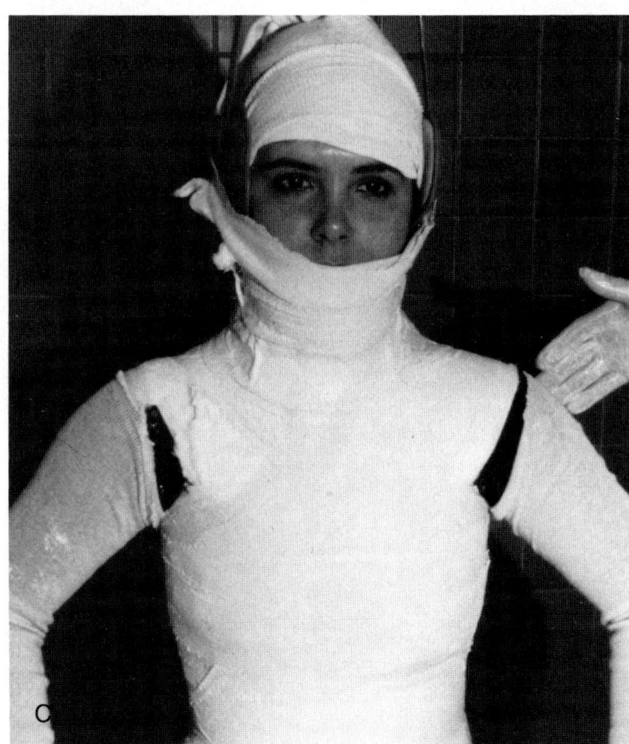

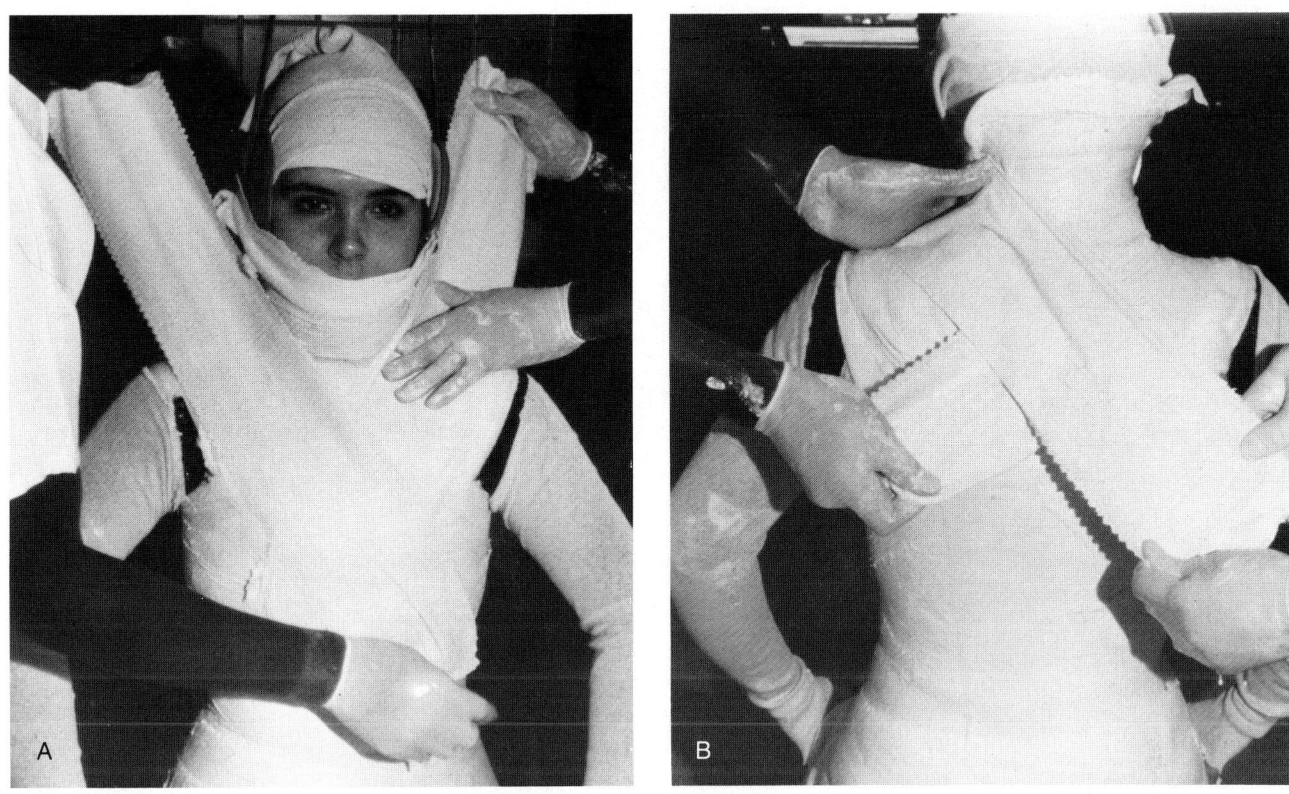

Fig. 11–32. *A, B,* Application of two plaster splints across the tops of the shoulders and diagonally across the upper part of the body.

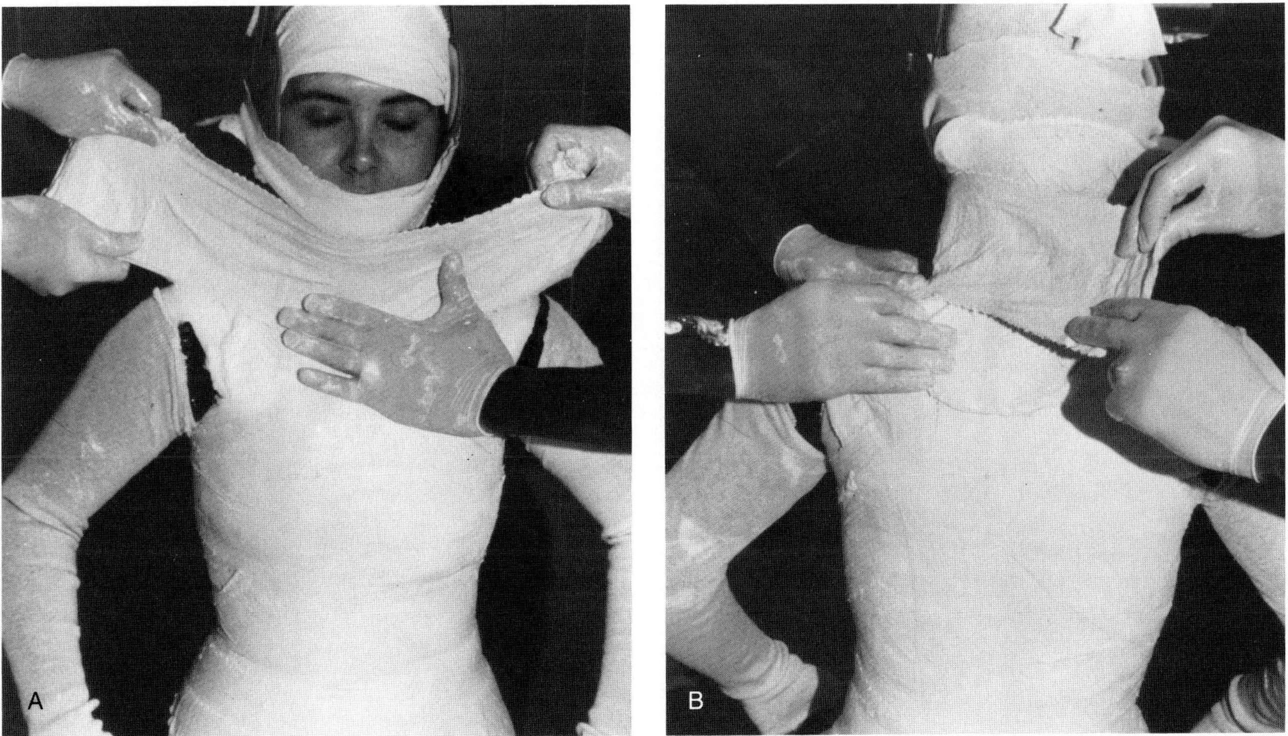

Fig. 11–33. *A, B,* Application of a plaster splint around the neck and the base of the skull.

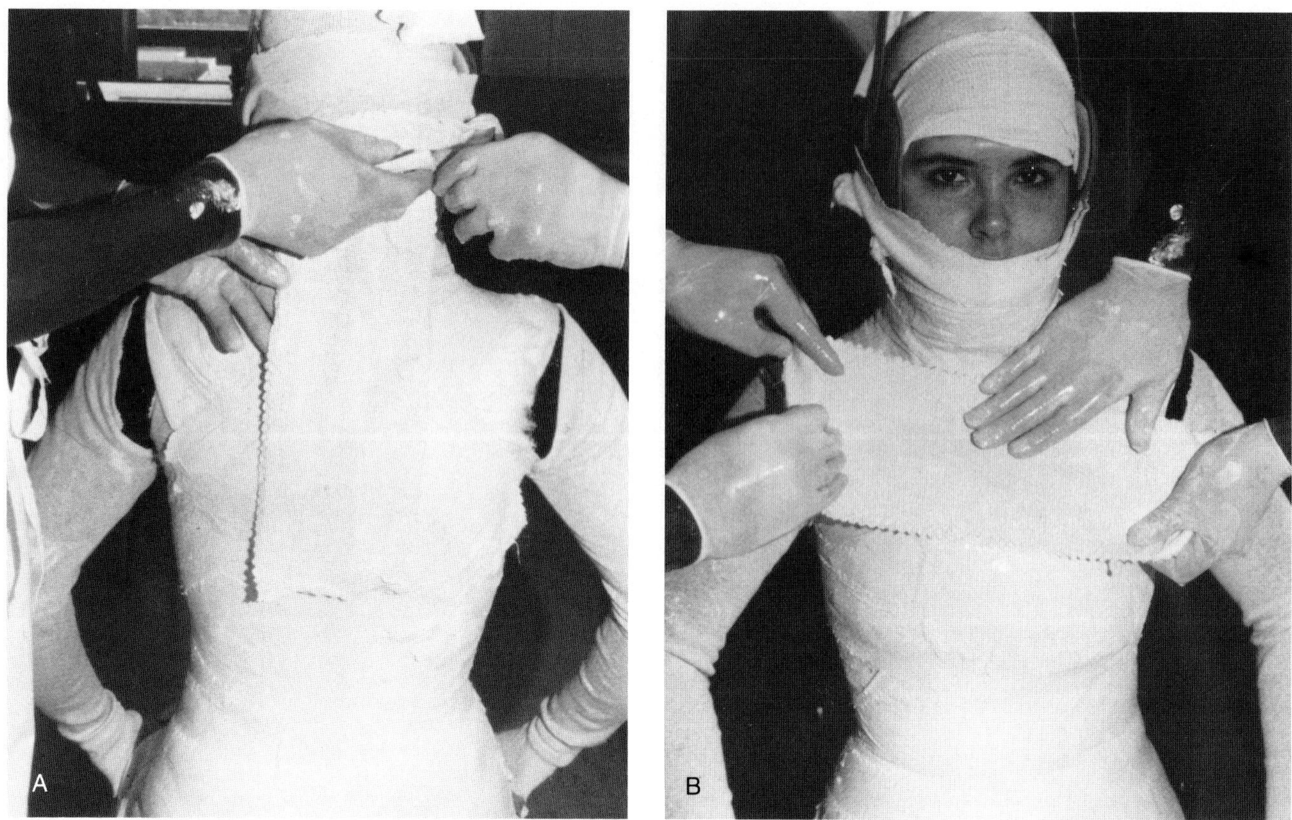

Fig. 11–34. *A, B,* Application of plaster splints to the upper part of the spine and chest.

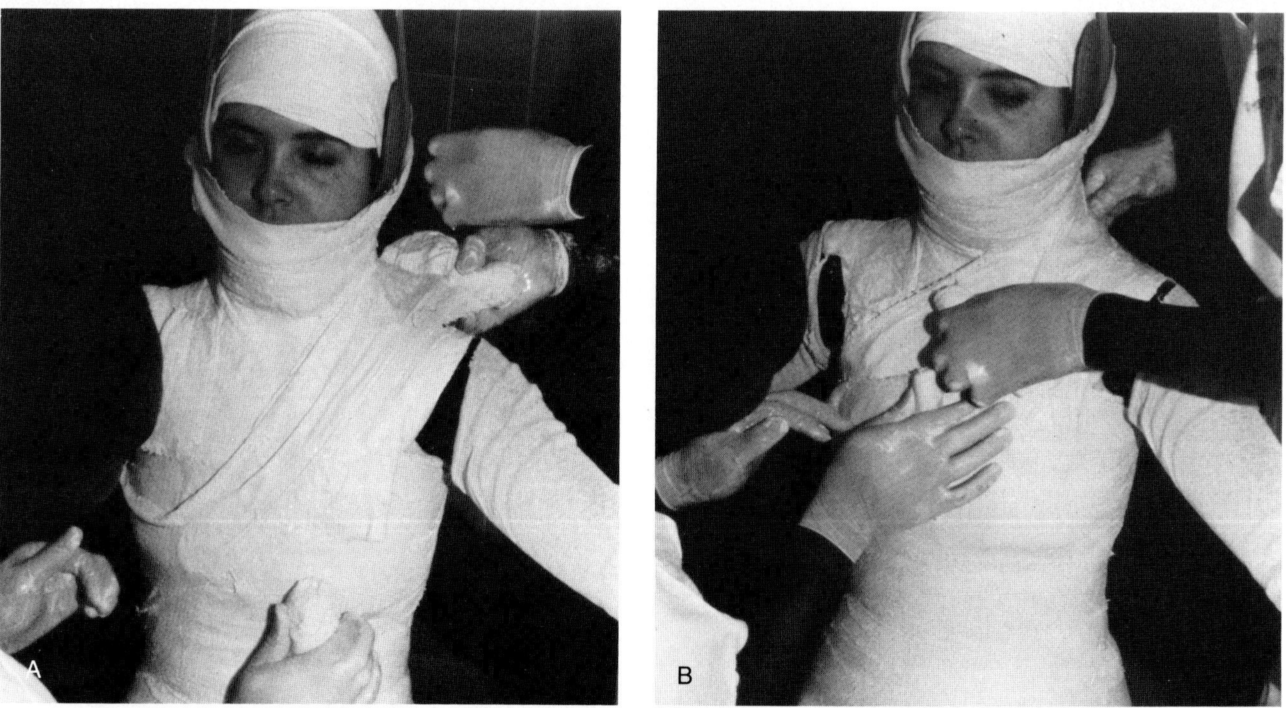

Fig. 11–35. *A, B,* Covering all the plaster splints around the body with 2 rolls of 6″ plaster bandage.

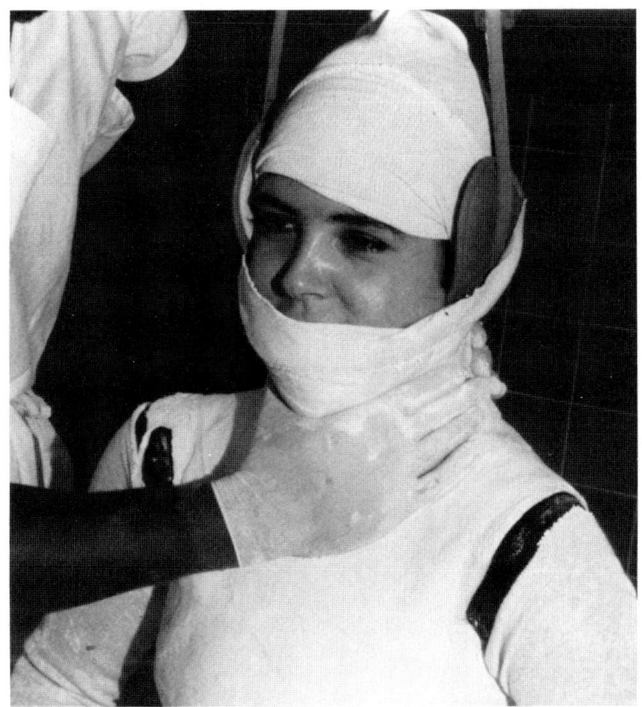

Fig. 11–36. Application of 4″ plaster bandages to the neck, chin, mandible, and base of skull.

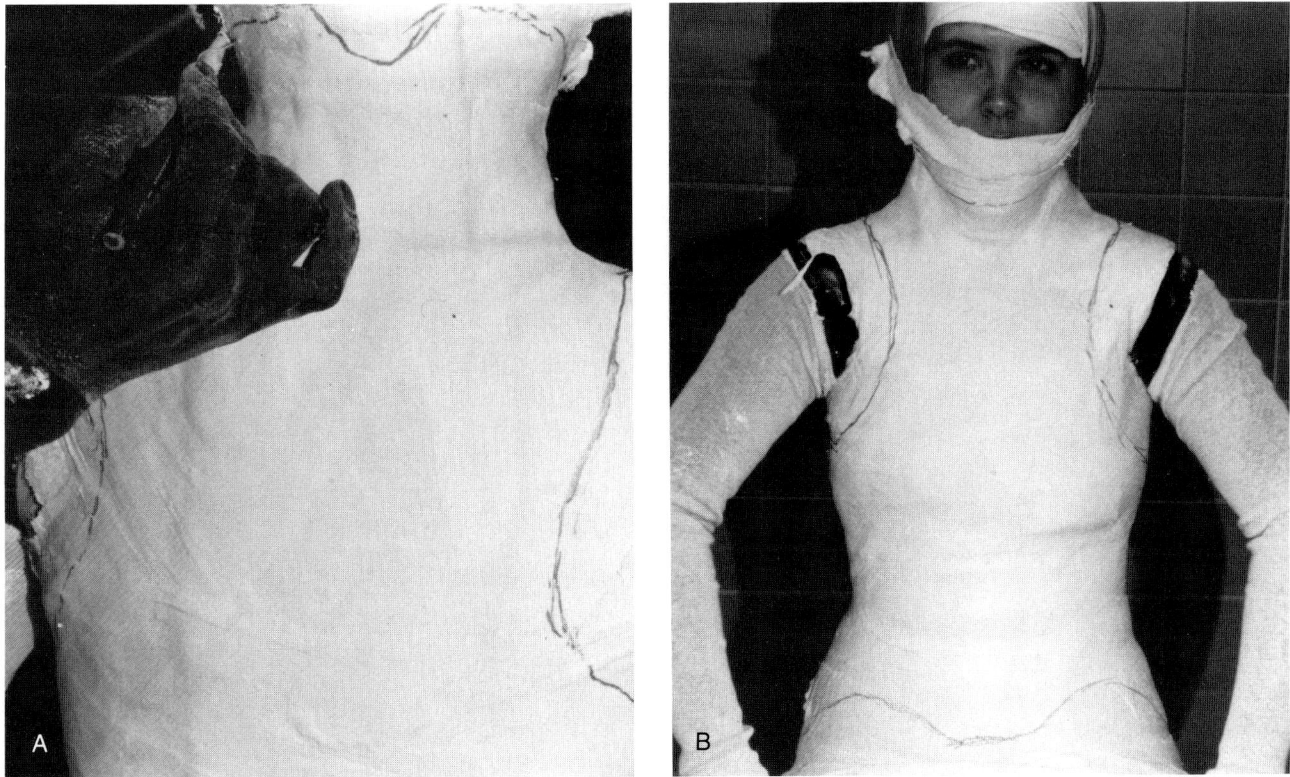

Fig. 11–37. *A, B,* Marking the proximal and distal margins and the two shoulder openings of the cast with a wax pencil.

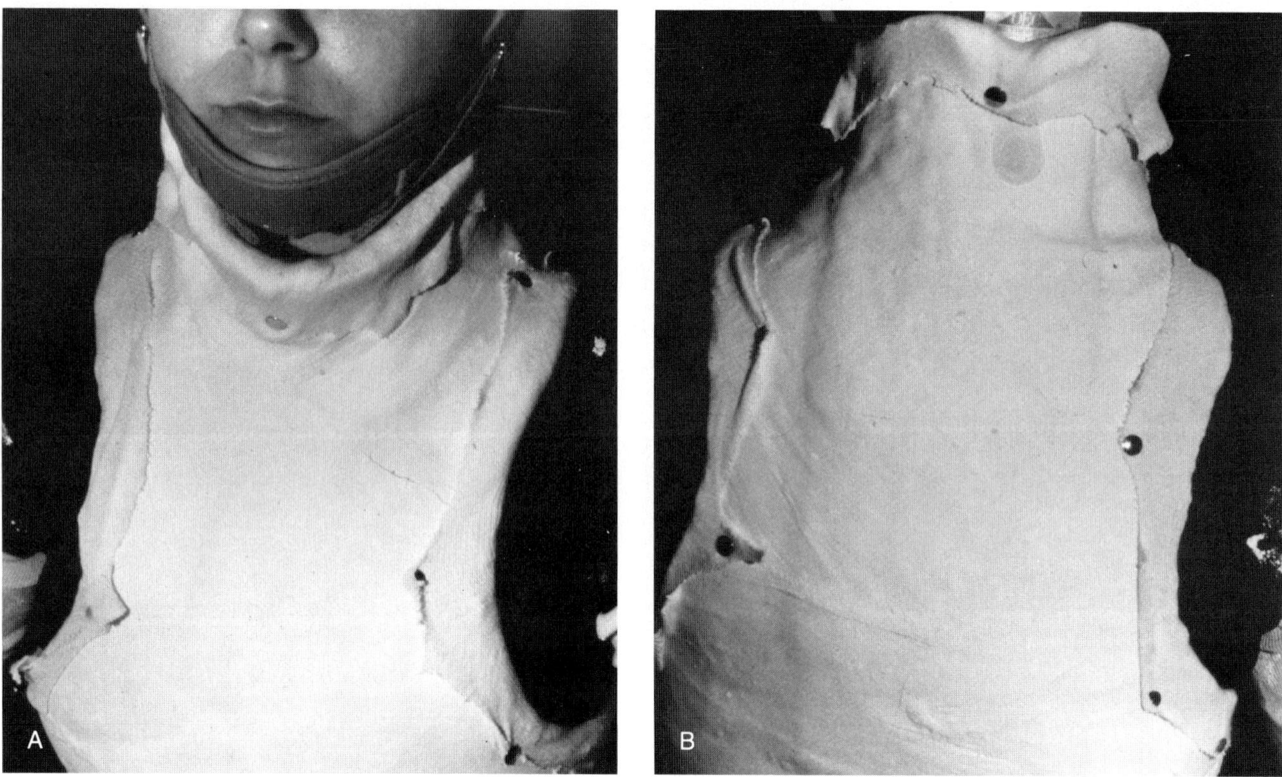

Fig. 11–38. *A, B,* The proximal end and the two shoulder openings of the cast have been trimmed, and the stockinet ends have been fixed to the cast with thumbtacks.

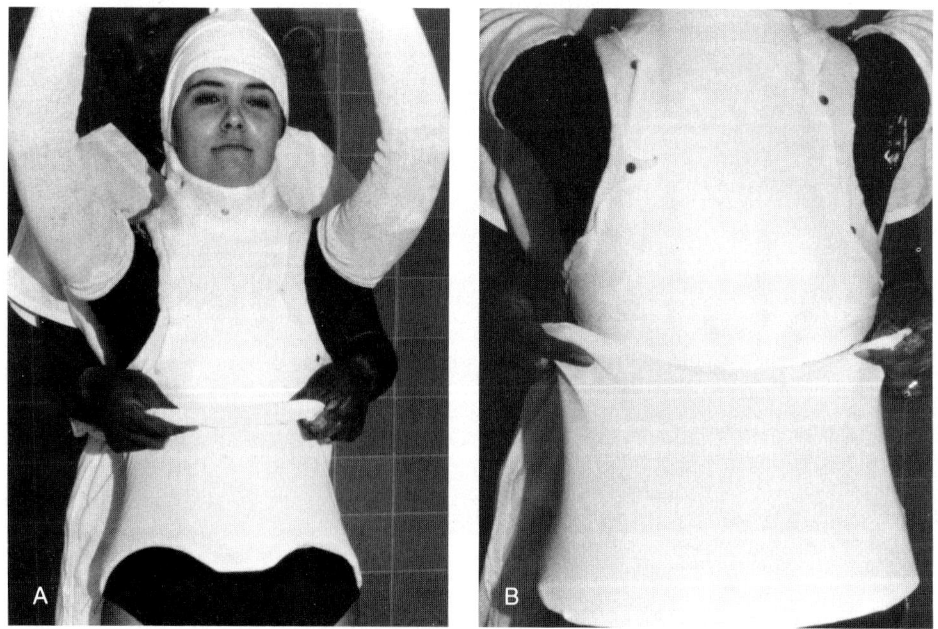

Fig. 11–39. *A, B,* The distal end of the cast has been trimmed, and the distal end of the stockinet is being folded over it.

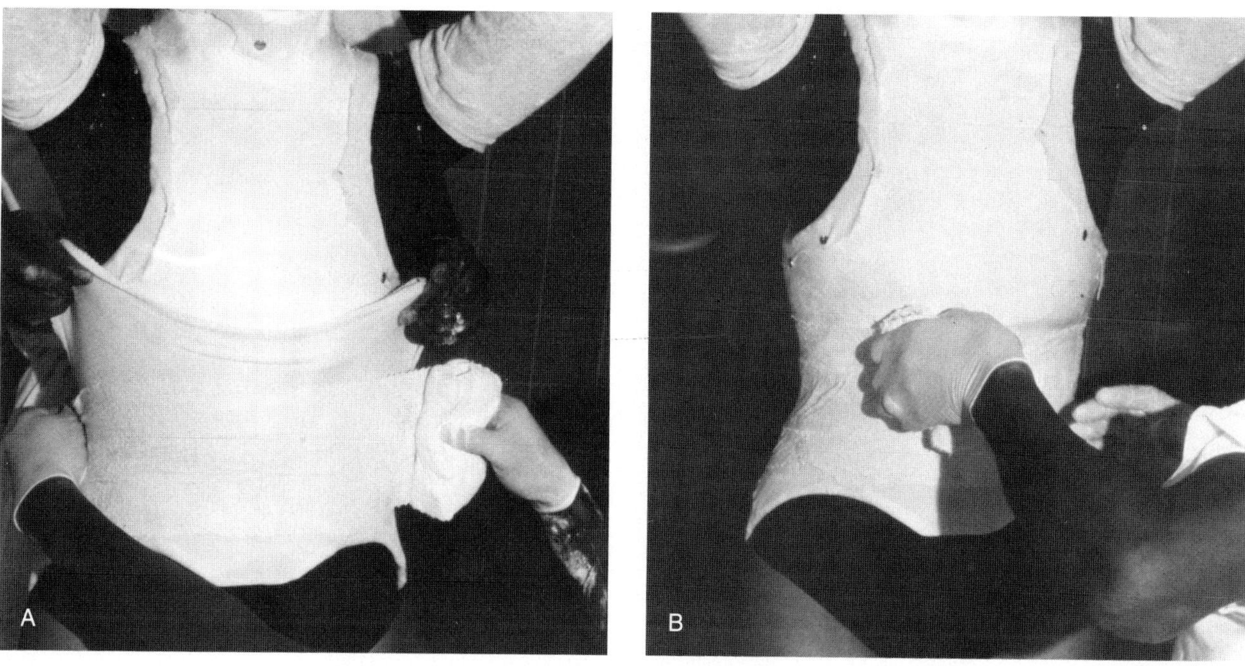

Fig. 11–40. *A, B,* The upturned distal stockinet end is covered with 1 roll of 6″ plaster bandage.

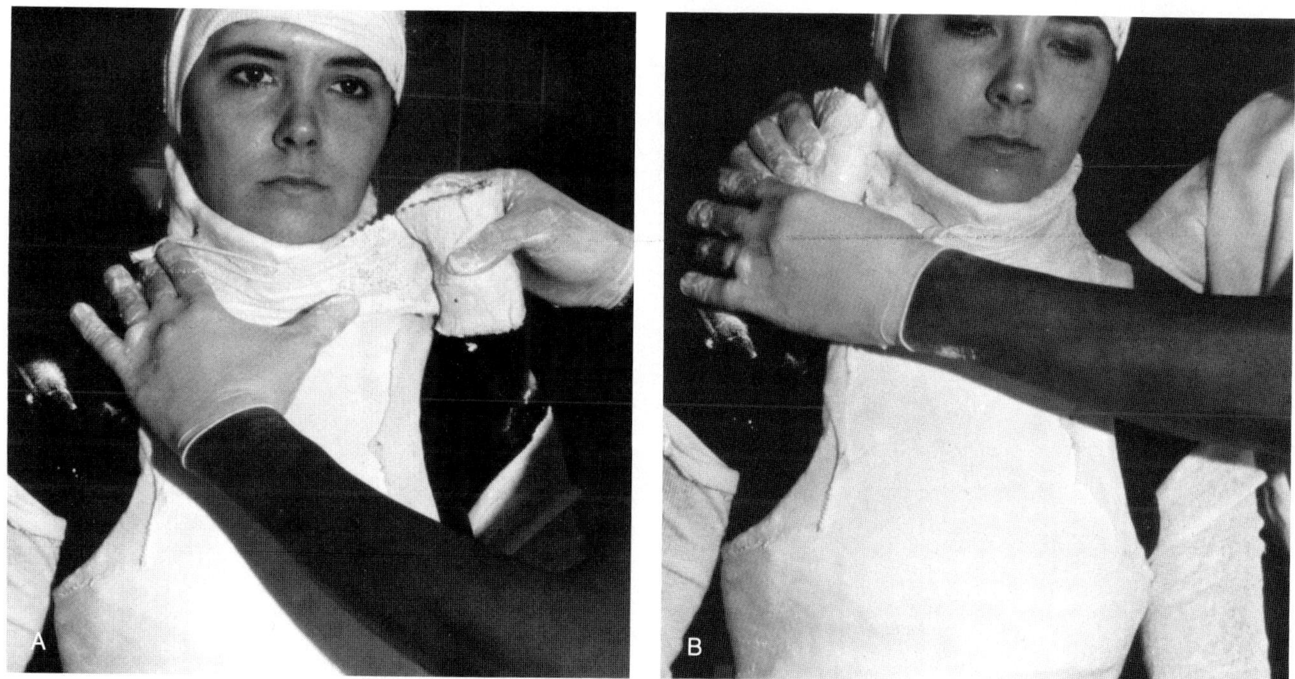

Fig. 11–41. *A, B,* The stockinet end at the neck opening is covered with a 4″ plaster bandage.

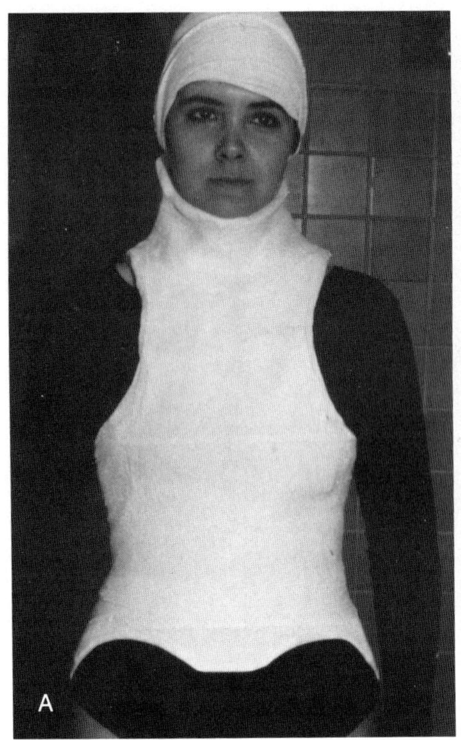

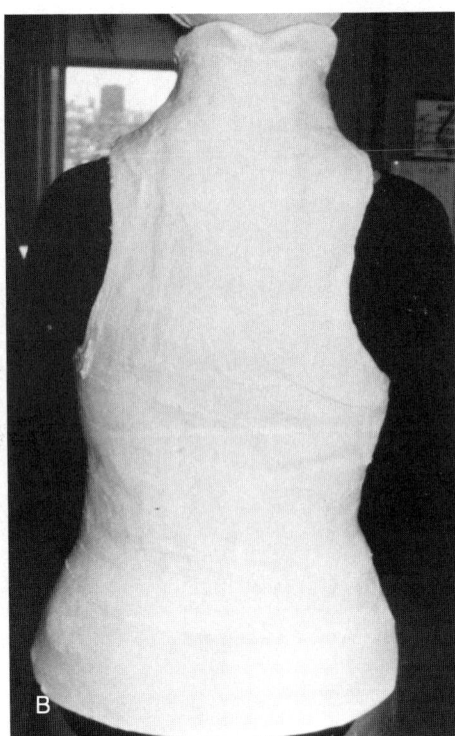

Fig. 11–42. Anterior (*A*) and posterior (*B*) views of a finished Risser cast after the stockinet ends at the shoulder openings have been fixed to the cast with 4″ plaster bandages. Note the small notch under the external occipital protuberance.

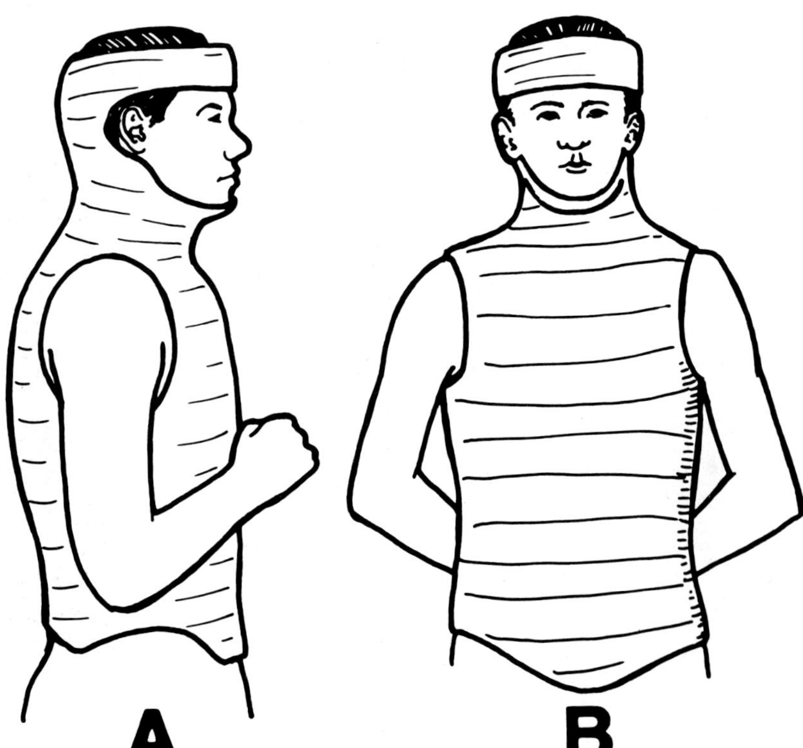

Fig. 11–43. Lateral (*A*) and anterior (*B*) views of a Minerva cast.

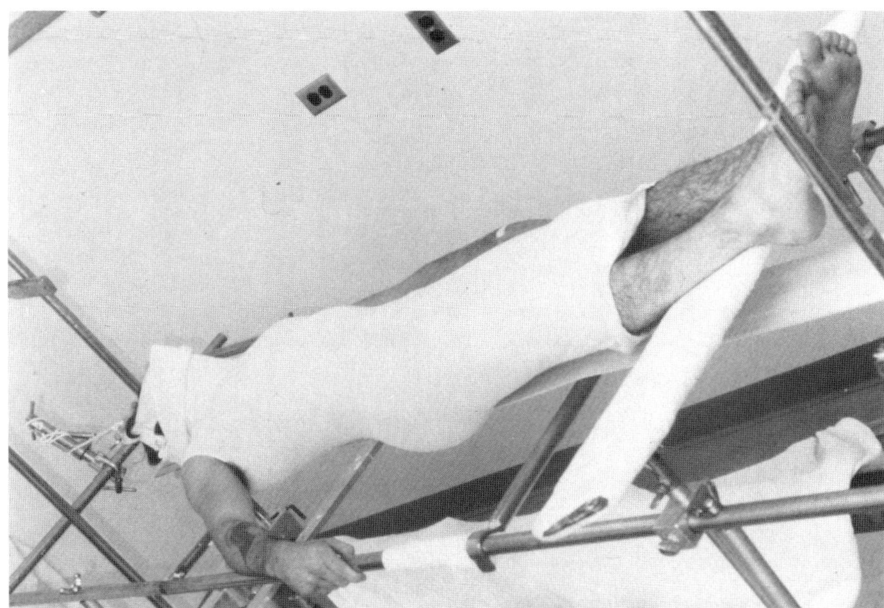

Fig. 11–44. Placement of a patient with an odontoid cervical fracture on a fracture table with head halter traction prior to application of a Minerva cast.

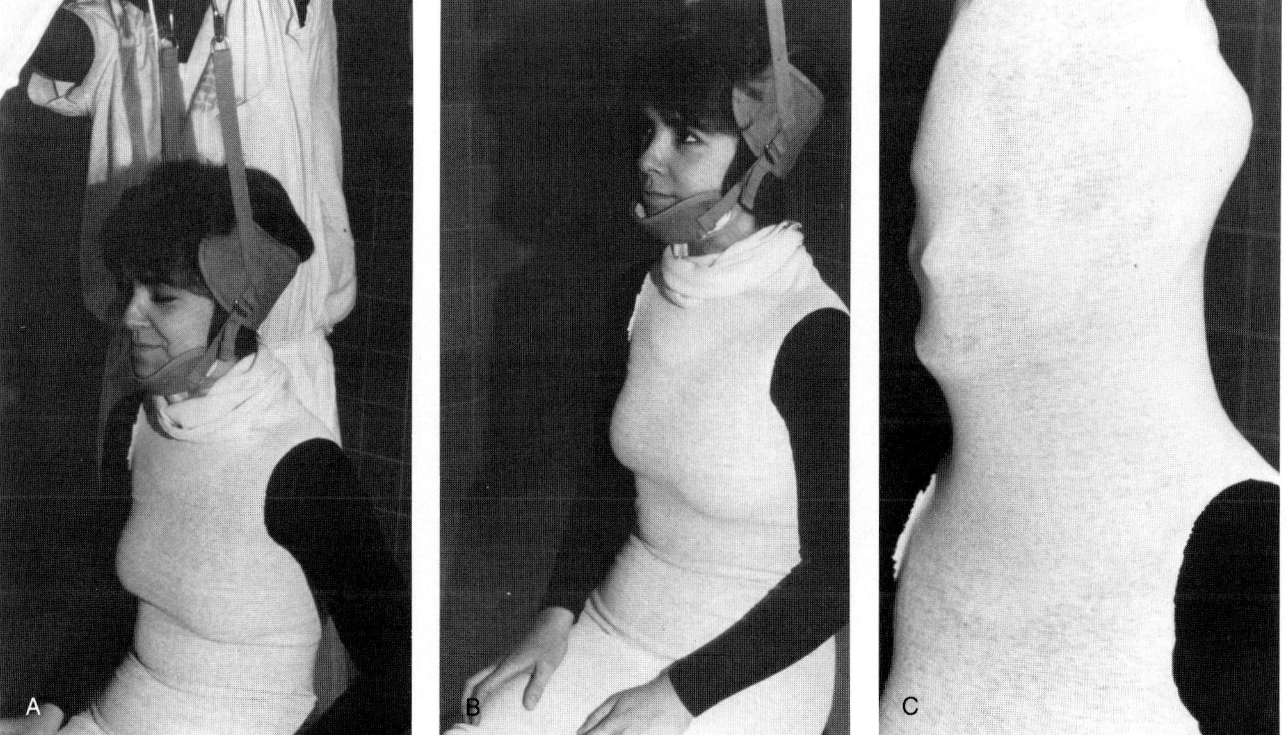

Fig. 11–45. *A, B, C,* Application of a piece of body stockinet from the mid-thigh level to the top of the head with patient in sitting position under head halter traction.

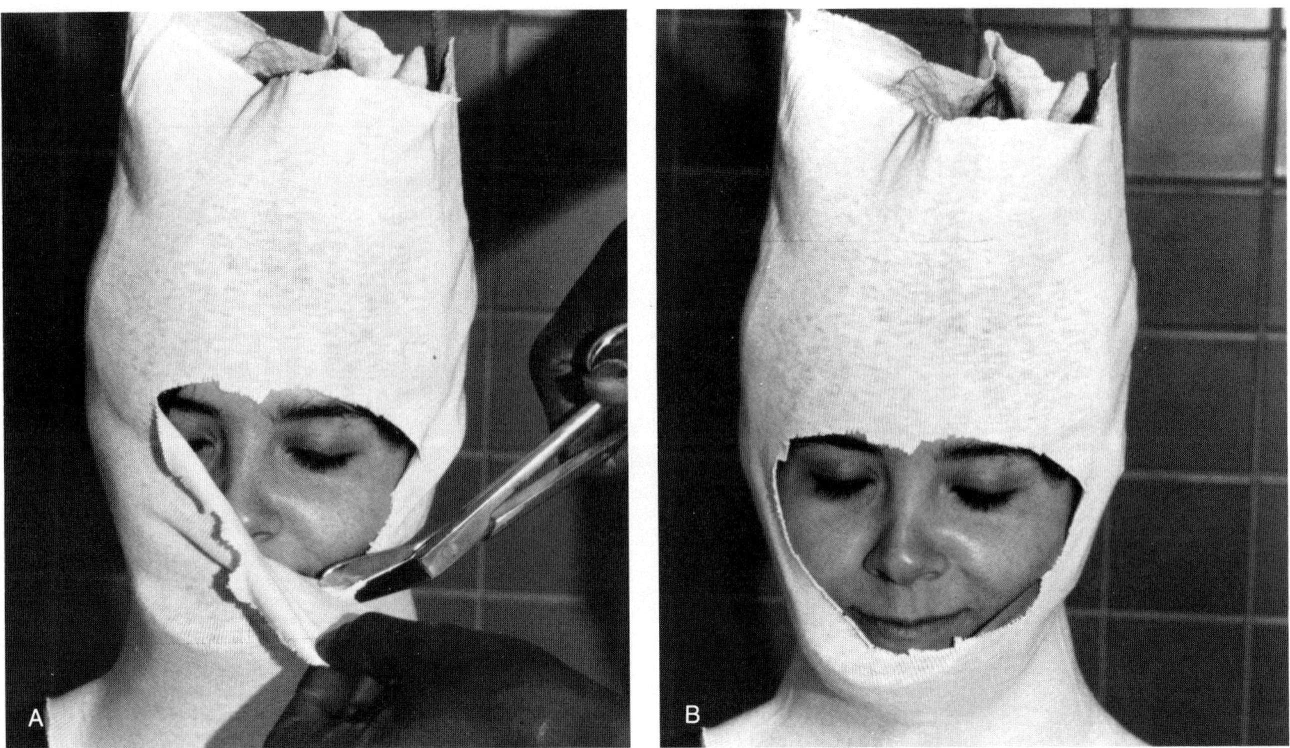

Fig. 11–46. *A, B,* Removal of the stockinet over the face to expose the eyes, nose, cheeks, and lips.

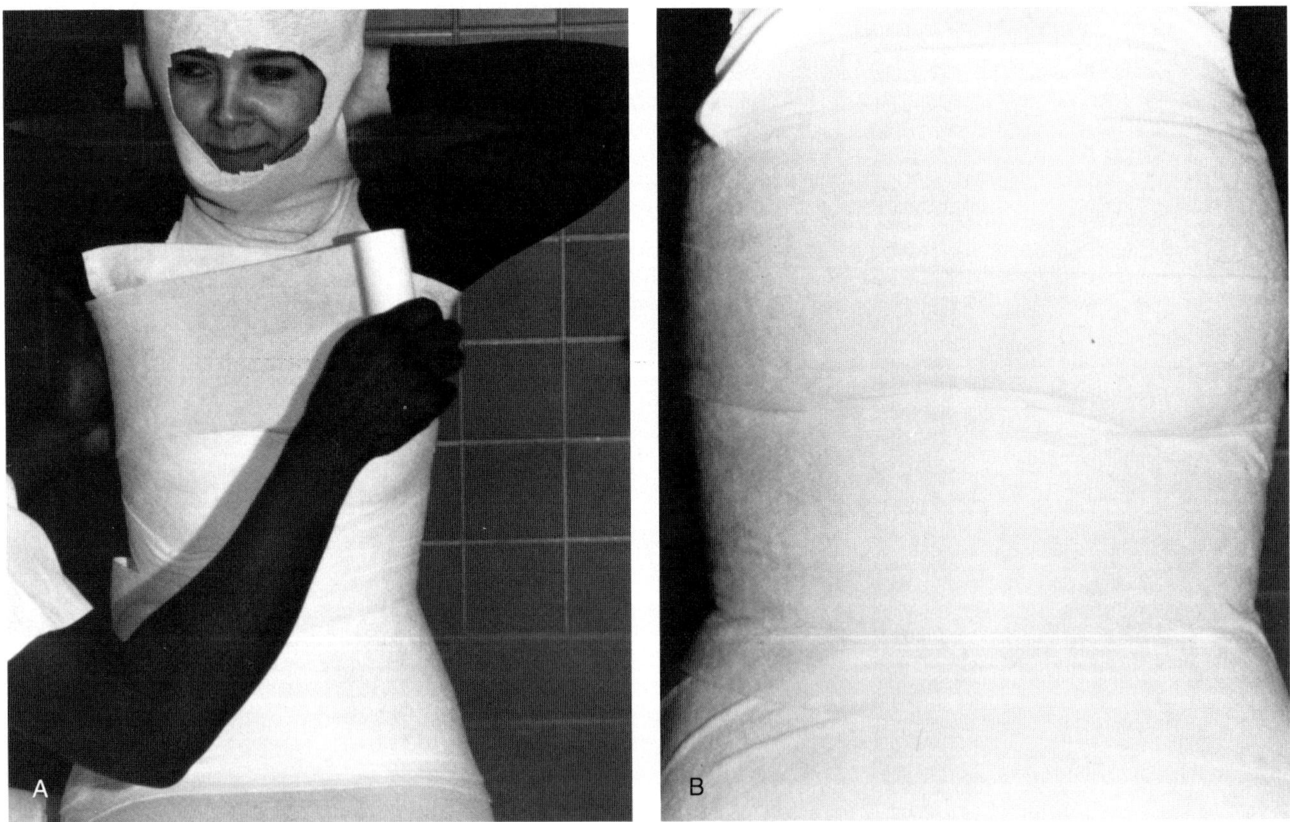

Fig. 11–47. *A, B,* Covering the body from the level of the greater trochanters to the upper axillary level with 4 rolls of 6″ Webril bandage.

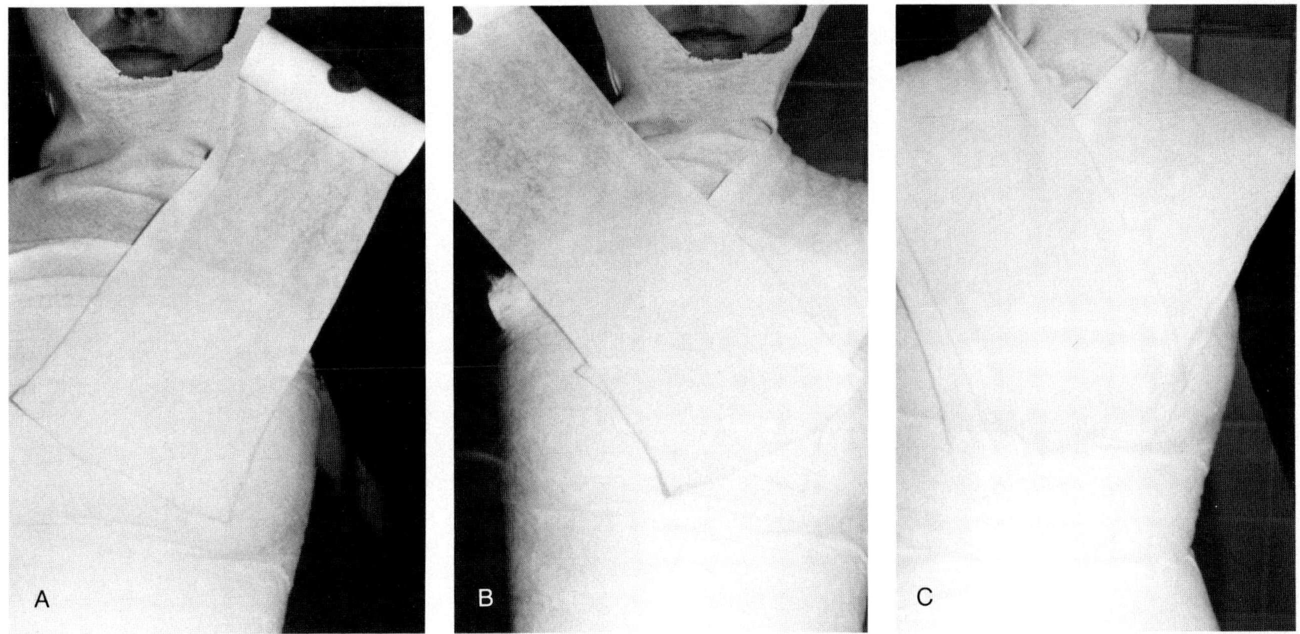

Fig. 11–48. *A, B, C,* Covering the shoulders and upper part of the body with 8 strips of 6″ Webril bandage.

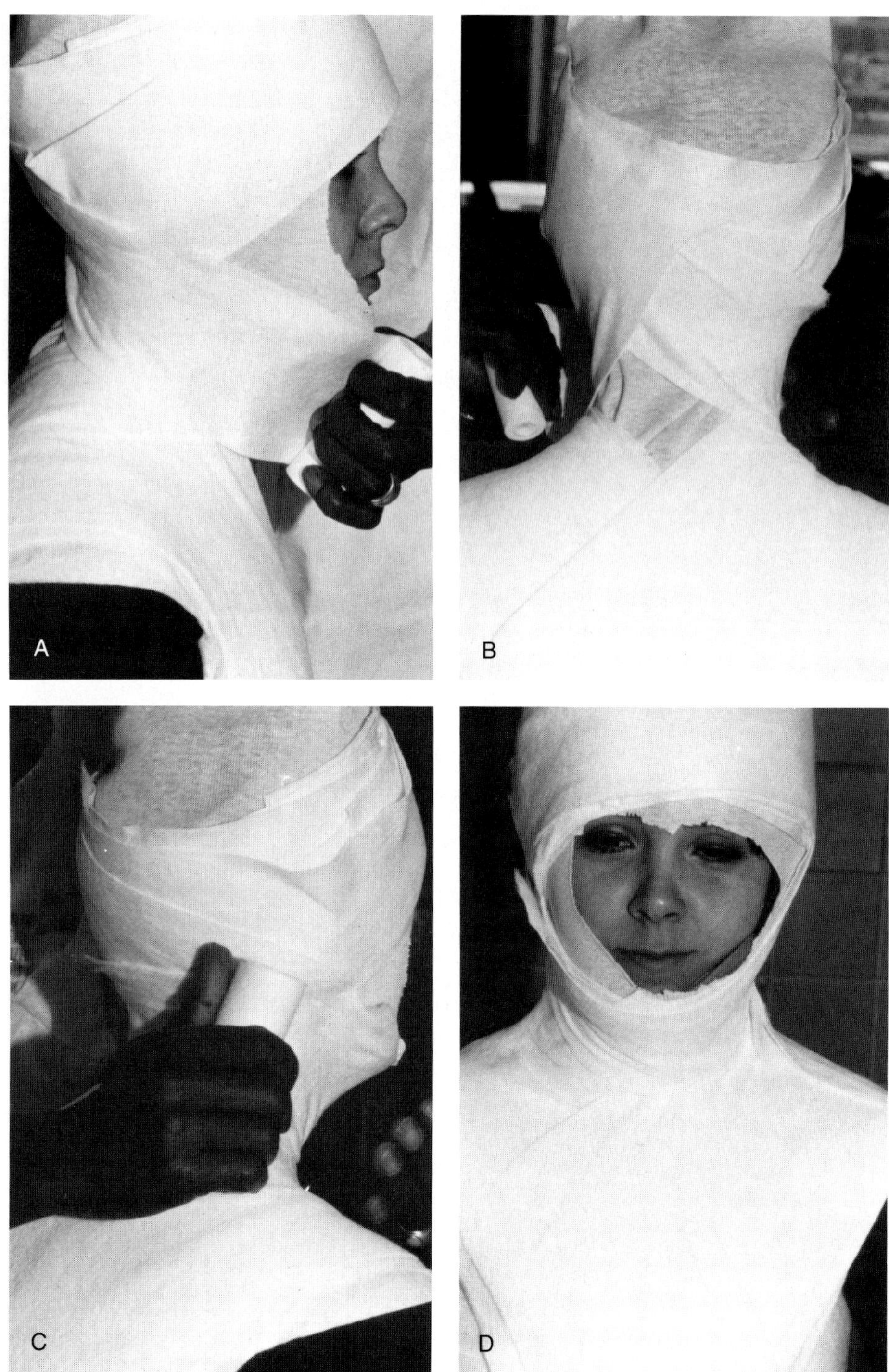

Fig. 11–49. *A–D*, Application of 3″ and 4″ Webril bandages to cover the head and neck region.

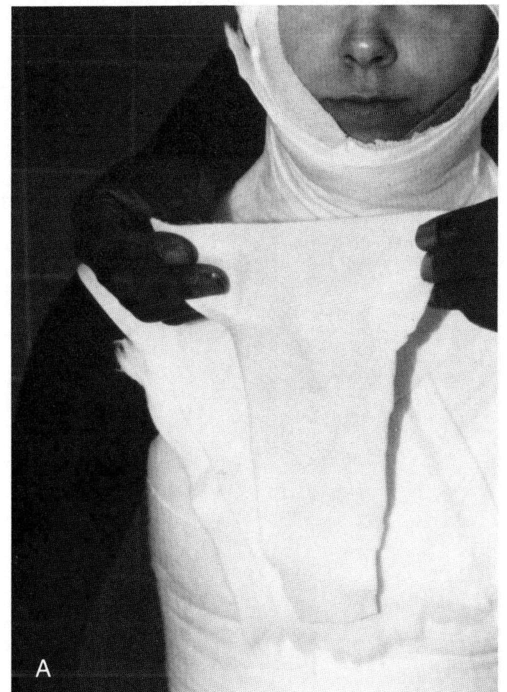

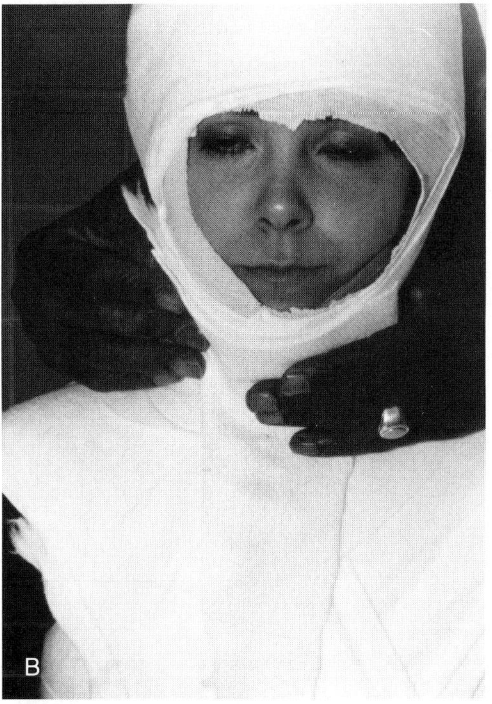

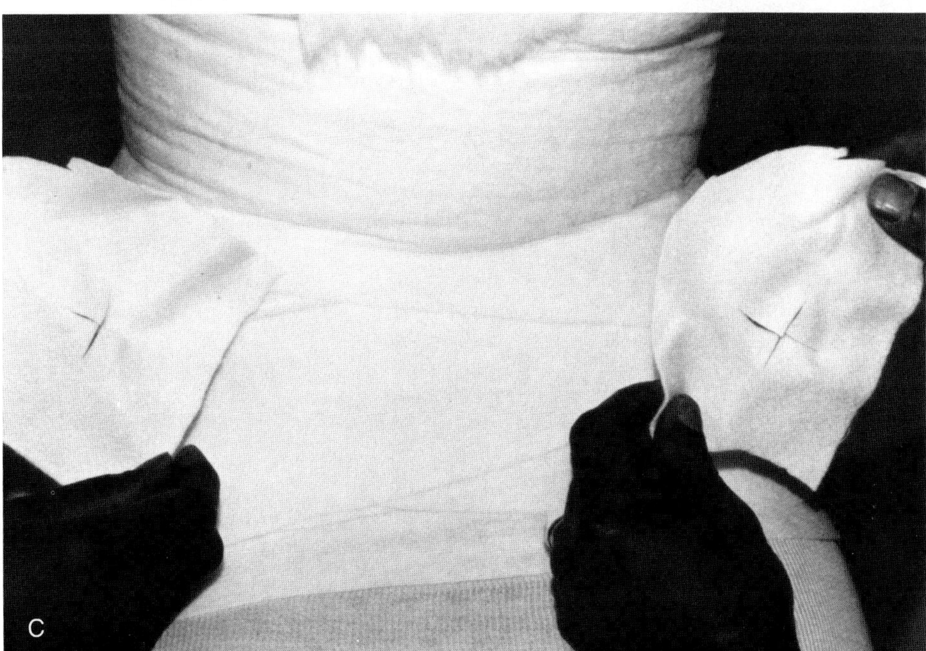

Fig. 11–50. *A, B, C,* Application of felt pads to the forehead, chin, and anterior superior iliac spines.

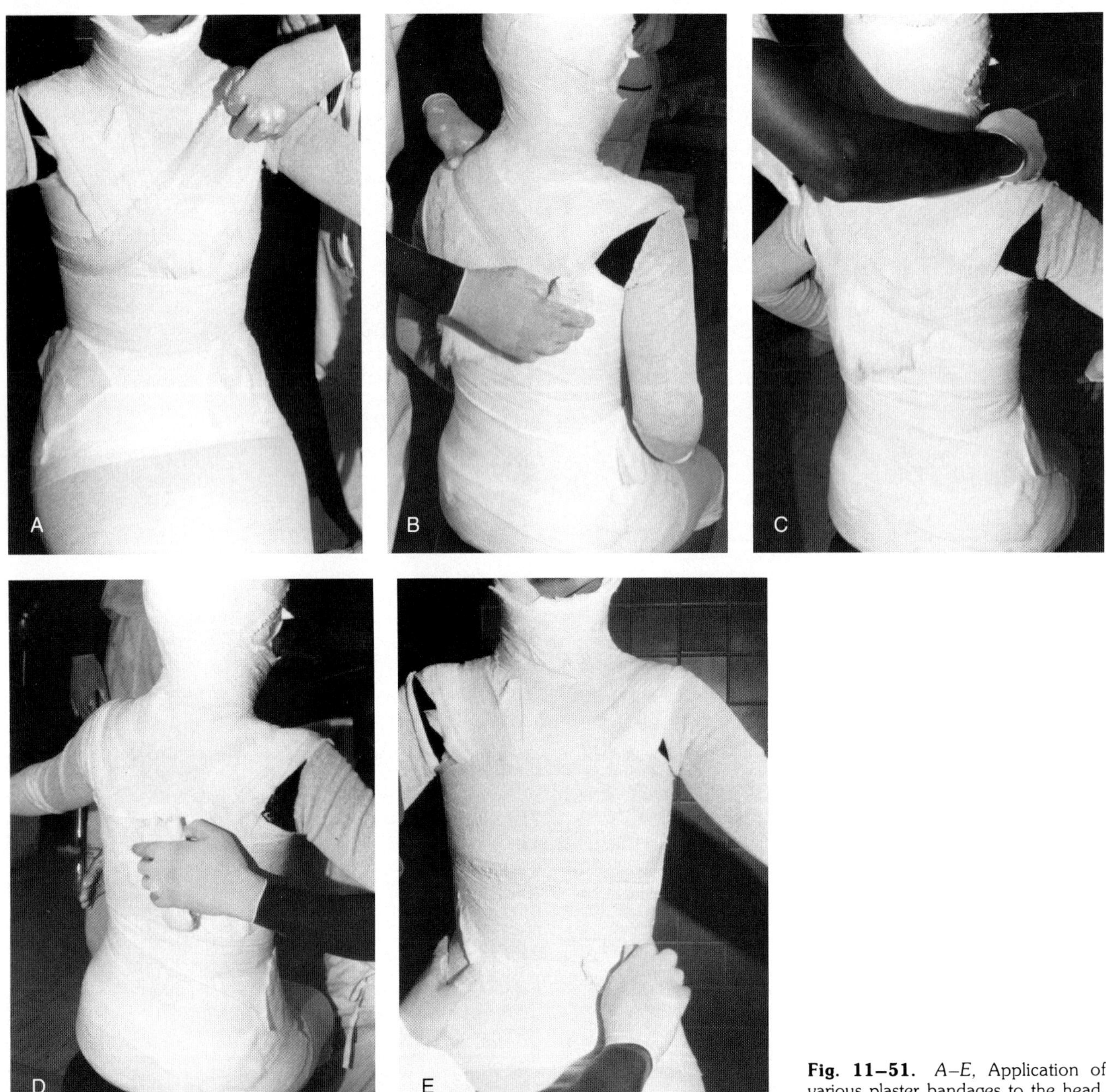

Fig. 11–51. *A–E*, Application of various plaster bandages to the head, neck, and body.

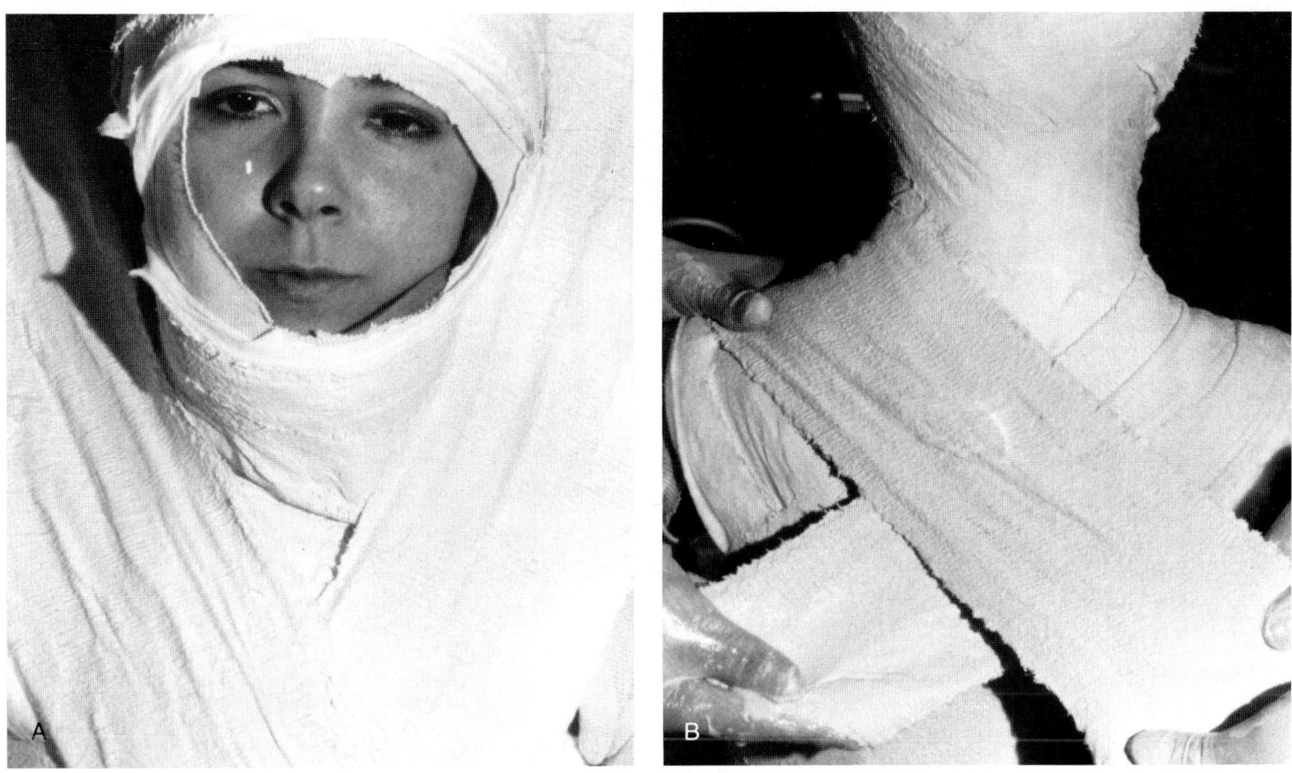

Fig. 11–52. *A, B,* Application of plaster splints from tops of both shoulders obliquely across the upper chest and back.

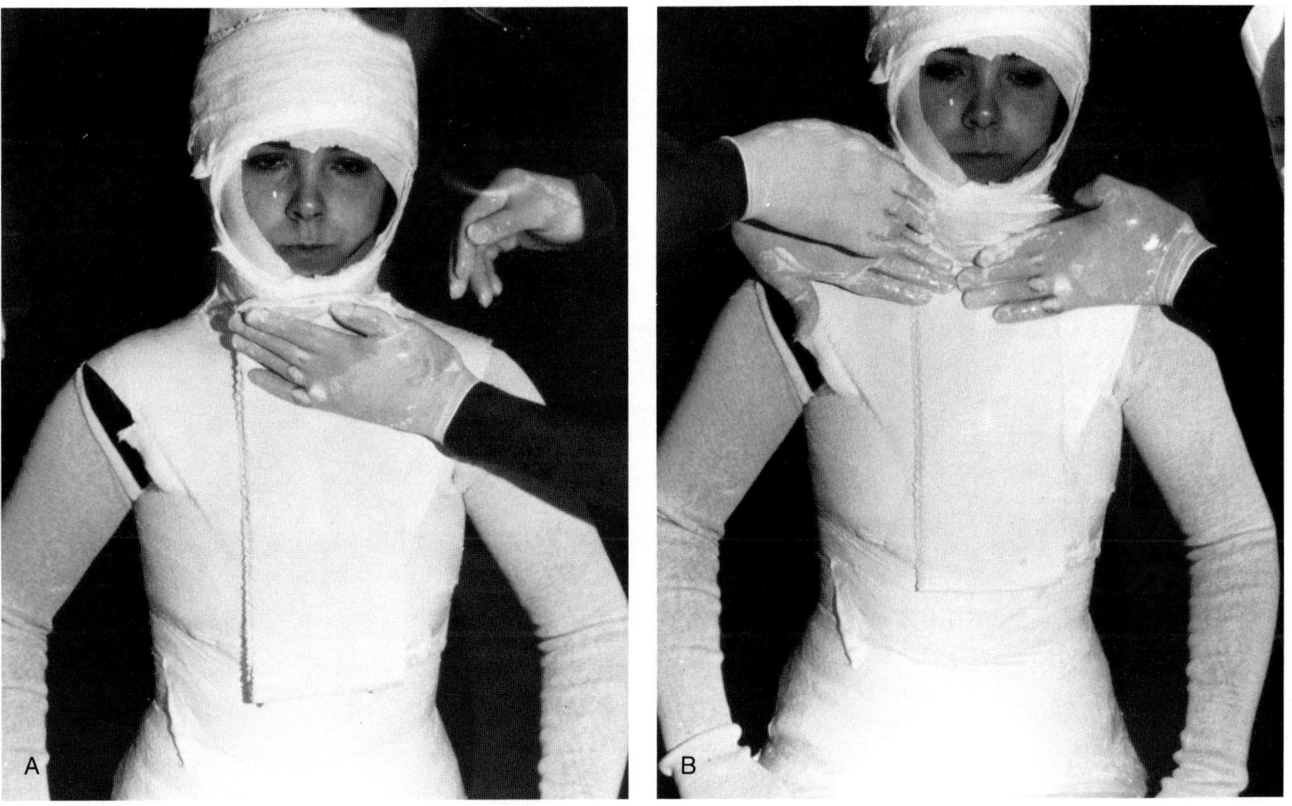

Fig. 11–53. *A, B,* Application of a plaster splint from the chin to the upper abdominal region.

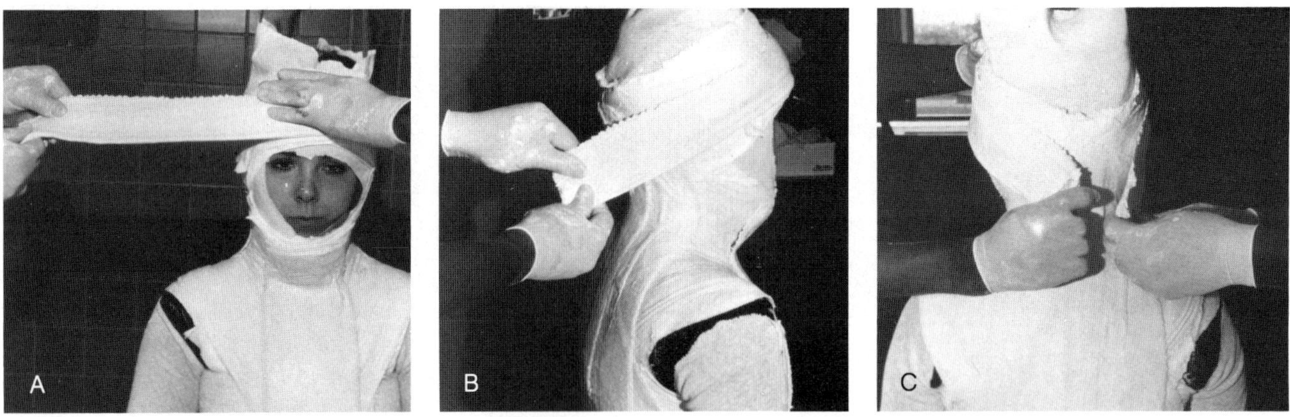

Fig. 11–54. *A, B, C,* Application of a longitudinally folded plaster splint around the headband.

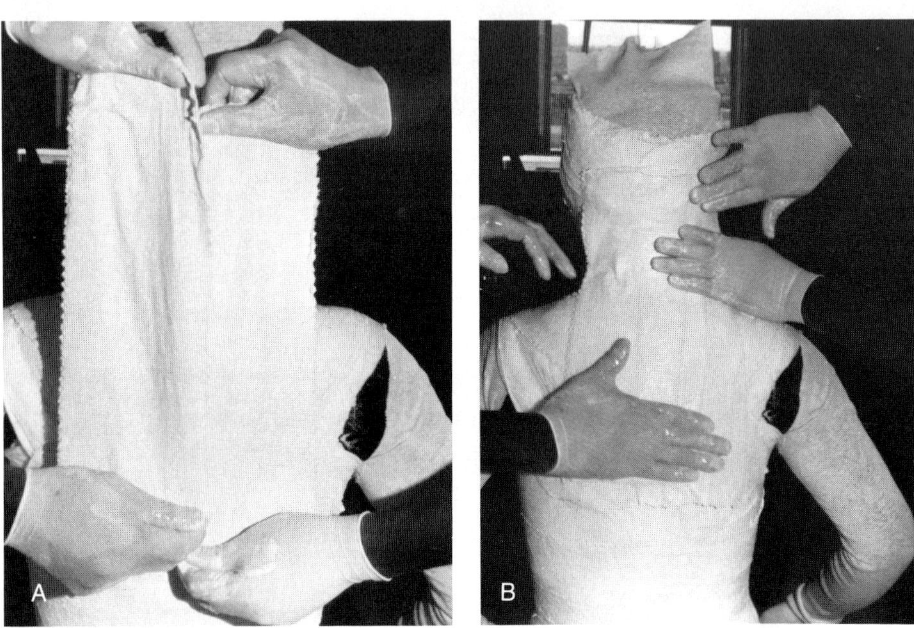

Fig. 11–55. *A, B,* Application of two plaster splints from the mid-level of the headband to the mid-back region.

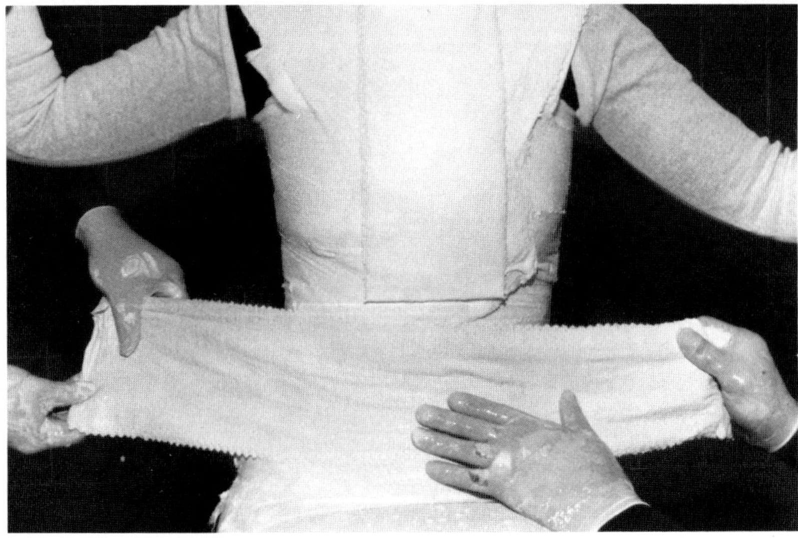

Fig. 11–56. Application of plaster splints to the lower part of the body in a circular and slightly overlapping manner.

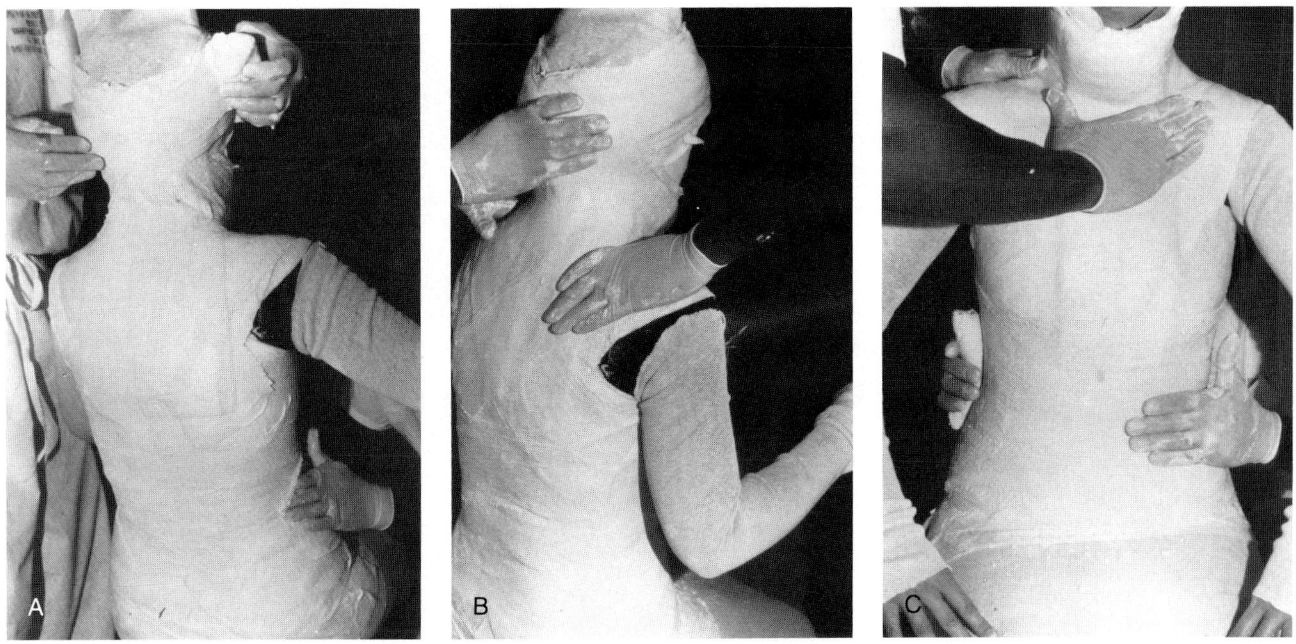

Fig. 11–57. *A, B, C,* Covering the plaster splints around the head and neck region with 4″ plaster bandages and covering the body portion with 6″ plaster bandages.

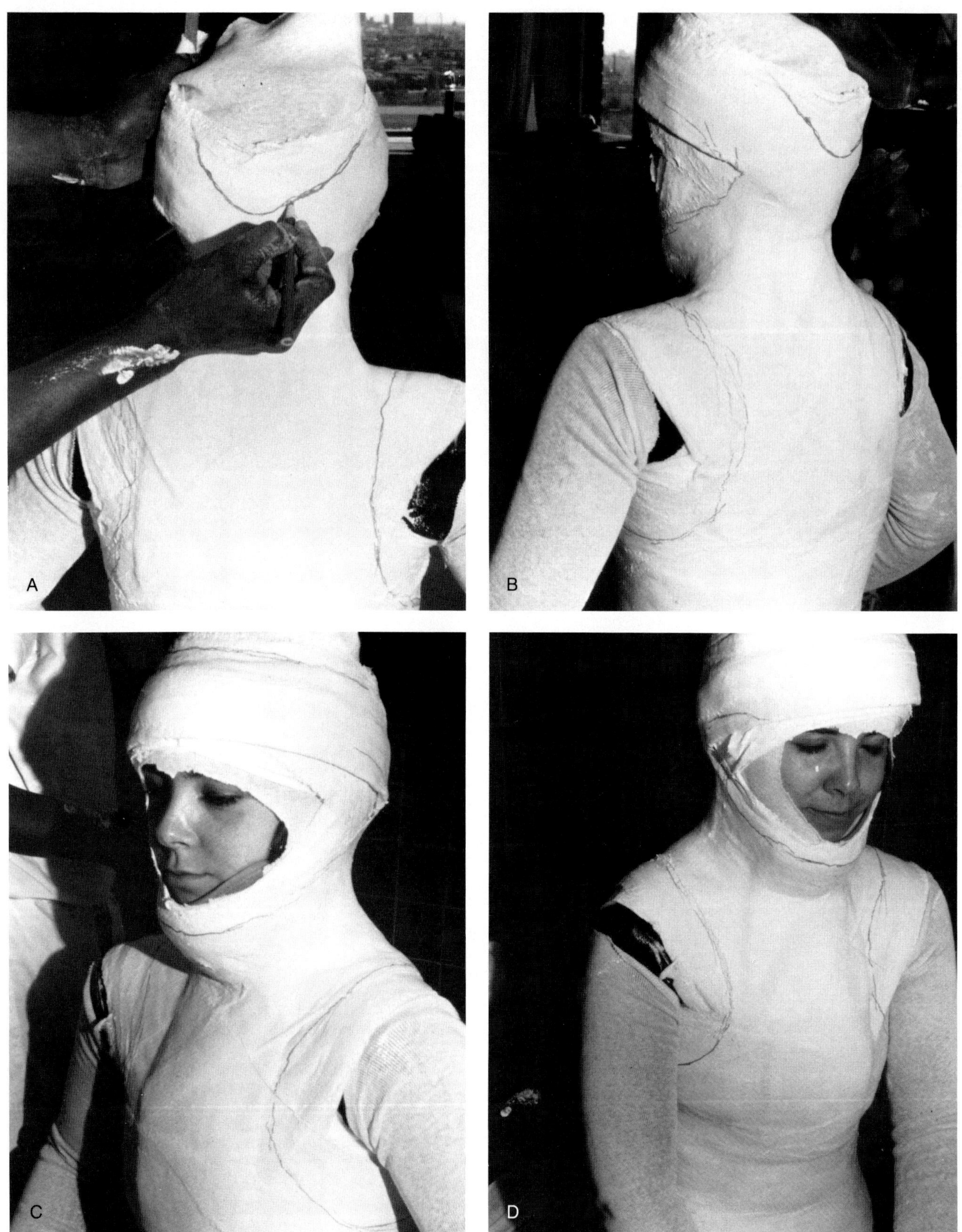

Fig. 11–58. *A–D,* Marking the final margins of the headband and face and shoulder openings of the cast with a wax pencil.

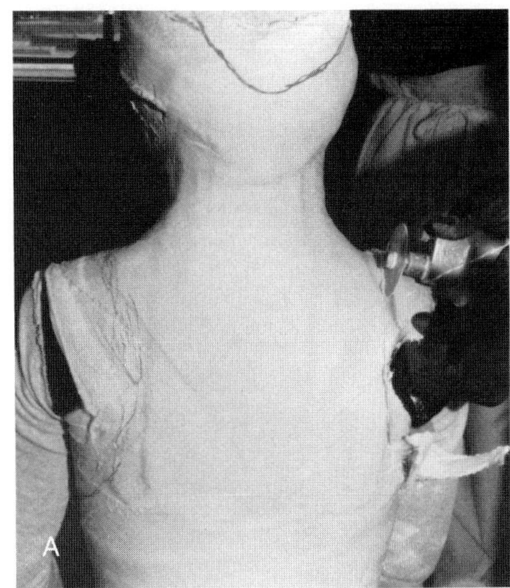

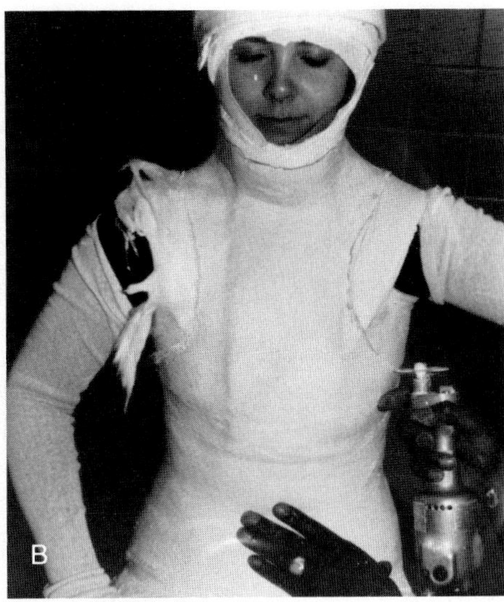

Fig. 11–59. *A*, *B*, Removal of excess plaster from the shoulder openings.

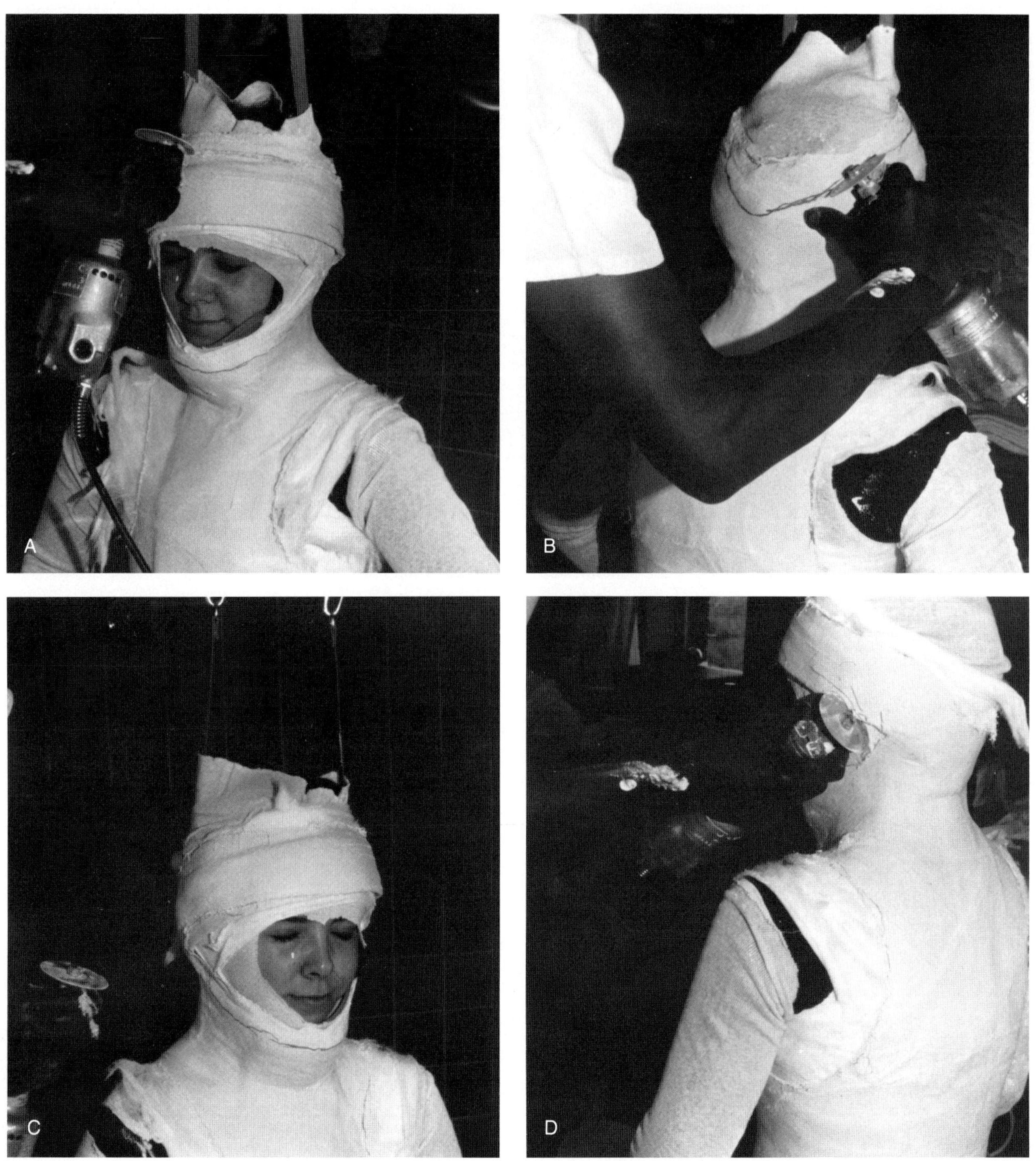

Fig. 11–60. *A–D*, Removal of excess plaster from the headband.

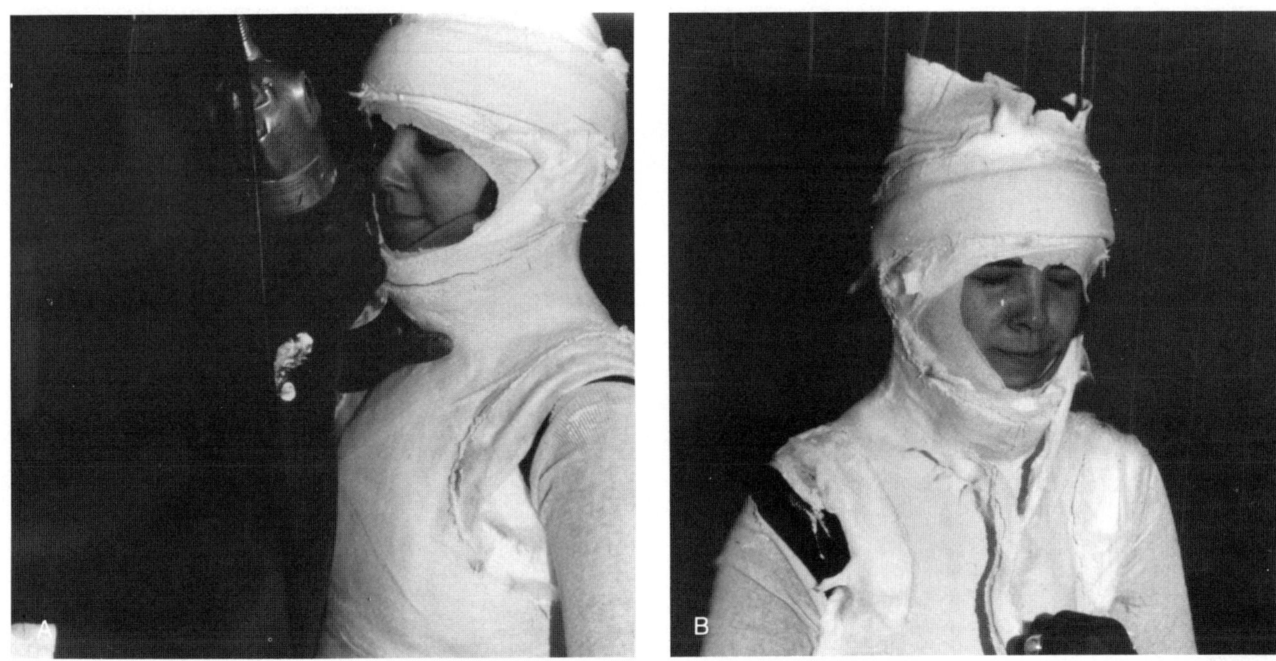

Fig. 11–61. *A, B,* Removal of excess plaster from around the face.

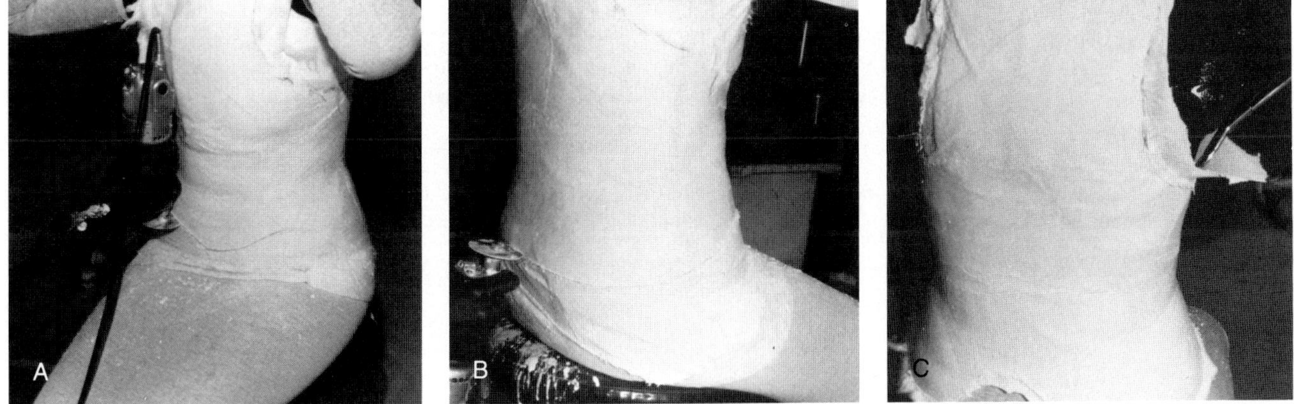

Fig. 11–62. *A–C,* Trimming lower end of the cast to allow good hip flexion and prevent pressure sores.

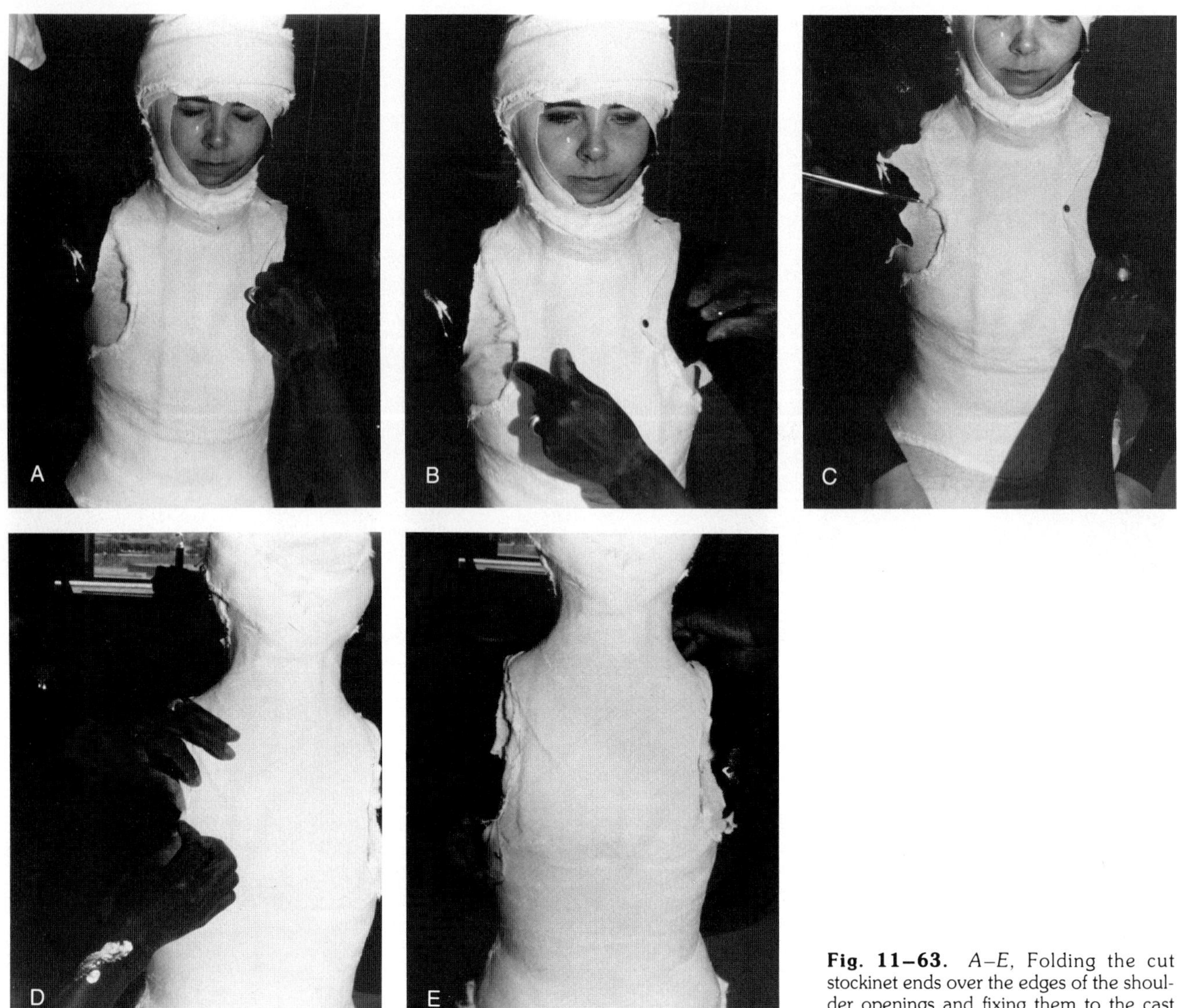

Fig. 11–63. *A–E*, Folding the cut stockinet ends over the edges of the shoulder openings and fixing them to the cast surface with thumbtacks.

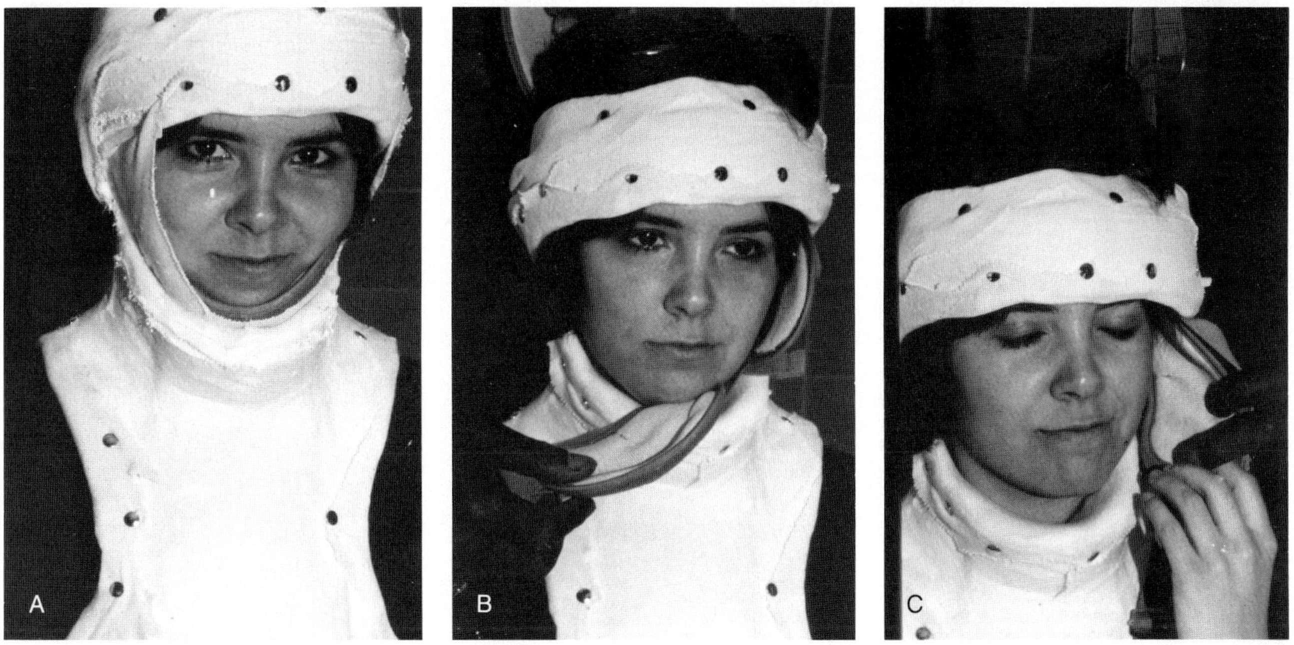

Fig. 11–64. *A, B, C,* Folding the proximal stockinet end and the stockinet at the margins of the face opening over the cast edges and fixing them to the cast with thumbtacks.

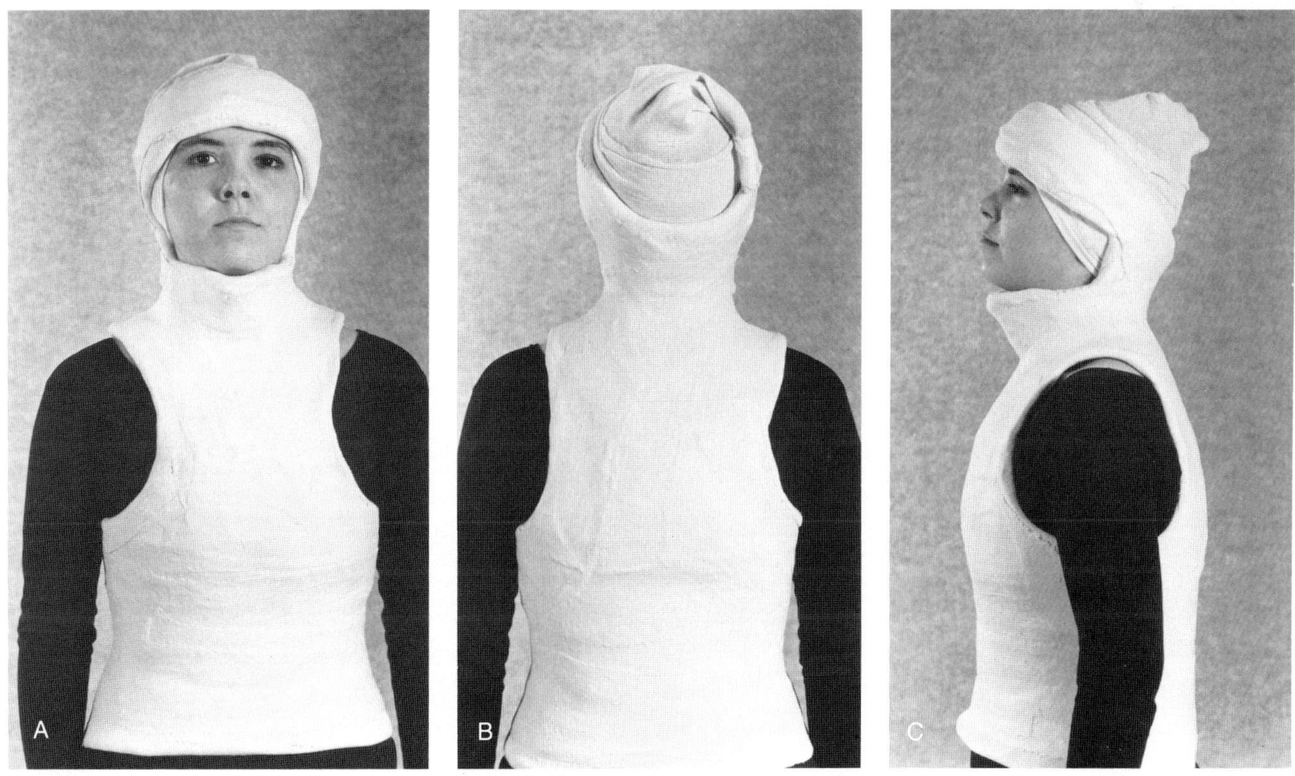

Fig. 11–65. Anterior (*A*), posterior (*B*), and lateral (*C*) views of the finished Minerva cast after the stockinet ends have been fixed to the cast with plaster bandages.

Index

Page numbers in *italics* indicate figures; numbers followed by *t* indicate tables.